Radiolabeled Blood Elements

Recent Advances in Techniques and Applications

NATO ASI Series

Advanced Science Institutes Series

A series presenting the results of activities sponsored by the NATO Science Committee, which aims at the dissemination of advanced scientific and technological knowledge, with a view to strengthening links between scientific communities.

The series is published by an international board of publishers in conjunction with the NATO Scientific Affairs Division

A	**Life Sciences**	Plenum Publishing Corporation
B	**Physics**	New York and London
C	**Mathematical and Physical Sciences**	Kluwer Academic Publishers
D	**Behavioral and Social Sciences**	Dordrecht, Boston, and London
E	**Applied Sciences**	
F	**Computer and Systems Sciences**	Springer-Verlag
G	**Ecological Sciences**	Berlin, Heidelberg, New York, London,
H	**Cell Biology**	Paris, Tokyo, Hong Kong, and Barcelona
I	**Global Environmental Change**	

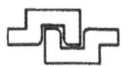

Series A: Life Sciences

Radiolabeled Blood Elements

Recent Advances in Techniques and Applications

Edited by

J. Martin-Comin

Department of Nuclear Medicine
CSUB Hospital "Princeps d'Espanya"
Barcelona, Spain

M. L. Thakur

Division of Nuclear Medicine
Thomas Jefferson University Hospital
Philadelphia, Pennsylvania

C. Piera

Department of Nuclear Medicine
Hospital Clinic
Barcelona, Spain

M. Roca

Department of Nuclear Medicine
CSUB Hospital "Princeps d'Espanya"
Barcelona, Spain

and

F. Lomeña

Department of Nuclear Medicine
Hospital Clinic
Barcelona, Spain

Springer Science+Business Media, LLC

Proceedings of a NATO Advanced Research Workshop on
Radiolabeled Blood Elements: Recent Advances in Techniques and Applications,
held November 23–27, 1992,
in Barcelona, Spain

Library of Congress Cataloging-in-Publication Data

Radiolabeled blood elements : recent advances in techniques and
    applications / edited by J. Martin-Comin ... [et al.].
        p.   cm. -- (NATO ASI series. Series A, Life sciences ; v.
    262)
    "Published in cooperation with NATO Scientific Affairs Division."
    "Proceedings of a NATO Advanced Research Workshop on Radiolabeled
Blood Elements: Recent Advances in Techniques and Applications, held
November 23-27, 1992, in Barcelona, Spain"--T.p. verso.
    Includes bibliographical references and index.
    ISBN 978-0-306-44700-6   ISBN 978-1-4615-2462-5 (eBook)
    DOI 10.1007/978-1-4615-2462-5
    1. Radiolabeled blood cells--Congresses. 2. Radiolabeled blood
platelets--Congresses. I. Martin-Comin, J. II. North Atlantic
Treaty Organization. Scientific Affairs Division. III. NATO
Advanced Research Workshop on Radiolabeled Blood Elements: Recent
Advances in Techniques and Applications (1992 : Barcelona, Spain)
IV. Series.
    [DNLM: 1. Blood Cells--radionuclide imaging--congresses.
2. Antibodies, Monoclonal--diagnostic use--congresses. 3. Isotope
Labeling--methods--congresses. 4. Radioisotopes--diagnostic use-
-congresses.   WH 140 R129 1994]
RC78.7.R43R33   1994
616.07'575--dc20
DNLM/DLC
for Library of Congress   94-8028
                                                               CIP

ISBN 978-0-306-44700-6

© 1994 Springer Science+Business Media New York
Originally published by Plenum Press, New York in 1994

PREFACE

Scintigraphic imaging with radiolabeled blood elements has continued to be a useful diagnostic modality. The major trust of recent investigation has been in simplifying labeling techniques and developing new agents that will label blood elements selectively in vitro. The VI Symposium of the International Society of Radiolabeled Blood Elements was held in Barcelona (Spain) during November 23 to 27, 1992.The conference was sponsored by the NATO Scientific Affairs Division, the USA Department of Energy and the Spanish National Health Service.

This monograph comprises articles that represent most of the 85 papers (70 oral and 15 posters) presented during the symposium. The meeting was attended by 110 investigators hailed from 21 countries.

Although 111In-oxine and 99mTc-HMPAO remain the choice agents for labeling blood components for routine applications, there was heavy emphasis on developing new labeling agents that will either simplify the in vitro labeling procedure, or, even better, will label blood components selectively in vivo, by injecting the radioactive agents directly into patients. The degree of success in imaging target lesions in humans by using these agents has been excellent.

In the ensuing chapters, a number of monoclonal antibodies specific for human neutrophils have been described. These have been labeled with 99mTc by instant kit preparation, administered to patients intravenously and abscesses have imaged in most cases within 6 hours post-injection. Although more studies comparing these results with WBC labeled in vitro may be warranted, the radiolabeled antibodies have offered results with high sensitivity and specificity. None of the patients receiving the protein has been reported with any serious reaction and less than 15% have been found to have elevated HAMA titer.

A nonspecific 111In or 99mTc labeled human polyclonal immunoglobulin has also emerged that by the virtue of its simplicity and ready availability makes a very attractive agent for imaging inflammatory foci. The mechanism by which this agent accumulates in the lesion is discussed and some of the clinical results are described.

For platelets, the fibrin binding glycoprotein IIb.IIIa complex has been the target of many antibodies developed. Certain peptides and molecular recognition units derived from antibody complementary determining region (CDR) have been also used to label activated platelets. Some promising results can be found in the monograph.

Renewed attention has been drawn to the applications and in vivo labeling of T Lymphocytes. 99mTc labeled W3/25 and MAX 16H5 have been used to target the CD4 receptor on lymphocytes where 99mTc-OKT3 has been used to label the CD3 receptors. 99mTc labeled IL-2 is also being investigated. A limited number of clinical results are given.

Three years after the V Symposium in Vienna, this meeting established the usefulness of "old" agents and opened new horizons in the field of radiolabeled blood components.

Overall it was clearly evident that the merger of new technologies has presaged an exciting period in the field of diagnostic imaging with radiolabeled blood components. We expect that the scientific program of the next meeting, to be held in August 1995 at the Yale University School of Medicine in New Haven, Connecticut, USA, will be even more exciting.

The Editors
Barcelona, October 1993

ACKNOWLEDGEMENTS

The collaboration and help received from our colleagues in the Nuclear Medicine Depts. from the "CSUB Hospital Princeps d'España" and from the "Hospital Clinic" is truly appreciated. Special thanks are deserved by the residents of both departments whose efficacy and help was invaluable.

The suggestions, ideas and support received from members of the ISORBE executive committee is also acknowledged. Prof. Rausell-Colom and Prof. Sertorio from the NATO Scientific Affairs Division gave us not only economic support but also advice and the human touch from NATO.

Finally Mrs. A. Pavia's technical assistance has been essential in preparing the manuscript.

CONTENTS

ADVANCES IN BLOOD CELL LABELING: PRETARGETING

D.A. Goodwin, C.F. Meares, M. McTigue, W. Chaovapong, C. Ransone, O. Renn, M.J. McCall and M. Studer

Nuclear Medicine Service, Veterans Admin. Medical Center, Palo Alto Stanford Univ. School of Medicine and Department of Chemistry University of California, Davis CA

The high sensitivity and specificity of the 111In labeled WBC method make it the "gold standard" against which all the new methods must be measured. However the 111In WBC method requires laborious separation, labeling and reinjection of 111In oxine labeled autologous leukocytes. With the increasing incidence of AIDS there is now the possibility of misadministration of HIV infected cells with disastrous consequences. Radiation exposure from a diagnostic misadministration pales into insignificance by comparison. There is also a small but finite chance of self-infection from a needle stick. These reasons, along with simplicity, are all persuasive arguments for the continued development of kit preparations wherever possible. Thus new approaches amenable to kit formulations, such as human polyclonal immuno-globulin and anti-leukocyte MABs[a] labeled with either 99mTc or 111In are very attractive alternatives.

111In or 99mTc labeled human non-specific polyclonal immunoglobulin technique has received much attention from publication of successful clinical trials showing both simplicity and sensitivity[1, 2]. However, other radiolabeled proteins have not been given comparable clinical trials; and because of logistic difficulties, it has not been possible to use them as the appropriate controls in these IgG studies. The necessary lack of controls in these clinical studies has given easy acceptance of the idea that IgG has some specificity through the Fc receptor on granulocytes. This hypothesis has never been rigorously demonstrated to be true, and there are numerous reasons why it is probably not the mechanism of localization[3]. The mechanism of uptake of the non-specific proteins remains obscure but it is likely that increased capillary permeability, which is a hallmark of inflammation causing the redness and swelling, probably plays the major role. Methods based on anti-leukocyte monoclonal antibodies rather than non-specific IgG are more attractive because of their potential for high specificity, equal to 111In WBCs. Clinical results from the use of polyclonal IgG, anti granulocyte and anti CD4 (T helper lymphocyte) MAbs were reported at this symposium and are discussed elsewhere in this volume.

---

[a]Behringwerke BW 250/183; Immunomedics IMMU-MN3.

To put the various non-specific methods mentioned above in perspective, it is instructive to review a carefully controlled animal study carried out by McAfee et al[3]. This work focused on the degree to which a variety of non-specific radioactive agents mimicked the biodistribution of 111In labeled mixed autologous leucocytes. These workers used the same animal model (dogs with acute soft tissue E. coli abscesses and an acute arthritic lesion) to evaluate eight agents: 67Ga citrate, human and canine polyclonal immunoglobulin, rabbit anti-dog polyclonal IgG, serum albumin, monoclonal antibody TNT-1 F(ab')$_2$ against nuclear antigens, 57Co porphyrin and serum albumin nanocolloid. Pure leucocytes were harvested from the joint effusion enabling the stability and association of the label with leucocytes to be measured *in vivo*. The advantage of 111In -WBCs was striking: none of the other agents achieved abscess concentrations approaching those obtained with labeled leucocytes which were almost 10 fold higher. The target to background ratios were also much lower with the non-specific agents. Nevertheless the search for agents capable of direct i.v. injection, preferably labeled with 99mTc, is very important until one is found with lesion concentration and contrast comparable to 111In WBC.

All of the antibody methods suffer from high circulating background activity at the time of imaging. To circumvent this problem we have developed a three step immuno-scintigraphy method in which the antibody and the radiolabel were administered separately[4, 5]. We[6] and others[7] have further suggested that bivalent haptens would improve *in vivo* binding to pretargeted antibody due to enhanced "functional affinity". This effect has already been demonstrated in other multivalent antigen-antibody binding systems[8]. In a mouse tumor model these "Janus" haptens increased the tumor uptake compared to the original method using monovalent haptens[5], but maintained the same high tumor to background ratios[6]. Other strategies employing avidin and biotin for pretargeting have also been described[9]. Avidin and biotin, have affinities much higher than antibodies (10^{15}), and Hnatowitch et al and others have demonstrated improved bio-distribution in mice with this system[10, 11].

Paganelli et al have recently reported excellent human colon cancer images in 20 patients with 1 mg pretargeted biotinylated MAB followed by Avidin and then 111In biotin-chelate conjugate[12]. The images showed increased tumor contrast with low background especially in the liver (2%). Tumors and metastases (including liver) were seen in 3 hrs in all patients. The excellent quality of the scans and high tumor to blood (5.5/1) and tumor to liver (6.7/1) ratios were compelling evidence that pretargeting will be a significant improvement over conventional immunoscintigraphy. The increasing interest in pretargeting technology was shown at the recent 39th Annual Society of Nuclear Medicine meeting in Los Angeles (June 9-12, 1992) where 11 abstracts were presented concerning various aspects of the application of biotin and avidin for pretargeting.

Rapid *in vivo* clearance and biodistribution of the radiolabeled biotin derivatives is crucial in producing a high target to background ratio in 3 hrs or less following i.v. injection. We studied the 24 hr whole body retention (WBR) and 3 hr organ distribution of six biotin-chelate conjugates in tumor mice, with and without avidin[13]. Biotin-chelate derivatives formed stable, high specific activity (1000 Ci/mM) complexes with 111In and 88Y. Endogenous biotin did not block *in vivo* biotin-chelate binding. None of the conjugates of benzyl-EDTA, DTPA or DOTA concentrated selectively in any organ (other than kidney and gut - the major routes of excretion) or in mouse tumor or human tumor xenografts. Avidin and de-glycosylated avidin cleared rapidly from the circulation into the liver where it was not available for targeting biotin. Streptavidin circulated much longer, 30% clearing into the kidney where ~15% was available for targeting of injected biotin activity, making it the highest background organ. We showed pretargeting of a streptavidin-anti IA^k (B lymphocyte determinant) MAB conjugate in antigen positive C3H

STEP 1. 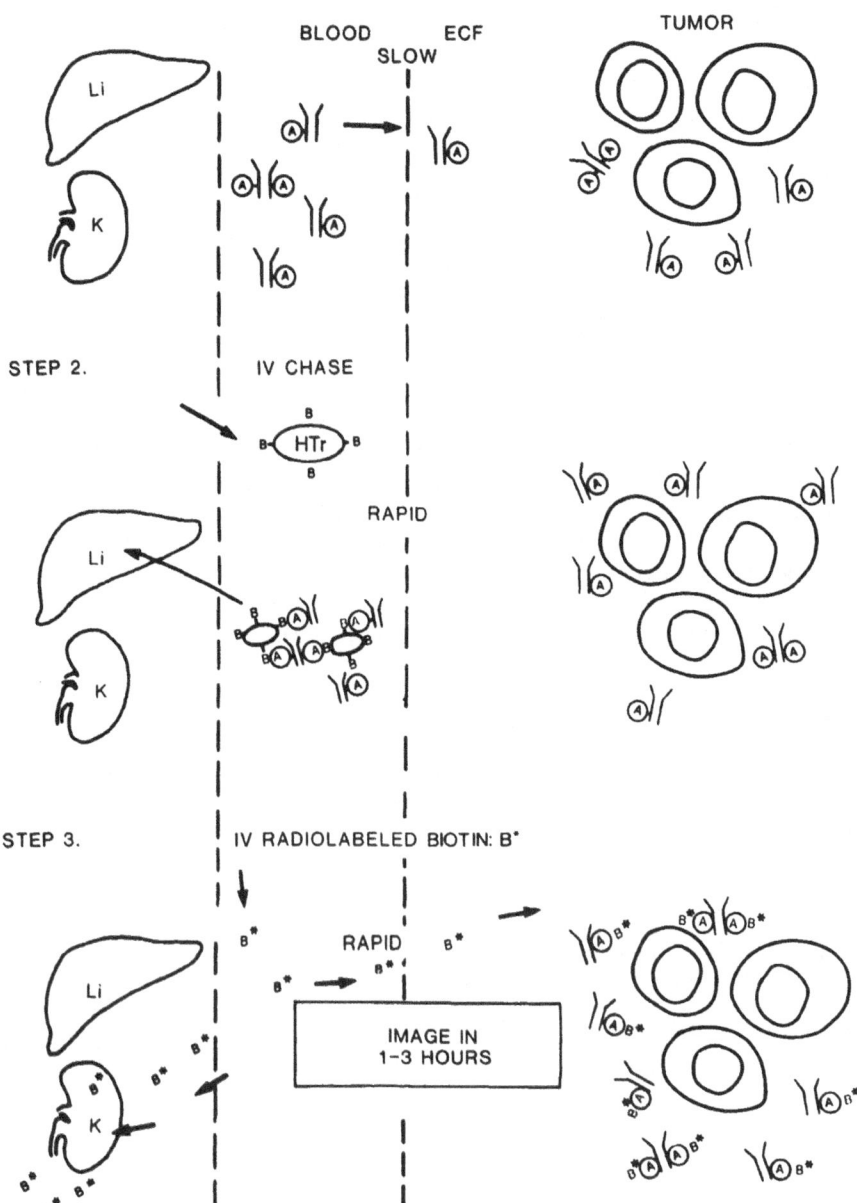   IV AB-AVIDIN : WAIT TIL LOCALIZE 1-4 DAYS

Figure 1. Scheme for pretargeted immunoscintigraphy.

    The dashed columns represent the capillary walls, with the major excretory organs the liver and kidney on the left and the tumor (or abscess) target surrounded by extracellular fluid (ECF) on the right. In this case an avidinated MoAb is injected and slowly diffuses to the target. The chase is biotinylated human transferrin, shown cross-linking the avidin. Radiolabeled biotinylated chelate diffuses rapidly througout the ECF and binds to the avidin in the target.

    By permission of The Journal of Nuclear Medicine and Antibody, Immuno-conjugates, and Radiopharmaceuticals.

mice (spleen=65%/gm) versus antigen negative balb/c (spleen=19%/gm) mice with high target to background ratios[11].

Ruskowski et al[14, 15], reasoning that the protein streptavidin will diffuse through leaky capillaries in a similar fashion to nonspecific polyclonal IgG, have proposed to use it for pretargeted localization of inflammation. These workers have shown encouraging results in their mouse model with E Coli infection in one thigh. Six hour uptake of 111In IgG, 111In streptavidin and 6 hr pretargeted streptavidin (the latter sampled 3 hr post 111In biotin) all showed equivalent uptake, but with target/blood ratios 3 fold higher for pretargeted streptavidin. This finding is in accordance with the view that most proteins will have approximately the same uptake in inflammatory lesions via the common mechanism of leaky capillaries. It is in this situation of equivalent target uptake that the low background obtainable with pretargeting is a great advantage, as shown in this study. The much lower affinity of the biotin chelate used here: EB_1 ($K_A = 10^8$), in the antibody-hapten range, decreased the target concentration, but increased the tumor to background ratios, since normal tissue concentrations also decreased.

Thus the avidin-biotin system promises to be useful for constructing bispecific MABs having both target specific sites, and radiolabel binding sites, for use in either leukocyte specific, clot specific or tumor specific pretargeted immunoscintigraphy[10, 11]. A diagram of the proposed pharmacokinetics is shown in Figure 1. This schema includes a chase step of polybiotinylated protein, capable of cross-linking and thus removing circulating avidin conjugates into the liver, prior to injecting labeled biotin. We have found this greatly reduces blood and liver background.

The widening interest and excellent results with the pretargeting technologies makes it likely that it will be applied in one form or another to cell labeling.

REFERENCES

1. Fischman AJ, Rubin RH, Khaw BA, et al. Detection of acute inflammation with 111In-labelled non-specific polyclonal IgG. *Semin Nucl Med*; 18:335-344 (1988).
2. Buscome JR, Lui D, Ensing G, de Jong R, Ell PJ. 99mTc-human immunoglobulin (HIG) - first results of a new agent for the localization of infection and inflammation. *Eur J Nucl Med*; 16:649-655 (1990).
3. McAfee JG, Gagne G, Subramanian G, and Schneider RF. The localization of Indium-111-leucocytes, Gallium-67-Polyclonal IgG and other radioactive agents in acute focal inflammatory lesions. *J Nucl Med*; 32: 2126-2131 (1991).
4. Reardon DT, Meares CF, Goodwin DA, et al: Antibodies against metal chelates. *Nature*;316:265-268 (1985).
5. Goodwin DA, Meares CF, McCall MJ, McTigue M, Chaovapong W. Pre-targeted immunoscintigraphy of murine tumors with indium-111 labeled bifunctional haptens. *J Nucl Med*; 29: 226-234 (1988).
6. Goodwin DA, Meares CF, McCall MJ, Chaovapong W, McTigue M, Diamante CI: Pretargeted immunoscintigraphy with In-111, Ga-67 and Ga-68 labeled bivalent ("Janus") haptens. *J Clin Nuc Med* 13:9Sp10 (Abstract A3) (1988).
7. Le Doussal J-M, Martin M, Gautherot E, Delaage M, and Barbet J. In vitro and in vivo targeting of radiolabeled monovalent and divalent haptens with dual specificity monoclonal antibody conjugates: enhanced divalent hapten affinity for cell-bound antibody conjugate. *J Nucl Med*; 30:1358-1366 (1989).
8. Karush F. Multivalent binding and functional affinity. *Contemp Top Mol Immunol*; 5: 217 (1976).
9. Goodwin DA. Strategies for antibody targeting. *Antibody, Immunoconjugates, and Radiopharmaceuticals*; 4(4):427-434 (1991).
10. Hnatowitch DJ, Virzi F, and Ruskovski M. Investigations of avidin and biotin for imaging applications.*J Nucl Med*; 28:1294-1302 (1987).
11. Goodwin DA, Meares CF, McCall MJ, McTigue M. An avidin-biotin chelate system for imaging tumors. *J Nucl Med*; 28:722 (abst) (1987).
12. Paganelli G, Magnani P, Zito F, et al. Three-step monoclonal antibody tumor targeting in carcinoembryonic antigen-positive patients. *Ca Res*; 51: 5960-5966 (1991).

13. Goodwin DA, Meares CF, McTiue M, Caovapong W, Ransone C, Renn O, McCall MJ, Studer M. Pharmacokinetics of biotin-chelate conjugates for pretargeted avidin-biotin immunoscintigraphy. *J Nucl Med*; 33: 880 [abstract] (1992).
14. Rusckowski M, Paganelli G, Hnatowich DJ, Virzi F, Fogarasi M, Fazio F. Imaging infection/inflammation in patients with streptavidin and radiolabeled biotin: preliminary observations. *J Nucl Med*; 33: 924 [abstract] (1992).
15. Ruskovsky M, Fritz BS, Hnatowich DJ. Localization of infection using streptavidin and biotin: an alternative to nonspecific polyclonal IgG. *J Nucl Med*; 33: 1810-1815 (1992).

A NEW DIRECT METHOD OF CELL-LABELING IN WHOLE BLOOD BY ADMINISTRATION OF 111In LABELED ANTI-SENSE OLIGONUCLEOTIDE PROBE: EVALUATION OF RADIOLABELED PROBES FOR NONINVASIVE IMAGING OF INFLAMMATION AND INFECTION

M.K. Dewanjee[3], A.K. Ghafouripour[3], W. Mallin[3], A.N. Serafini[3], G.N. Sfakianakis[3], R.K. Werner[3], A.T. Samy[3], A. Krishan[3], S.D. Glenn[1], R.K. Gupta[1], M. Subramanian[2] and M.G. Hanna[2]

[1]Division of Coulter Immunology, Hialeah, FL 33010
[2]Organon Teknika Corp., Rockville
[3]Division of Nuclear Medicine, Department of Radiology, Department of Biochemistry and Molecular Biology, Department of Oncology
University of Miami, School of Medicine, Miami, FL 33101

ABSTRACT

The antisense oligonucleotide probes were labeled with 111Indium for determination of metabolic fate by in vitro and in vivo systems. We optimized the conditions of the chelation e.g. concentration of reactants, pH, time and temperature. The 25-mer nucleotide sequence (sense and antisense) for histone4-mRNA was modified by coupling with aminohexyl group (AHON) and conjugated with DTPA-isothiocyanate (1/10); 50 μg of DTPA-AHON were chelated with 37-370 MBq (1-10 mCi) of 111In chloride with high specific activity 30-100 μCi/μg and labeling efficiency (60-80)%. Incubation of radiolabeled probe with murine leukemic cells (P388) and neutrophils demonstrated probe-stability in plasma and minimum essential media and high permeability, cellular extraction and retention; 0.1 μg/ml of IN-AHON was found optimal for cell-labeling. The histone4 probe showed higher specificity for neutrophils than platelets and red cells. The blood-clearance in Beagle dogs and biodistribution studies in Yorkshire pigs were carried out after injection of In-AHON or In-AHON labeled neutrophils, imaged with a gamma camera and sacrificed for biodistribution; (75±5)% of radioactivity stayed in blood at 720 hours after injection. Margination in lung and pooling in spleen and liver were observed after injection of labeled neutrophils. These results suggested that cells in blood could be labeled directly and could be imaged non-invasively for blood-pool and infection.

INTRODUCTION

The cellular elements of blood had been radiolabeled with a variety of radionuclides for turnover, survival time and imaging blood pool and myocardial contractility (red cells), the sites of infection and inflammation (leukocytes) and thrombosis (platelets). The chemical forms of the tracers were designed to take the opportunity of permeability of anions e.g. 51Cr-chromate, 99mTc-pertechnetate[1], or lipid-soluble metal-complexes, e.g. 111In-oxine or 111In-tropolone, 99mTc-HMPAO[2 - 7] and binding to extracellular membrane-antigens with radiolabeled monoclonal antibodies. Previous cell-labeling procedures were time-consuming and needed separation of blood cells and misadministration of HIV blood products in other bacteria-infected products was catastrophic. In the past, cell-labeling without isolation of cells of interest was possible only with radiolabeled monoclonal antibody against the antigens of the platelets and white-cells.

The base-pairing of adenine with thymine or cytosine with guanine essential for maintaining the stability of duplex DNA, provided the basis for the specificity of the hybridization of synthetic oligonucleotides (antisense) to the complementary DNA or RNA molecules (sense). This specificity has led to the synthesis of 15-50 mer oligonucleotides for using them as tools for molecular biologists for the identification and isolation of specific gene sequences in bacteria, insects, animal models and human genetic diseases. The 5'-OH end of a oligonucleotide can be labeled to a very high specific activity with polynucleotide kinase and [γ-P-32] ATP and S-35 ATP and used in hybridization assays[9 - 11].

Aminolink-2, permits introduction of a primary amine at the 5'-end of the oligonucleotide[12], which can react with biotin, fluorescent dyes, EDTA and DTPA for labeling with 111In, hydroxyphenyl succinimide or activated benzene ring for radioiodination with 125I and 123I[18].

The ß-emitting antisense oligonucleotide probes (radioactive with P-32, S-35) and non-radioactive probes labeled with biotin and digoxin are used widely in in vitro hybridization experiments. The abundance and half-life of some of the mRNAs and DNA-binding proteins, e.g. are sufficiently long; in addition, DTPA-derivatization may stabilize the molecules against nuclease degradation. We presumed that mRNAs and DNA-binding proteins could be localized by permeable radiolabeled probe and noninvasive imaging in a live animal[14]. We have developed the radioiodinated oligonucleotide probes[18] of high specific activity and the techniques of thin-layer and high performance chromatography for the separation, purification and characterization of these labeled probes. Our experience with radiodination with paramethoxyphenyl-isothiocyanate-conjugated aminohexyl oligonucleotide (PMPITC-AHON) helped us in optimizing the reaction conditions of other isothiocyanate with oligonucleotide. The labeling of diethylenetriamine-pentaacetate-(DTPA)-conjugated monoclonal antibodies with 111In radionuclide had been perfected by several investigators[19, 20]. In this study, we describe the techniques of development of sensitive hybridization probes labeled with gamma-emitting radionuclide of indium-111 by direct chelation of DTPAITC-conjugated aminohexyloligonucleotide. During biodistribution studies, we found that some of these 111In labeled oligonucleotides labeled cellular elements of blood by direct intravenous administration.

Considering the possibility the repeated thrombosis and infections in the life-time of a patient and the human anti-mouse response, this new cell-labeling approach with radiolabeled oligonucleotides may be more appropriate and provided a new avenue for blood-pool imaging studies and potential diagnosis of infection.

MATERIALS AND METHODS

The sterile techniques with sterile solutions, plastic-ware and glass-ware were carried out in the laminar flow-hood to prevent the bacterial nuclease-degradation of the precursors and radiolabeled probes. The synthesis of the antisense oligonucleo-tide specific for histone4 mRNA, derivatization with hexylamine, chelation of DTPAITC and conjugation with the oligonucleotide are described below:

Synthesis of Aminohexyl-Conjugated Oligonucleotides

The base sequence of the 25-mer anti-sense oligonucleotide probe, specific for the histone4 mRNA was selected from the nucleic acid data-base (GenBank, University of Wisconsin, Madison). This oligonucleotide carrying an aminohexyl group at their 5'-end was synthesized on a DNA synthesizer with the dimethoxytrityl nucleoside phosphoramidite triester coupling method[13] on a 10 μM solid support column (Applied Biosystems, 3-column 380 B), deprotected and purified by ion exchange HPLC column (Zorbax Bioseries Oligo column). The general formula of AHON, DTPA-AHON, 111In DTPA-AHON and specific sequences (25-mer) of AHON probe for binding histone4 mRNA are as follows:

5'-NH$_2$-(CH$_2$)$_6$-OPO$_3$-OLIGONUCLEOTIDE-OH-3'.
5'-DTPA-CSNH-(CH$_2$)$_6$-OPO$_3$-OLIGONUCLEOTIDE-OH-3'.
5'-In-111-DTPA-CSNH-(CH$_2$)$_6$-OPO$_3$-OLIGONUCLEOTIDE-OH-3'.
5'-H$_2$N-(CH$_2$)$_6$-OPO$_3$-CT-TTG-CCA-AGG-CCC-TTC-CCG-CCT-TT-OH-3'.

The aliquots of purified oligonucleotide were stored frozen in a microfuge tube at -80°C and used as needed.

The conditions of conjugation of DTPAITC with amino-hexyl-oligonucleotide (AHON) were evaluated and the optimization of chelation of AHON were carried out with triplicate samples, at different stoichiometry of DTPAITC/AHON, time, temperature and pH.

Conjugation of DTPA-isothiocyanate with Aminolink-2 Oligonucleotide and Chelation with 111In Radionuclide

The radiolabeling by chelation was carried in two steps: conjugation of DTPA-isothiocyanate (DTPAITC) with aminohexyl-oligonucleotide and direct chelation with 111In. Like the labeled antibody and other proteins, the primary amino group on this aminohexyl-oligomer was then conjugated with the isothiocyanate group of DTPAITC. DTPAITC was synthesized by the method of Mirzadeh et al.[20] and aliquots of 1 mg were transferred to the 1.5 ml polypropylene microfuge tube and stored at -80°C before coupling.

The freeze-dried preparation of DTPAITC (1 mg) was dissolved in 1 ml of 0.1 M Na-acetate buffer (pH=7.95) at room temperature; AHON (200 μg) was added at a stoichiometry of 1/10 and incubated at 45°C for 24 hours. Uncoupled DTPAITC was separated by the Sephadex G-25 (2X20 cm) column with 0.1 M Na-acetate. The DTPAITC-AHON in the void volume is checked by absorbance at 254 nm; the aliquots were combined and 50 microgram aliquots were freeze-dried and stored at -28°C. The 10-50 μg aliquot was dissolved in 100 μl of metal-free 0.1M Na-acetate buffer (pH=5.0); 0.5-1.0 mCi of 111In chloride was mixed with 100 μl of 1M Na-acetate, added to DTPA-AHON and pH was adjusted to 5.5 with 1 M NaOH solution. Unbound 111In was separated by gel-filtration (2X20 cm G-25 column) using 0.1 M Na-acetate buffer and stored at -4°C before use. The chelation with 111In was carried out with the DTPA-isothiocyanate conjugated aminohexyloligonucleotide.

Localization of 111In DTPAITC-aminohexyloligonucleotide Probe in P388 Murine Monocytic Leukemic Cells (P388s) in Tissue Culture

Murine leukemic cells (triplicate), 4.2×10^6 in log and plateau phase were incubated with 111In AHON probes for histone4 and cyclin2 in minimum essential media, at a specific activity of 1 μCi/μg of probe to evaluate probe-stability, permeability and cellular retention of probe. Cells were washed with minimum essential media and radioactivity in supernatant and washings were measured with a gamma counter. The percent of retained radioactivity per million P388 cells were determined.

Labeling of Neutrophils, Platelets and Red Cells with 111In DTPAITC-aminohexylolgonucleotide

The PMN granulocytes were separated according to the method of Chowdhury et al.[5]; 130 mL of blood were collected in 20 mL of ACD anticoagulant solution (NIH-A Fenwal Laboratory) from dogs (conditioned Beagle), pigs (Yorkshire) and non-smoking healthy human volunteers. The PMN granulocytes were separated by Volex sedimenation and Ficoll-Hypaque double-density differential centrifugation and were washed with ACD-saline. Aliquots of platelets, neutrophils and red cells were incubated with variable amounts of 111In labeled sense and antisense probes. The free 111In was removed by centrifugation at 1500G for 10 minutes and cell-bound and washings-associated radioactivity was determined with a gamma counter.

Blood Clearance of 111In Labeled DTPAITC-aminohexyloligonucleotide in Beagle Dogs

Serial blood samples (6 ml each, 3 ml for determination of free radionuclide and 3 ml for measurement of radioactivity in whole blood) were withdrawn post-IV injections (150-200 μCi/20μg) from Beagle dogs (jugular vein) in preweighed and heparinized tubes at 10, 30, and 60 minutes, 2, 3, 4, 6, 8, 24 and 48 hours post-injection. The radioactivity in plasma and cell-pellet were measured after centrifugation at 1650g for 10 minutes.

Biodistribution in Yorkshire Pigs with Labeled 111In DTPAITC-aminohexyloligonucleotide

The Yorkshire pigs were immobilized with ketamine and imaged at 2, 6, 24 and 48 hours with a gamma camera fitted with a medium energy parallel-hole or pin-hole collimator (Siemens Phogamma V). They were sacrificed with an overdose of potassium chloride after anesthetizing with sodium pentobarbital; tissue samples (muscle, blood, fat, marrow) and viscera were harvested and weighed in a microbalance. The tracer distribution in the viscera, blood, marrow and muscle was determined with a gamma counter (Packard Inc., Cobra II) in the 140-470 keV window to include the 171-, 245- and the sum peak at 416 keV of the 111In radionuclide. The mean and standard deviation values of relative radioactivity ratios of blood/muscle, percent of injected dose/gram and percent of injected dose were calculated for each pig with the LOTUS-123 software and IMB PS/2 computer.

RESULTS AND DISCUSSION

Although several 25-mer nucleotide sequence selected for binding ß-actin, myosin, histone2 and histone4 were evaluated for cell-labeling, only 111In labeled oligonucleotide selected for binding histone4 mRNA showed highest affinity for labeling cellular elements of blood, mainly neutrophils; this partial selectivity was observed with neutrophils from mouse, dog, pig and human blood.

The optimal conditions of conjugation and radiolabeling were established. The cojugation of DTPAITC with AHON at a ratio 10/1 for 18-20 hours at a temperature of 40°C gave an coupling yield of 85-95%. The incubation of 111In chloride with DTPAITC-AHON at a ratio 10/1 for 30 minutes gave an yield of 85-90%. The optimum pH of chelation of DTPAITC-AHON probe with 111In was 6.5; on the other hand, the pH of coupling of DTPAITC with AHON was 8.5.

The majority of radioactivity after intravenous administration in dogs and pigs were not excreted. The HPLC analyses demonstrate the presence of smaller fragments of oligonucleotides in plasma sample at 3 hours. DTPA-coupling stabilized the AHON. The instant labeling and higher ratio of blood/muscle and blood/fat permitted early immediate blood-pool imaging.

The steady-state concentrations of an mRNA are determined by 3 factors: (i) rate of transcription, (ii) efficiency of processing and transport to cytoplasm, and (iii) half-life in the cytoplasm. The degradation of histone mRNA depends on the nucleotide sequence, the efficiency of 3'-end formation, the level of nuclease and the signals regulating the nuclease[17]. Marzluff and Graves[14] indicated that in mice, the histone genes are present in 2 clusters on chromosomes 3 and 13 and both sets are regulated coordinately during S phase. The histone mRNAs have simple structures with 5' cap , short 5'- and 3'-untranslated regions of nucleotides for probe-hybridization. The synthesis of major histone proteins in mammalian cells is directly related to DNA synthesis. The concentrations of the histone mRNAs increase rapidly 30-50 fold during the DNA synthesis; the half-life of histone mRNA in S phase is about 45-60 minutes but decreases to 10-15 minutes at the end of S phase. This level and time of mRNA retention in cytoplasm may be sufficient for hybridization, retention of labeled probe and non-invasive imaging. The mRNA target for the labeled oligonucleotide is shown in Figure 1. The exact role of histone4 mRNA and DNA-binding proteins in the binding of 111In labeled oligonucleotides and cellular retention is not known.

The permeability and probe-stability are two issues of concern. We believe that these probes of smaller size after intravenous administration has high permeability and permitted higher signal/ratio sufficient for non-invasive imaging of blood-pool. Homogenization of cells, separation of organelles and TCA precipitation demonstrated that 70-80% of 111In radioactivity was bound to macromolecules.

Binding with P388 cells in log phase with more mRNA copies is higher than that of plateau phase cells. Similar values were obtained with 25-mer cyclin2 probes (Figure 2). Incubation of probe in plasma media, followed by HPLC separation showed 85-90% of probe was stable for a period of 24 hours. The cellular-uptake reached a saturation value at 30 minutes. The results of homogenization and TCA precipitation demonstrated 60-70% of the probe insoluble and possibly bound to mRNA of histone4, nucleic acids and DNA-binding proteins. The DTPA-coupling probally inhibited the exonuclease and ribonucleaseH degradation to a certain extent permitting the receptor-dependent uptake of these probes[16]. Dorsch observed uptake of iodine-labeled single-stranded DNA (SSDNA) in platelets[15]; this uptake could be blocked by carrier SSDNA. Loke et al. found that the oligonucleotide localized in the cells by receptor-dependent endocytic process[16].

Unlike cell-labeling with radiolabeled monoclonal antibody, one specific radiolabeled AHON could be used specific for all animals and patients and there is no possibility of adverse reaction due to anti-mouse antibody. The antisense oligonucleotide was found useful for therapy of leukemia[21]; the midsection of this probe was found to have common sequence with that of In-DTPAAHON. The acute toxicity[21] of the oligonucleotide in mice and rats was found acceptable (LD_{50} = 50-60 mg/kg). These probes could be prepared without cloning and enzymatic treatment. Considering the nuclease-resistance of the DTPA-AHON, we believe that the 111In and 99mTc labeled derivative of oligonucleotide probes may be more useful than conventional radioactive tracers and associated reagents. Further studies are in progress for understanding the fate of radiolabeled oligonucleotide probes and screen nucleotide sequence to increase further the leukocyte-binding in whole blood for potential use in the diagnosis of infection. In addition, we are finding novel applications for measurement of amplified oncogenes (c-myc and c-myb) in malignant tissues in animal models.

As oligonucleotides are increasingly being used in understanding the DNA-turnover in normal cell function, cell pathology (SLE), diagnosis and therapy of various diseases, 111In labeled oligonucleotides will promote exploration of these areas in both in vitro and in vivo systems.

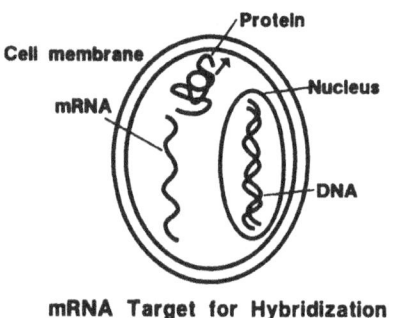

Figure 1. Mechanism of cellular in situ hybridization for the binding and retention of 111In labeled antisense oligonucleotides with specific mRNA signal.

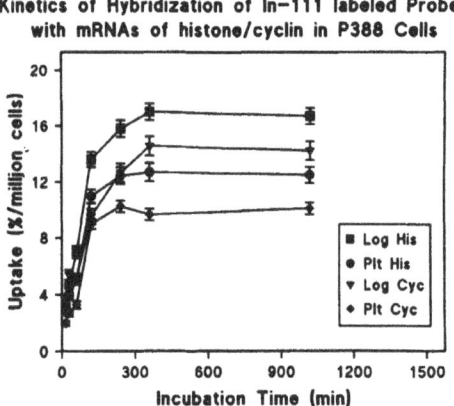

Figure 2. Normalized values of extraction of 111In labeled antisense aminohexyl-oligonucleotide for histone4 and cyclin2 by P388 cells in log and plateau phase.

ACKNOWLEDGEMENT

The authors highly appreciate the supports of DOE DE-FG05-88ER60728, NIH HL47201, Baxter Healthcare Corporation and Florida High Tech Industry Council. The technical assistance was provided by Mansoor Kapadvanjwala, Sarat Chandarlapaty, Maryam Minhaj and Larry Willems.

REFERENCES

1. Eckelman WC, Richards P, Hauser W, et al. Technetium-labeled red cells. *J Nucl Med* 11: 22-24 (1971).
2. Dewanjee MK. The binding of technetium(IV)-99m ion to hemoglobin. *J Nucl Med* 15: 703-706 (1974).
3. McAfee JG and Thakur ML. Survey of radioactive agents for in vitro labeling of phaogocytic leukocytes. I. Soluble agents. *J Nucl Med* 17: 480-487 (1976).
4. Dewanjee MK, Rao SA and Didisheim P: 111Indium tropolone, a new high-affinity platelet label: Preparation and evaluation of labeling parameters. *J Nucl Med* 22: 981-987 (1981).
5. Chowdhury S, Brown ML, Dewanjee MK, Forstrom LA, Katzman JA. Labeled polymorphonuclear leukocytes: a comparison of methodology. *Int J Nucl Med Biol Part B*. 15 (5), 5111-5114 (1988).
6. Dewanjee MK. Cardiac and vascular imaging with labeled platelets and leukocytes. *Sem Nucl Med* 14: 154-187 (1984).
7. Peters AM, Danpure HJ, Osman S, et al: Clinical experience with 99mTc hexamethylpropyleneamineoxime for labeling leukocytes and imaging inflammation. *Lancet* 946-949, Oct. 25 (1986).
8. Dewanjee MK, Ghafouripour AK, Werner RK, Ganz WI, Glenn SD, Gupta RK, Serafini AN, Sfakianakis GN. Development of 111In labeled mRNA probes by conjugation of DTPA-isothiocyanate with antisense oligonucleotides specific for actin and histone. *J Nucl Med* 32: 1048 (1991).
9. Sambrook J, Fritsch EF, Maniatis T. Synthetic oligonucleotide probes. Chapter 11, In Molecular Cloning, A Laboratory Manual. (Cold Spring Harbor Laboratory Press, New York, 1989), Vol 2, p. 11.3.
10. Smith LM, Sanders JZ, Kaiser RJ, Hughes P, Dodd C, Connell CR, Heiner C, Kent SBH and Hood LE. Fluorescence detection in automated DNA sequence analysis. *Nature* 321: 674-678 (1986).
11. Doel MT and Smith M. The chemical synthesis of deoxyribo-oligonucleotides complementary to the lysozyme gene of phage T4 and their hybridization to phage specific RNA in phage DNA. *FEBS Lett* 34: 99-102 (1973).
12. Connolly BA. The synthesis of oligonucleotides containing a primary amino group at the 5'-terminus. *Nucl Acid Res* 15(7): 3131-3139 (1987).
13. Matteucci MD, Caruthers MH. Synthesis of deoxyoligonucleo-tides on a polymer support. *J Amer Chem Soc* 103:3185-3191 (1981).
14. Marzluff WF, Pandey NB. Multiple regulatory steps control histone mRNA concentrations. *Trends Biochem Sci* 13: 49-52 (1988).
15. Dorsch CA. Binding of single-strand DNA to human platelets. *Throm Res* 24: 119-129 (1981).
16. Loke SL, Stein CA, Zhang XH, Mori K, Nakanishi M, Subasinghe C, Cohen JS, Neckers LM. Characterization of oligonucleotide transport into living cells. *Proc Natl Acad Sci* 86: 3474-3478 (1989).
17. Dudding LR, Harington A, Mizrahi V. Endoribonucleolytic cleavage of RNA: oligonucleotide hybrids by the ribonuclease H activity of HIV-1 reverse transcriptase. *Biochem Biophys Res Commun* 167: 244-250 (1990).
18. Dewanjee MK, Ghafouripour AK, Werner RK, Serafini AN, Sfakianakis GN. Development of sensitive radioiodinated anti-sense oligonucleotide probes by conjugation technique. *Bioconjugate Chemistry* 2: 195-200 (1990).
19. Hnatowich DJ, Layne WW, Childs RL, et al: Radioactive labeling of antibody: a simple and efficient method. *Science* 220: 613-615 (1983).
20. Mirzadeh S, Brechbiel MW, Atcher RW, Gansow OA. Radiometal labeling of immunoproteins: Covalent linkage of 2-(4-isothiocyanatobenzyl) diethylenetriaminepentaacetic acid ligands to immunoglobulin. *Bioconjugate Chem* 1, 59-65 (1990).
21. Agrawal S. Antisense oligonucleotides: a possible approach of chemotherapy of aids. In Prospects for Antisense Nucleic Acid Therapy of Cancer and Aids. E. Wickstrom, Ed. Wiley-Liss, New York, 1991, pp. 143-158.

TRANSCHELATION OF 114mIn FROM IgG-DTPA TO ABSCESS-RELATED PROTEINS

A.J. Carlson, D. Sasso, and R.E. Weiner

Department of Nuclear Medicine
University of Connecticut Health Center
Farmington CT

INTRODUCTION

Human, polyclonal, nonspecific IgG labeled with 111In has shown clinical utility for inflammation detection[1], but the process by which 111In localizes in an abscess is little understood. While breakdown in the endothelial barrier may explain the initial localization process, it cannot explain the retention over 24 or 48 hr of the clinical time frame. We have suggested that factors at the abscess site, e.g., high concentrations of Lactoferrin (LF) or Ferritin (FE) and low molecular weight mediators e.g., ATP, permit 67Ga to be translocated to these proteins and aid in the continual accumulation of radionuclide[2,3]. This general model can be applied to the localization of 111In-IgG and is shown in Figure 1. In this study we have examined the details of the transfer of 114mIn from IgG-DTPA to LF and transferrin (TF).

METHODS

Influence of Mediators and pH on 114mIn Transfer from DTPA to Protein

A 20 μM LF solution in 50 mM MES buffer containing, 100 mM NaCl, 5 mM NaHCO$_3$, and 0.02 % N$_3$ (MES/HCO$_3$ buffer) pH 6.7 or a 20 μM TF solution in 50 mM TRIS buffer containing, 78 mM NaCl, 30 mM NaHCO$_3$, and 0.02 % N$_3$ pH 7.4, was split into 400 μL samples, and an aliquot of a stock 114mIn-DTPA solution and an aliquot of buffer as a control, or a stock of PP$_i$, glutathione, L-cysteine, or ATP solution was added to each sample to yield 0.1 and 1 mM PP$_i$ or 1 mM of the other mediators. At various times between 0-50 hr for TF and 0-390 hr for LF the protein-bound activity was determined by G-50 chromatography as described[2] except that the chromatography was performed at $\sim$20°C and 0.02% N$_3$ was included in the buffer. To test the effect of pH, a 20 μM LF solution in MES/HCO$_3$ buffer was adjusted to pH 5.3, 6.0 and 6.7, an aliquot of stock 114mIn-DTPA solution was added to each and at 0, 24, 140 and 325 hr protein bound activity was determined as described. In the above experiments the final concentration was: LF or TF = 20 μM, 0.4 μM DTPA, 450-600 μM Citrate and 114mIn = 1-4 X 10^5 CPM/mL, 113In = 0,2 - 0,4 μM and incubations at 37°C.

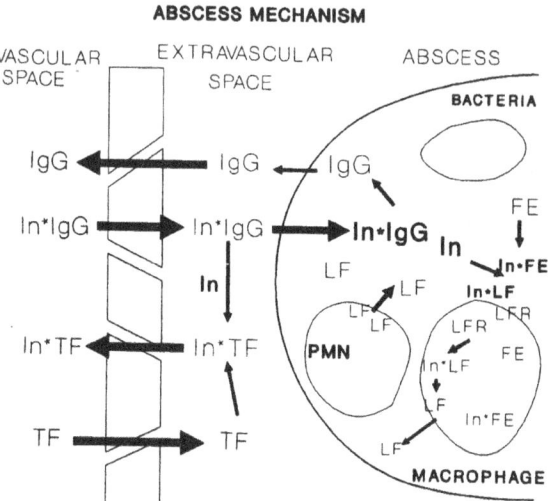

Figure 1. Model for the translocation of 111In from IgG-DTPA to Lactoferrin (LF), Ferritin (FE) or transferrin (TF), in the presence of polymorphonuclear leukocytes (PMN), and subsequent binding of 111In*LF complex to LF macrophage receptor (LFR) and incorporation of the 111In to intracellular FE.

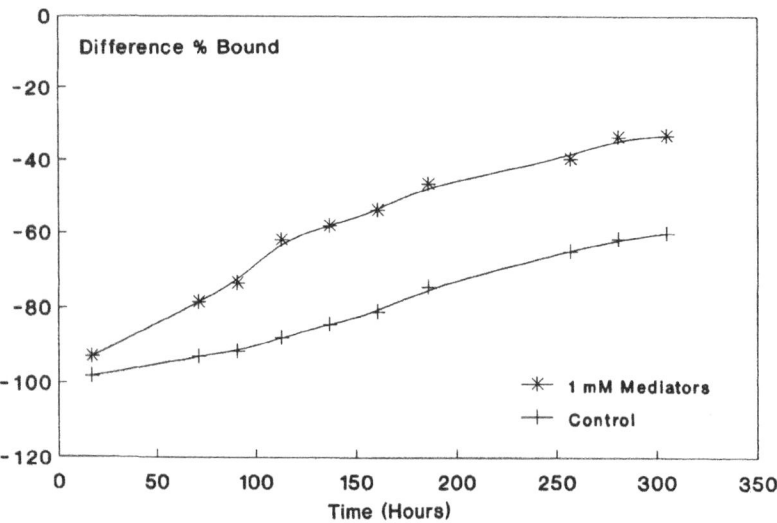

Figure 2. Influence of mediator mixture on the transfer of 114mIn from 0.4 μM IgG-DTPA (~0.8 DTPA/IgG) to 20 μM LF using equilibrium dialysis. The samples were incubated at 37°C in the presence of buffer (+) and (*) 1 mM ATP, PP$_i$, glutathione and L-cysteine. Other conditions given in the text. Points represent means of at least duplicate samples.

Effect of Mediators on Translocation of 114mIn from IgG to LF

The coupling of cyclic anhydride DTPA (cDTPAA) to IgG was performed according to Paik et al.[4]. Briefly, cDTPAA in anhydrous DMSO was added to a human polyclonal IgG (Calbiochem) solution (~ 16 mg/ml) in a 30-50:1 ratio. To remove unbound DTPA, 100-200 μL of the IgG-DTPA solution was washed 3 times with 2 mL of 50 mM Pipes buffer containing 100 mM NaCl (Pipes buffer) pH 6.5 using a Centricon-30 microconcentrator. To add 114mIn to the IgG-DTPA, an In-NTA solution was made by titrating the acidic 114mInCl (Dupont 47-128 mCi/mg), NTA solution with HCO_3^- to the desired pH and incubating for 30 min at 80°C. Then 5-50 μL of this mixture, ~ 1 mM NTA, was added to IgG-DTPA in Pipes buffer pH 6.7 and incubated for 1 hr at 37°C. Non-bound 114mIn was removed with 3 washes using the Centricon-30 microconcentrator. Control experiments showed that < 0.1% of added activity remained bound to IgG after this procedure. Translocation experiments were performed using dialysis technique as previously described[2]. Briefly, 1 mL of a 0.4 μM 114mIn*IgG solution in Pipes buffer pH 6.7, containing 1-4 x 10^5 CPM/mL and 113In = 0.16 μM, is placed in the left chamber while 1 mL of a 20 μM LF solution in the same buffer was placed in the right chamber of 5 dialysis cells. To test the influence of mediating agents, 100 μL of a mediator solution was added to right and left chambers of 3 cells and 100 μL of buffer was added to 2 of the cells. A relative amount of nuclide bound to LF was computed from Difference % Bound (D%B) = (R-L/R+L) x 100 where R is the activity in the right chamber and L is the activity in the left chamber.

RESULTS

Translocation of 114mIn from DTPA to LF and TF

While previous results had demonstrated that PP_i stimulated translocation from IgG to LF and TF[5], PP_i concentration had no influence on binding of activity to LF at pH 6.7 but PP_i inhibited 114mIn binding to TF at pH 7.4 and did not stimulate transfer as might be expected. After an incubation of 20 hr, the % of TF-bound nuclide was 86, 65 and 30 for 0, 0.1 and 1 mM PP_i, respectively. Because a number of phosphoryl containing compounds stimulated 67Ga translocation, various intracellular compounds were examined that could be present at the abscess site due to cell damage. ATP and thiol-containing mediators dramatically stimulated movement of nuclide from DTPA to LF at pH 6.7. After 380 hr of incubation, LF bound 58% of the activity in the presence of ATP while the LF-bound 114mIn with added L-cysteine and glutathione, was 43% and 41% respectively, compared to 15% in the control. Incubation pH profoundly effected transfer; as the pH was reduced the LF-bound 114mIn declined from 20% at pH 6.7, 1% at pH 6, to 0.1% at pH 5.3 (150 hr).

Effect of Mediators on 114mIn Transfer from IgG-DTPA to LF

Figure 2 shows that even in the presence of buffer at a slightly acidic pH 6.7, there is a slow movement of activity from IgG-DTPA to LF. After 113 hr of incubation, the D%B was -88±2% which corresponds to ~6% LF-bound activity. With the addition of a mixture of L-cysteine, glutathione, ATP and PP_i, the amount of 114mIn transferred to LF significantly ($P < 0.05$) increased as the experiment proceeds. At 113 hr, the D%B was -62±9% which corresponds to ~ 19% LF-bound nuclide.

CONCLUSIONS

PP$_i$ actually slowed the transfer of 114mIn from DTPA to TF; however when DTPA is coupled to IgG, PP$_i$ stimulated nuclide transfer[5]. This suggests that DTPA-IgG coupling enables PP$_i$ to bind to the antibody, properly position the mediator to attack the chelate and increase the off rate of the 114mIn from the DTPA. Other mediators did not act directly on IgG-DTPA but stimulated transfer by enhancing 111In binding LF and shifting the equilibrium toward the higher affinity LF. Reducing the pH reduced the binding of nuclide to LF but pH decline appeared to have the opposite effect on the translocation from IgG-DTPA to LF. At pH 6, after 120 hr of incubation in the absence of any mediators, LF bound 31% of the 111In activity[5] which is 3-fold greater than the value we observed at pH 6.7, ~8% (Fig. 2). This implies that the effect of pH on IgG-DTPA is rate limiting in the translocation reaction.

These experiments coupled with our previous data[5] demonstrate that even though 111In has a high affinity for DTPA, conditions at the abscess site can stimulate the removal of the nuclide and are consistent with data from an *in vivo* model. Claessens and co-workers[6, 7] have shown in a rat abscess model that if 99mTc, 111In, and 131I labeled IgG are compared, the 111In alone remains at the abscess and while the %ID/g of the other nuclides declines as a function of time. It is likely that both the 131I and 99mTc are stripped from the protein moiety by the conditions at the abscess site but cannot rebind to other abscess constituents and are removed by diffusion. In sum, after 111In*DTPA-IgG passes into an abscess site via a disrupted endothelial cell barrier the 111In is translocated to LF, FE or proteins at the site, allowing the 111In to remain.

REFERENCES

1. Oyen WJG, Claessens RAMJ, van Horn JR, et al. Scintigraphic detection of bone and joint infections with indium-111-labeled nonspecific polyclonal human immunoglobulin G. *J Nucl Med*;31:430-412 (1990).
2. Weiner RE. The role of phosphate containing compounds on the transfer of 111In and 67Ga from transferrin to ferritin. *J Nucl Med*;24:608-614 (1989).
3. Weiner RE. The role of transferrin and other receptors in the mechanism of 67Ga localization. *Nucl Med Biol*;17:141-149 (1990).
4. Paik CH, Ebbert MA, Murphy PR, et al. Factors influencing DTPA conjugation with antibodies by cyclic DTPA anhydride. *J Nucl Med*;24:1158-1163 (1983).
5. Rayne D, Weiner RE. Exchange of In-111 between IgG and lactoferrin, transferrin and ferritin. *J Nucl Med*;32:1099 (1991).
6. Oyen WJG, Claessens RAMJ, van der Meer JWM, et al. Biodistribution and kinetics of radiolabeled proteins in rats with focal infection. *J Nucl Med*;31:403-412 (1992).
7. Claessens R, Oyen W, Koenders E, et al. Potential and pitfalls of In-labelled and iodinated proteins for scintigraphy of infectious disease and malignancy. *Nucl Med Commun*;13:628 (1992).

THE ANTIBODY APPROACH OF LABELING BLOOD CELLS

S.C. Srivastava

Medical Department
Brookhaven National Laboratory
Upton, New York 11973, USA

ABSTRACT

Although the science of blood cell labeling using monoclonal antibodies directed against specific cellular antigens is still in its early stages, considerable progress has recently been accomplished in this area. The monoclonal antibody approach offers the promise of greater selectivity and enhanced convenience since specific cell types can be labeled in vivo, thus eliminating the need for complex and damaging cell separation procedures. This article focuses on these developments with primary emphasis on antibody labeling of platelets and leukocytes. The advantages and the shortcomings of the recently reported techniques are critically assessed and evaluated.

INTRODUCTION

The important role of radiolabeled cellular blood elements in diagnostic nuclear medicine procedures is by now clearly well established. A variety of methods have been developed for labeling red blood cells (RBC), leukocytes (WBC) and platelets (P) with different radionuclides. Most techniques employ either 99mTc or 111In, and a number of kit methods are now available for the in-vitro labeling of the above cell types with these radionuclides. Technetium-99m-RBC and 111In-labeled WBC and platelets are now routinely used, for example in applications such as: cardiovascular blood pool imaging, detection of GI bleeding and hemangiomas, etc. (RBC); localization of inflammatory lesions (WBC); and for thrombus detection (P). In-vivo cell kinetics and survival in health and disease can be studied using longer-lived indium-111. Despite the proven usefulness of these methods in the clinical setting, however, research activity in the area of leukocyte and platelet labeling has continued with a view to developing newer and better techniques particularly those that overcome the serious disadvantage of cell separation before labeling.

The methodology for RBC labeling with 99mTc has matured to the point that available kit methods now assure highly reliable clinical data (Srivastava, 1990; Patrick, 1991). This is primarily a result of extensive mechanistic investigations of the uptake and binding of tin and technetium to various blood components which in turn have led to a clearer understanding of both in-vitro and in-vivo RBC labeling reactions (Srivastava, 1984). Non-specific cell labeling mechanisms such as the "pretinning" approach used for 99mTc-RBC when applied to leukocytes and platelets require prior cell separation (Srivastava, 1990). Cell separation methods are cumbersome, time consuming, and pose the likelihood of cell damage and thus a compromise in in-vivo cell function. Another nonspecific technique involves the use of lipophilic chelates that are taken up into the cells by passive diffusion. This mechanism is utilized in the classical 111In-oxine method (Desai, 1986), and more recently in 99mTc-HMPAO -labeling of both isolated leukocytes (Peters, 1986) and platelets. Following uptake into the cells, the radionuclide gets more strongly bound to intracellular components.

Specific cell labeling mechanisms include the in-vitro method for labeling leukocytes in whole blood based on the phagocytosis of tin-technetium colloids applicable to granulocytes and monocytes (Hanna, 1984; Srivastava, 1990), and the monoclonal antibody approach for labeling both leukocytes and platelets. Even though this latter approach is an evolving science that is still in its early stages, significant progress has been made during the last few years. These developments offer the promise to selectively label specific cell types in blood, in vitro or in vivo, thus overcoming the need for complex and damaging cell separation steps. Monoclonal antibodies directed against specific cellular antigens continue to be identified and developed (Buchegger, 1984; Bosslet, 1985; Coller, 1985; Thakur, 1987, 1988; McAfee, 1988a). A number of these have attracted considerable interest and are presently undergoing active investigation. This paper provides a brief review and assessment of the advantages and the shortcomings associated with these techniques that utilize cell-specific monoclonal antibodies, the focus being primarily on platelets and leukocytes.

PLATELETS

Since platelets play a crucial role in the formation of thrombi and other vascular lesions, much research has focused on the development of radiolabeled platelets for the scintigraphic localization of these lesions. Following adhesion to the damaged vessel wall, platelets undergo aggregation at these sites. These platelets also introduce biochemical changes that result in the release of various substances that accelerate fibrin production during thrombus formation. Platelets are not only important physiologic mediators of clot formation but they also make up for a significant portion of the mass of the clots. Conventional 111In-oxine labeled platelets, though useful for thrombus detection, are not ideal due to their high blood pool background. Since a monoclonal antibody directed against platelets would be expected to specifically bind to platelets in vivo, this approach has been investigated in detail for a number of years.

Coller et al (Coller, 1983) were the first to report the development of an antiplatelet antibody (7E3) directed against the fibrinogen receptor that consists of a glycoprotein IIb/IIIa complex on the platelet surface. Following further characterization of this antibody (Coller, 1985) studies were undertaken to develop chemical methods to label it with various radionuclides including 123I, 131I, 111In, and 99mTc. Binding of the labeled antibody with platelets in whole blood was investigated and these labeled blood samples were evaluated for imaging experimental thrombi and vascular lesions in dogs (Srivastava, 1984; Oster, 1985; Srivastava, 1988). The antibody 7E3 belongs to the IgG1 subclass and inhibits ADP-induced platelet aggregation, as well as the ADP-induced binding of fibrinogen to platelets. There are 5×10^4 antibody binding sites per human platelet, and 7.5×10^4 binding sites per dog platelet. In vitro studies with human and dog platelets showed that: there is only one type of binding site; greater than 90% tracer antibody dose binds to human platelets; ~70% of tracer dose binds to dog platelets; there is negligible binding to other blood components; virtually all platelet-bound 7E3 becomes incorporated into thrombin produced clots; 10 μg antibody/ml blood causes total inhibition of platelet aggregation; and 0.5-1 μg antibody/ml blood did not produce any significant change in platelet function (Srivastava, 1984). The antibody was iodinated by reacting 100 μg of 7E3 with radioiodine (123I, 131I) at a molar ratio of iodine to antibody of ~0.5, in the presence of 5 μg Chloramine T as the oxidant. The Iodogen technique was equally effective. Labeling yields (following purification) were 30-80% depending upon the reaction conditions, and the specific activity ranged between 20-300 μCi/μg (for 123I at an average of <0.5 iodine atoms per antibody molecule). Labeling with 111In was accomplished after conjugating DTPA to the antibody using the cyclic anhydride method

(Hnatowich, 1983). Labeling yields (using 100 μg antibody) were ~80% and the specific activity ranged between 10-40 μCi/μg at an average of 0.2 to 0.5 indium atoms per antibody molecule. Both iodine and indium labeled 7E3 displayed >90% binding specificity in the fibrinogen-coated bead assay (Coller, 1985).

Blood clearance in dogs of the 7E3-labeled platelets showed that the initial recovery was ~70%, very similar to indium-oxine-labeled platelets. Approximately 50% of injected activity remained in the blood at 30 min, dropped to 40-45% at ~60 min, and then remained fairly constant up to 4 hr. Both iodine- and indium-7E3-labeled platelets showed a very similar blood clearance; plasma levels of 111In were ~10% as opposed to ~5% for 123I. Total urinary excretion at 4 hr was less than 2%. Arterial and venous clots were produced in dogs either by thrombin injection into vein segments, by transcatheter placement of a copper coil into blood vessels, or by electrocoagulation. One to 3 hr post-injection of the 7E3 labeled blood sample, clots in the lung as well as carotid thrombi were visualized well. Clot-to-blood ratios in various imaging experiments ranged between 5 and 35. Early and clear images of experimental arterial and venous thrombi in these areas were obtained in all experiments without the need for blood pool subtraction (Oster, 1985). Thrombus localization using 131I-7E3-platelets was compared with the 111In-oxine-platelet technique in the same animals (Ezekowitz, 1986). The venous thrombi were clearly imaged within 5-30 min with 131I-7E3-platelets and in ~60 min with 111In-oxine-platelets. The clot to blood ratios were approximately twice as high as with 111In-oxine-platelets. Coronary thrombi were visible ex vivo but only one-third of the time in vivo at 3-4 hr after injection. 111Indium-oxine images at this time period were negative. It was concluded that more rapid blood clearance of 7E3-platelets, either through a manipulation of the degree of substitution of 7E3 on platelets, or through using antibody fragments, would be required for prompt and reproducible imaging of coronary thrombi (Ezekowitz, 1986; Srivastava, 1988).

Antibodies similar to 7E3 (glycoprotein IIb/IIIa antigen) have been investigated by other groups as well. In one study B 79.7 and B59.2 antibodies were labeled with 125I and 111In and shown to be effective for imaging experimental thrombi in animals (Thakur, 1987). The specific activities of 111In and 125I preparations averaged 5 and 2.4 Ci/μmol respectively. Scatchard analysis gave values of Kd for 111In-B79.7 and 125I-B79.7 as 83×10^{-9}M/L and 113×10^{-9}M/L respectively. MAb B59.2 reacted with canine platelets and at 50% antigen saturation, 49.5% of the 111In-DTPA-B59.2 was bound to platelets. The thrombus to blood ratios averaged 15.8, 2 hr following injection of the labeled platelets. Clinical evaluation of these antibodies remains yet to be carried out. Other publications discuss results on 111In and 99mTc-labeled P-256 antibody (whole IgG as well as Fab'$_2$) for imaging deep venous thrombi in patients (Peters, 1986a; Stuttle, 1988). In this study in six patients, DVT were imaged at 24 hr in three which had documented clots. Old thrombi were not detected. This is a current limitation of this approach since it images fresh clots where platelet adhesion is an active phenomenon. Prolonged circulation of labeled platelets is also a problem that needs to be resolved, as mentioned above.

Another antibody, 50H.19, that recognizes a low molecular weight tumor cell antigen and also cross-reacts with human platelets recognizing three proteinase-sensitive low molecular weight antigens was evaluated for thrombus imaging (Som, 1986). A kit method was used to label 50H.19 fragments with 99mTc with an average of 97 $\pm$ 6% labeling yield. Binding to platelets in vitro or in vivo averaged around 60%. Approximately 50% of the radioactivity was cleared from the blood in 3-6 min and 18-24% was excreted in urine within 3 hr. Experimental thrombi in dogs in peripheral veins and arteries, pulmonary arteries and the right ventricle could be visualized 2-3 hr following injection. Blood pool subtraction or delayed imaging were not necessary. Detailed investigation in patients, yet to be carried out, will determine the eventual clinical effectiveness of 99mTc-50H.19 for thrombus imaging.

Another promising approach has been the development of antibodies specific for an external membrane protein of activated platelets (Palabrica, 1989). These "anti-activated platelet" monoclonal antibodies would seem to provide greater contrast for thrombus imaging since their binding to the normal circulating platelet pool can be expected to be small or negligible. A recent study in animals with 99mTc-labeled S12 (Chouraqui, 1991a) has suggested the potential usefulness of this agent for imaging coronary and other arterial thrombi in humans. In this study, 19 out of 20 femoral clots and 3 out of 3 coronary thrombi were visualized immediately after injection and remained positive until more than one hour. Blood clearance was biphasic with a t½ of the two components of 36 and 96 min respectively. The uptake of 99mTc-S12 by arterial thrombi, however, was found to decline rapidly with the age of the thrombus. This points to a diminished effectiveness (e.g., only ~35% for 48 hr old thrombi) of this technique for in vivo imaging of aged thrombi (Chouraqui, 1991).

A number of antifibrin antibodies have been found to be useful for imaging fresh as well as aged thrombi with a varying degree of effectiveness (Knight, 1988; McAfee, 1988). A discussion of these systems is beyond the scope of this paper since the emphasis is primarily on antibodies that recognize and label cellular antigens.

LEUKOCYTES

Even though studies involving anti-leukocyte antibodies are still preliminary, some very promising results have been reported with the use of at least four antigranulocyte antibodies for the localization of abscesses and other inflammatory lesions (Table 1). The first report was by Locher et al (Locher, 1986) who presented data on imaging abscesses in humans with an 123I labeled anti-CEA MAb 47. This antibody was identified and developed by Mach's group in 1984 (Buchegger, 1984). The antibody is directed against a non-specific cross-reacting antigen (NCA 95) on the granulocyte surface, expressed particularly during the final stages of the development of these cells. Undifferentiated and rapidly proliferating early granulopoeitic cells do not bind the antibody. The only cross reaction was observed from CEA producing tumors. The antibody was iodinated with 123I using the Iodogen method, with a final activity concentration of 20-60 mCi/mg IgG (Andres, 1988). As with other granulocyte labels, 123I-AK-47 does not distinguish between abscesses and other types of inflammatory foci (Seybold, 1988). Hasler et al (Hasler, 1988) reported that 8-17% of the injected dose was associated with circulating granulocytes and the clearance of the antibody from the circulation fitted a biphasic model with effective half-lives of the components of 0.73 and 9.3 hr respectively. In five patients administered with 3.4-5.4 mCi of 123I-AK-47 (~120 μg antibody), clear images of the lesions were obtained at 30 min to 24 hr following injection. No HAMA was detectable in patients with small doses (<120μg) of the antibody. This antibody was also recently labeled with 99mTc using a new one-step method in which a free terminal amino group was utilized (Locher, 1991). When compared with 123I-AK-47 in same patients, the distributions and scan qualities were observed to be similar although diagnostically relevant differences were noted in some cases of chronic osteomyelitis. The accuracy, sensitivity, and specificity of both methods averaged greater than 90%. These investigators concluded that 99mTc-AK-47 is more advantageous for routine use although 123I-AK-47 is preferable in some cases of chronic infections (Locher, 1991).

A similar antibody, reported first by Bosslet et al (Bosslet, 1985) was later developed and produced as MAb BW-250/183 by Behringwerke AG, Germany (Table 1). It recognizes the same NCA-95 antigen on granulocytes and its in-vivo properties are very similar to MAb AK-47. Joseph et al (Joseph, 1988) were the first to label MAb BW 250/183 with 99mTc using the kit method of Schwarz and Steinsträsser (Schwarz, 1987; Steinsträsser, 1989). In a first step, free sulfhydryl groups are generated by reducing some of the disulfide bonds in the antibody using a thiol reagent (2-mercaptoethanol or others). Following column purification, 2mg of the reduced antibody is lyophilized in the presence of a pH 7.2 phosphate buffer. The second lyophilized reagent consists of stannous chloride and a phosphonate compound (usually pyrophosphate, methylene diphosphonate, or propanetetraphosphonic acid). The tin reagent is reconstituted with saline and an aliquot containing ~10 μg tin is added to the antibody vial, followed by the addition of 99mTc from the generator. Labeling yields are >95% and the labeled antibody can be injected without further purification.

Table 1. Monoclonal antibodies for in-vivo labeling of human granulocytes

Antibody	Antigen	Radiolabel(s) used	Kd,M/L (Antigens/cell)	References(s)
CEA-47 (AK-47)	NCA-95	123I 99mTc	6.8×10^{-9} (7.1×10^4)	Buchegger,1984 Andres,1988
BW-250/183	NCA-95	99mTc	2×10^{-9} (7.1×10^4)	Bosslet,1985 Becker,1989
MCA-480	Lacto-N-fuco-pentoase	99mTc, 111In	1.6×10^{-11} (5.1×10^5)	Thakur,1991
NCA-102	NCA-95	111In	9.1×10^{-10}(IgG) 5.3×10^{-9}(Fab'$_2$) (1.2×10^5)	Collet,1991

Technetium-99m-labeled BW 250/183 has been evaluated by a number of investigators. In one early study (Becker, 1989), 15 patients with suspected infections were studied. There was no change in the peripheral leukocyte count following the antibody injection. The recovery of 99mTc-MAb labeled granulocytes peaked at around 10%. There was a rapid binding of BW 250/183 with granulocytes in the bone marrow and spleen. The kinetics (with a typical lung and cardiac transit) were comparable with those of 111In-oxine or 99mTc-HMPAO labeled granulocytes although the early curves (first 5 min) were different due to the necessity of slow antibody injections. The recovery rates are significantly lower than those of 111In-oxine labeled granulocytes and this resulted in low lesion to background ratios with the use of the antibody. The general in-vivo behavior for both cases under normal and activated conditions, however, was quite comparable. The delayed localization of infections with the antibody was attributed to a slow antigen-antibody reaction. Because of the amounts (~ 200 μg) of the antibody used, all granulocytes, circulating as well as those in the bone marrow, were labeled. It was suggested that abscess targeting resulted from a chemotactic attraction of the MAb-labeled cells rather than from MAb targeting of granulocytes within the abscess (Becker, 1990). In a recent study in 56 patients (Becker, 1991), the percent sensitivity, specificity and accuracy of the method, respectively, were 57, 89 and 71 at 4 hr and 86, 89, and 88 at 20 hr after injection. The recommended time for best images was 20 hr following administration. In a recent report (Berberich, 1991), 19 patients with inflammatory lesions were studied with the simultaneous injection of both 99mTc labeled 250/183 and 111In-oxine labeled granulocytes. Two energy channels were used for simultaneous detection of 99mTc and 111In. Clearance of radioactivity from blood as well as from whole body was much faster with 99mTc-MAb than with 111In-oxine-granulocytes (31 and 11% remaining at 4 and 20 hr respectively in blood, vs 46 and 31% for 111In). Cell bound 99mTc-MAb ranged between 18-25% at 0.5 to 20 hr after administration. Localization in bone marrow was higher but lower in liver/spleen compared to 111In-oxine-granulocytes. Nearly all abscesses were localized within 4-6 hr post injection of the antibody. The statistical quality of 99mTc images, as expected, was superior. However, since a relatively larger number of cells get labeled with the antibody in vivo, especially in the bone marrow, results are somewhat impaired. Nonetheless, 99mTc-MAb 250/183 was found to be a very promising overall agent for imaging acute focal inflammatory lesions.

A yet another antibody (NCA 102) directed against the NCA 95 protein of granulocyte cell membrane was developed and investigated recently (Collet, 1991). F(ab')$_2$ fragments of this IgG1 antibody were produced and labeled with 111In-DTPA. Upon incubating 100 μg F(ab')$_2$ with 30 ml blood (1 hr, 37°C), 30-35% of the radioactivity was bound to PMN leukocytes. Following the injection of 250 μg fragment labeled with 0.5 mCi 111In, all infectious foci were imaged in five patients, and the lesion uptake corresponded well with 99mTc-HMPAO labeled leukocyte studies done 48 hr later.

A panel of ten monoclonal antibodies for human neutrophils was evaluated by Thakur et al (Thakur, 1988; 1990) in order to identify systems suitable for imaging inflammatory foci. Out of these, MCA-480, an IgM antibody reacting with the lacto-N-fucopentoase antigen, was found to be the most attractive for further development (Thakur, 1990, 1991) (Table 1). This antibody was labeled with 99mTc using the reduced antibody method (Thakur, 1990a) and with 99mTc and 111In using the cyclic DTPA dianhydride method (Hnatowich, 1983). Greater than 70% of the labeled antibody was found to bind to fresh human neutrophils in a saturable fashion. This antibody does not bind to granulocytes from the commonly used animal species and therefore its evaluation had to proceed directly in humans. In recent preliminary clinical studies (Thakur, 1991), the overall distribution of 99mTc-MCA-480 was found to be similar for both radiolabeling methods. Average percent distribution of radioactivity in blood 3 hr following injection (4 patients) was as follows: 36 $\pm$ 14 (PMN); 2.6 $\pm$ 1.3 (platelets); 9.4 $\pm$ 1.7 (lymphocytes); 1.5 $\pm$ 0.7 (RBC); and 51.6 $\pm$ 10.8 (plasma) (Thakur, 1991). Intestinal or thyroid uptake was absent in the 3-4 hr images. The radioactivity in the liver and spleen was, however, persistent as is also found to be the case with 111In-oxine-WBC. Positive localization of administered 99mTc-MCA-480 was observed in patients with osteomyelitis and appendicitis. The exact mechanisms have not yet been elucidated (Thakur, 1991). The preliminary results look sufficiently promising to warrant further evaluation.

LYMPHOCYTES

Very little work has been reported on the development of anti-lymphocyte monoclonal antibodies. There is, however, some interest in radiolabeled lymphocytes for the study of transplant rejection as well as for determining cellular kinetics and migration. Indium-111-oxine labeling imparts significant damage to the radiation sensitive lymphocytes since this agent is taken up into the cell and binds to intracellular components. Monoclonal antibodies that bind to lymphocyte surface antigens may offer an improvement in this regard. Preliminary results on labeling lymphocytes using monoclonal antibodies directed against cell surface antigens CD-2 and CD-4 have been reported recently. Immunoscintigraphic detection of transplant rejection (Baum, 1990), and the imaging of rheumatoid arthritis (Becker, 1990a) were investigated.

CONCLUSION

Blood cell labeling using monoclonal antibodies directed against specific cellular antigens is an area that has undergone exciting progress during the last five years. Even though the results thus far are preliminary, the technique does offer substantial future promise for the in-vivo labeling of various cells including leukocytes and platelets. In-vivo labeling would be a major advantage since it will eliminate the undesirable step of cell separation that is required in existing methods. In-vivo labeled cells will be expected to better maintain viability and thus produce good localization. Also, a number of good imaging isotopes such as 99mTc, 123I, and others can be used as labels for monoclonal antibodies (Srivastava, 1991). The whole body and organ doses are expected to be much less compared to In-oxine labeled cells. In principle, it would also be possible to differentiate between different types of lesions and infections. Despite these advantages and future promise, however, a number of problems and concerns remain yet to be addressed. Development of chimeric and human antibodies may eliminate or minimize the HAMA problem that is frequently experienced with the use of murine antibodies. Normal tissue cross reactivity could be overcome with the identification and development in the future of antibodies with higher specificity and avidity for particular cell surface antigens. Future prospects for such improvements indeed look very promising at this point.

ACKNOWLEDGEMENTS

This work was performed under the auspices of the Office of Health and Environmental Research, U.S. Department of Energy, Contract #DE-AC02-76-CH00016. Thanks are due to Ms. Susan Cataldo for excellent secretarial assistance in the preparation of this manuscript.

REFERENCES

Andres RY, Seybold K, Tiefenauer L, et al (1988) Radioimmunoscintigraphic localization of inflammatory lesions: Concept, radiolabeling and in vitro testing of a granulocyte antibody. *Eur J Nucl Med* 13:582

Baum RP, Hentel A, Bosslet K, et al (1990) First use of Tc-99m labeled monoclonal antibody directed against the T cell receptor for immunoscintigraphic detection of transplant rejection. *Eur J Nucl Med* 16:163 (abstr)

Becker W (1990) Immunoscintigraphy of infectious lesions. In: Immunoscintigraphy: Facts and Fictions, edited by D.L. Munz and D. Emrich, Elsevier, Amsterdam, pp. 159-171

Becker W, Borst U, Fischbach W, et al (1989) Kinetic data of in-vivo-labelled granulocytes in humans with a murine Tc-99m-labelled monoclonal antibody. *Eur J Nucl Med* 15:361

Becker W, Horneff G, Emmrich F, et al (1990a) Tc-99m labeled anti CD-4 helper (lymphocytes) antibody scans for imaging of rheumatoid arthritis. *Eur J Nucl Med* 16:401 (abstr)

Becker W, Saptogino A, Wolf F (1991) Diagnostic accuracy of a late single Tc-99m-granulocyte antibody scan in inflammatory or infectious diseases. *J Nucl Med* 32:1002 (abstr)

Berberich R, Sutter M, Oberhausen E (1991) Inflammation detection with Tc-99m labeled monoclonal antibody for granulocytes. Dialogos (Siemens), 3/91: pp. 6-11

Bosslet K, Lüben G, Schwarz A, et al (1985) Immunohistochemical localization and molecular characteristics of three monoclonal antibody - defined epitopes detectable on carcinoembryonic antigen (CEA). *Int J Cancer* 36:75

Buchegger F, Schreyer M, Carrel S, et al (1984) Monoclonal antibodies identify a CEA crossreacting antigen of 95 kD (NCA-95) distinct in antigenicity and tissue distribution from the previously described NCA of 55 kD. *Int J Cancer* 33:643

Chouraqui P, Davidson M, Thomas C, et al (1991) Effect of thrombus age on uptake of Tc-99m labeled anti-activated platelet monoclonal antibody. *J Nucl Med* 32:1013 (abstr)

Chouraqui P, Maddahi J, Fung P, et al (1991a) Rapid in vivo imaging of arterial thrombi by Tc-99m labeled anti-activated platelet monoclonal antibody. *J Nucl Med* 32: 1005 (abstr)

Coller BS (1985) A new murine monoclonal antibody reports an activation-dependent change in the conformation and/or microenvironment of the platelet glycoprotein IIb/IIIa complex. *J Clin Invest* 76:101

Coller BS, Peerschke EI, Scudder LE, et al (1983) A murine monoclonal antibody that completely blocks the binding of fibrinogen to platelets produces a thrombasthenic-like state in normal platelets and binds to glycoproteins IIb and or IIIa. *J Clin Invest* 72:325

Collet B, Moisan A, Maros S, et al (1991) A new In-111 labeled F(ab')₂ antigranulocyte antibody for imaging focal sites of infection: In vitro studies and preliminary results. *J Nucl Med* 32:1051 (abstr)

Desai AG, Thakur ML (1986) Radiolabeled blood cells: Techniques and applications. *CRC Critical Rev Clin Lab Sci* 24:95

Ezekowitz MD, Coller B, Srivastava SC (1986) Potential application of labeled antibodies for thrombus detection. *Nucl Med Biol* 13:407

Hanna R, Braun T, Levendel A, et al (1984) Radiochemistry and biostability of autologous leucocytes labeled with 99mTc-stannous colloid in whole blood. *Eur J Nucl Med* 9:216

Hasler PH, Seybold K, Andres RY, et al (1988) Immunoscintigraphic localization of inflammatory lesions: Pharmacokinetics and estimated absorbed radiation dose in man. *Eur J Nucl Med* 13:594

Hnatowich DJ, Layne WW, Childs RL, et al (1983) Radioactive labeling of antibody: A simple and efficient method. *Science* 220:613

Joseph K, Höfken H, Bosslet K, et al (1988) In vivo labelling of granulocytes with 99mTc anti-NCA monoclonal antibodies for imaging inflammation. *Eur J Nucl Med* 14:367

Knight LC, Maurer AH, Ammar IA, et al (1988) Evaluation of indium-111 labeled anti-fibrin antibody for imaging vascular thrombi. *J Nucl Med* 29:494

Locher JT, Frey LD, Seybold K, et al (1991) Dual isotope immunoscintigraphy of infections. *Eur J Nucl Med* 15:555 (abstr)

Locher JT, Seybold K, Andres RY, et al (1986) Imaging of inflammatory lesions after injection of radioiodinated monoclonal antigranulocyte antibodies. *Nucl Med Commun* 7:659

McAfee JG, Grossman ZD, Rosebrough SF, et al (1988) Monoclonal antibody against human fibrin for imaging thrombi. In: Radiolabeled Monoclonal Antibodies for Imaging and Therapy, Edited by S.C. Srivastava, Plenum, New York, pp. 807-815

McAfee JG, Gagne G, Subramanian G (1988a) Radioactive monoclonal antibodies against cell surface antigens for labeling leukocyte subpopulations. In: Radiolabeled Monoclonal Antibodies for Imaging and Therapy, Edited by S.C. Srivastava, Plenum, New York, pp. 795-805

Oster ZH, Srivastava SC, Som P, et al (1985) Thrombus radioimmunoscintigraphy. An approach using monoclonal antiplatelet antibody. *Proc Natl Acad Sci* USA 82:3465

Palabrica TM, Furie BC, Konstam MA, et al (1989) Thrombus imaging in a primate model with antibodies specific for an external membrane protein of activated platelets. *Proc Natl Acad Sci* USA 86:1036

Patrick ST, Glowniak JV, Turner FE, et al (1991) Comparison of in vitro RBC labeling with the UltraTag[R] RBC kit versus in vivo labeling. *J Nucl Med* 32:242

Peters AM, Lavender JP, Danpure H, et al (1986) Clinical experience with Tc-99m HMPAO for labeling leukocytes and imaging inflammation. *Lancet* 2:946

Peters AM, Lavender JP, Needham SG, et al (1986a) Imaging thrombus with radiolabeled monoclonal antibody to platelets. *Brit Med J* 293:1525

Schwarz A, Steinsträsser A (1987) A novel approach to Tc-99m-labeled monoclonal antibodies. *J Nucl Med* 28:721

Seybold K, Locher JT, Coosemans C, et al (1988) Immunoscintigraphic localization of inflammatory lesions: Clinical experience. *Eur J Nucl Med* 13:587

Som P, Oster ZH, Zamora PO, et al (1986) Radioimmunoimaging of experimental thrombi in dogs using technetium-99m labeled monoclonal antibody fragments reactive with human platelets. *J Nucl Med* 27:1315

Srivastava SC, Mease RC (1991) Progress in research on ligands, nuclides and techniques for labeling monoclonal antibodies. *Nucl Med Biol* 18: 589

Srivastava SC, Meinken GE (1988) Radiolabeled antiplatelet monoclonal antibodies for the scintigraphic localization of in vivo thrombi and vascular lesions. In: Radiolabeled Monoclonal Antibodies for Imaging and Therapy, Edited by Srivastava SC, Plenum, New York 1988, pp. 817-830

Srivastava SC, Meinken GE, Som P, et al (1984) Evaluation of 123I and 111In labeled monoclonal antiplatelet antibody for the scintigraphic localization of in-vivo thrombi. *J Nucl Med* 25:P65 (abstr)

Srivastava SC, Straub RF (1990) Blood cell labeling with 99mTc: Progress and perspectives. *Semin Nucl Med* 20: 41

Srivastava SC, Straub RF, Richards P (1984a) Mechanistic aspects of the technetium-99m-RBC labeling reactions. *J Labeled Compds Radiopharm* 21:1055

Steinsträsser A, Berberich R, Schwarz A, et al (1989) Strahlenexposition bei der Szintigraphie mit Tc-99m-Antigranulozyten-Antikörpern. *Nuklearmedizin* 28:148

Stuttle AWJ, Peters AM, Loutfi I, et al (1988) Use of an anti-platelet monoclonal antibody F(ab'), fragment for imaging thrombus. *Nucl Med Commun* 9:647

Thakur ML (1990) Immunoscintigraphic imaging of inflammatory lesions: Preliminary findings and future possiblities. *Semin Nucl Med* 20:92

Thakur ML (1991) Cell labeling in radiopharmacy: What can radiolabeled monoclonal antibodies offer? Proceedings 4th European Symposium on Radiopharmacy and Radiopharmaceuticals, Baden, Switzerland, May 1-4, 1991, Westera G. and Schubiger, PA, editors, Kluwer Academic Publishers, Dordrecht, NL (In press)

Thakur ML, DeFulvio J, Richard MD, et al (1990a) Technetium-99m labeled monoclonal antibodies: Evaluation of reducing agents. *Nucl Med Biol* 18:227

Thakur ML, Richard MD, White FW III (1988) Monoclonal antibodies as agents for selective radiolabeling of human neutrophils. *J Nucl Med* 29:1817

Thakur ML, Thiagarajan P, White F, et al (1987) Monoclonal antibodies for specific cell labeling: Considerations, preparations, and preliminary evaluation. *Nucl Med Biol* 14:51

QUALITY CONTROL OF RADIOLABELLED WHITE CELLS

A.M. Peters

Department of Diagnostic Radiology
Hammersmith Hospital
London, United Kingdom

INTRODUCTION

White blood cells are now being labelled by an increasing variety of agents, including 111In oxine, 111In tropolone, 99mTc HMPAO and monoclonal antibodies to granulocytes. Of major concern is the effect of these procedures on granulocyte viability and function, and in particular, on their ability to localise at inflammatory sites. Tests of granulocyte function can be divided into *in vitro* and *in vivo* tests. The latter particularly concern the ability of cells to recirculate and to distribute and survive normally.

IN VITRO TESTS

In vitro tests examine the granulocyte's ability to release enzymes and superoxide in response to activation, their ability to migrate in response to chemoattractants, and their morphology in terms of shape change. A fundamental difficulty with several of these techniques is that the test itself activates the granulocyte and cannot therefore discriminate between a non-activated cell and one that has been activated as a result of *in vitro* manipulation. Activation is as undesirable as cell damage, the two effectively being indistinguishable as far as ultimate capacity to migrate into inflammatory foci is concerned.

There have been very few attempts to correlate the status of radiolabelled granulocytes on *in vitro* testing, with their subsequent *in vivo* kinetics. Haslett et al[1] have compared several methods of 111In labelling of granulocytes with respect to shape change, chemotaxis, and superoxide and lysozyme release in response to activation with the cytokine FMLP. They demonstrated that evidence of cell activation could be reproduced with trace concentrations of bacterial lipopolysaccharide (LPS). Granulocytes isolated on Ficoll-Hypaque gradients were clearly activated, but not those isolated on plasma-Percoll gradients. They also demonstrated that erythrocyte lysis with ammonium chloride resulted in change of shape, which could be reproduced with LPS, and which was greater than the activation demonstrated after red cell lysis with hypotonic saline.

Radiolabeled Blood Elements, Edited by J. Martin-Comin
Plenum Press, New York, 1994

These authors[2] then went on to demonstrate the effects *in-vivo* of LPS pretreatment on 111In labelled granulocytes. Cells exposed to increasing doses of LPS *in vitro* showed increasing pulmonary retention when subsequently re-injected. In contrast to the behavior of labelled granulocytes activated *in vitro* by isolation and labelling in saline, the lung released the LPS pretreated cells slowly, such, that even by four hours, the lung signal was greater than that for control cells not pretreated with LPS. The same pattern of kinetics could be reproduced by intravenous injection of LPS. The increased pulmonary retention was accompanied by a markedly reduced recovery of cells in the circulating blood.

IN VIVO TESTS

When radiolabelled granulocytes are damaged or activated, they fail to circulate normally. This is largely the result of sequestration in the lung microvasculature by a mechanism that is poorly understood. Granulocytes might be capable of migrating into inflammatory foci following labelling and activation *in vitro*, except that as a result of their activation, they transit the lung slowly and are rapidly removed from the circulation by the reticuloendothelial system. It seems that the cells are activated prematurely in the test tube, rather than appropriately in the circulation in the presence of a chemotactic stimulus at the site of an inflammatory focus.

Cell hold-up in the lung may also involve a mechanical factor. Physiologically, granulocytes have a longer transit time through the lung capillaries compared with red cells. Vital microscopy can readily demonstrate native granulocytes apparently stuck in lung capillaries[3]. Pulmonary capillaries far outnumber the granulocytes attempting to negotiate them, so these delayed granulocytes have no effect on the transit time of red cells because they can be bypassed via unobstructed capillaries.

Granulocytes activated *in vitro* are probably stiffer than native granulocytes, and this would be expected to prolong their transit time. Worthen et al[4] developed a tool called the "cell poker", which can measure the deformability of individual granulocytes. 111In labelled cells exposed to FMLP demonstrated reduced deformability and underwent prolonged transit time through the lungs compared with 111In labelled cells not exposed to FMLP. Radiolabelled granulocytes pretreated with cytochalasin B, a toxin which interferes with the actin/myosin function of the cell, did not become stiff or undergo prolonged transit through the lung after exposure to FMLP. Cell stiffness may be an important factor in the artefactual sequestration seen following injection of cells activated during labelling.

Granulocytes isolated on saline-based density gradient columns, such as saline-Percoll, and labelled in saline with 111In, show marked initial hold-up in the lung, whereas granulocytes isolated on gradients made up with autologous plasma and labelled in plasma transit the lungs rapidly, albeit more slowly than red cells. Even these relatively normal granulocytes demonstrate an element of artefactual hold-up in that their mean transit time through the lung gradually falls after injection, reaching a stable value about 30-40 minutes after injection[5]. This strongly suggests a reversible element causing initial mild lung hold-up.

Cells that have undergone marked initial lung retention are all soon released from the lung, so that the lung counts fall to a low level by one to one-and-a-half hours after injection. Indeed, frequent blood sampling during this period will demonstrate a progressively rising, although small, amount of circulating cell-bound 111In, consistent with release of previously sequestered cells. These cells do not circulate normally; their preactivation leaves them exposed to rapid removal into the reticuloendothelial system, and as a consequence, the liver and to a lesser extent the spleen, become prominent from an early time after injection. Interestingly, bone marrow is not prominent at this or any other stage. This suggests that the splenic uptake is due to sinusoidal trapping rather than to reticuloendothelial phagocytosis, similar to the splenic retention of heat damaged red cells (which, incidentally, are also stiff).

In contrast, cells not showing undue activation after labelling, and which transit the lung normally, recirculate normally and enter physiological marginating pools. Whereas activated cells give liver and splenic time-activity curves which parallel each other and which are mirror images of the "lung release" curve, normal cells give time-activity curves of the liver and spleen which have quite different shapes from each other. This is because the cells enter and equilibrate in the various marginating pools at different rates, depending on the blood flow to the pool and the transit time through it. The time-activity curve over the liver in the optimal state shows a peak at 2 to 5 minutes and then declines in parallel with the fall in blood activity. Splenic activity on the other hand, continues to rise for 20 minutes or so, on account of the longer transit time through the spleen and its relatively small blood flow.

These kinetic features combine to determine the so-called radiolabelled granulocyte recovery. This can be defined as the fraction of injected labelled granulocytes that are circulating in blood at any specified time after injection. Because of substantial and widespread physiological margination, the maximum recovery is probably about 50 %. It falls to less than 5 % when the cells are severely activated or damaged. The normal recovery values, about 35 %, are essentially the same for 99mTc HMPAO labelled cells and 111In tropolone labelled cells, provided plasma is not excluded from the incubation media at any stage[6]. It is also interesting that the recovery is not appreciably less in patients with inflammatory disease, who presumably have an expanded marginating granulocyte pool at the site of infection[6]. Nevertheless, the recovery represents the most sensitive and meaningful quality control procedure for radiolabelled granulocytes. It can readily be performed by retaining a small aliquot of the injectate, which along with the injectate itself, are carefully weighed as a comparative measure of respective radioactivity doses. This standard is then diluted in several hundred ml of saline. Samples from the diluted standard can then be compared with blood samples taken following injection, and recovery calculated from an estimate of the patient's total blood volume based on height and weight. If mixed leucocytes are injected rather than pure granulocytes, then the recovery can still be relatively easily measured by isolating granulocytes on Percoll-saline columns from the pre-diluted standard and post-injection blood samples in order to determine what fraction of the injected and sampled radioactivity is granulocyte-associated.

The effects of anti-granulocyte monoclonal antibodies on granulocyte function *in vivo* have not been widely studied. This is partly because few granulocytes are actually labelled by these monoclonal antibodies, most of the dose labelling granulocyte precursors in the bone marrow. Antibodies are in dynamic equilibrium between their antigen and plasma, and so, because of the large mass of bone marrow myeloid cells contributing to this equilibrium, the percentage of circulating radioactivity bound to granulocytes is, in general, well below 50 % and closer to 10 %. Nevertheless, this value may rise slowly over several hours following injection. As a result, the hallmarks of normal granulocyte distribution are rather difficult to identify.

CONCLUSION

In conclusion, the most sensitive and practical means of quality control of radiolabelled granulocytes are based on their *in vivo* distribution following injection. The useful tests are dynamic imaging over the lungs, measurement of recovery at 45 minutes after injection and simple visualisation of the distribution of activity between the liver, lungs and spleen in the images obtained at one hour (if taken) and three hours (mandatory). Dynamic imaging, and especially recovery, need not be performed with every preparation, but are useful tests of cell integrity when first setting up a white cell labelling service or changing technical personnel.

REFERENCES

1. Haslett C, Guthrie LA, Kopaniak MM, Johnston RB, Henson PM. Modulation of multiple neutrophil functions by preparative methods or trace concentrations of bacterial liopopolysaccharide. *Am J Pathol* 119: 101-110 (1985).
2. Haslett C, Worthen GS, Giclas PC, Morrison DC, Henson JE, Henson PM. The pulmonary vascular sequestration of neutrophils in endotoxemia is initiated by an effect of endotoxin on the neutrophil in the rabbit. *Am Rev Resp Dis* 136: 9-18 (1987).
3. McNee W, Selby C. Neutrophil Kinetics in the lung. *Clin Sci* 79: 97-107 (1990).
4. Worthen GS, Schwab B, Elson EL, Downey GP. Mechanics of stimulated neutrophils: cell stiffness induces retention in capillaries. *Science* 245: 183-186 (1989).
5. Peters AM, Allsop P, Stuttle AWJ, Arnot RN, Gwilliam M, Hall GM. Granulocyte margination in the human lung and its response to strenuous exercise. *Clin Sci* 82: 237-244 (1992).
6. Peters AM, Roddie ME, Danpure HJ, Osman S, Zacharopoulos GP, George P, Stuttle AWJ, Lavender JP. 99mTc HMPAO labelled leucocytes: comparison with 111In tropolonate labelled granulocytes. *Nucl. Med Commun* 9: 449-463 (1988).

GRANULOCYTE CELL LABELING WITH TcN-NOET

A. Moisan[1], R. Pasqualini[2], A. Devillers[1], A. Trichet[1], S. Maros[1],
V. Quillien[1], L. Dazord[1] and P. Bourguet[1]

[1]CAC, Rennes
[2]CIS-bio international, Gif sur Yvette
France

The TcN-NOET bis (N-ethoxy, N-ethyldithiocarbamate) nitrido technetium (99mTc) is a new complex containing a Tc^V nitrogen multiple bond. This compound showed high myocardial uptake in various animal species and in humans[7, 8, 10].

Blood cell labeling was carried out with this neutral and lipophilic complex and especially, granulocyte labeling, used in diagnostic nuclear medicine for the detection of inflammatory lesions[1].

MATERIALS AND METHODS

I - Preparation of TcN-NOET

The synthesis of dithiocarbamate ligand is obtained by the reaction between a secondary amine with a carbon disulfide in presence of NaOH.

The lateral chains can be alkyl groups.

When $R = C_2H_5O$ and $R' = C_2H_5$, the ligand is called NOET.

The TcN-NOET is prepared in 2 steps. New pharmaceuticals based on the $[Tc \equiv N]^{2+}$ core have been investigated first by Baldas (2). The $(Tc^V \equiv N)$ intermediate is prepared from $Tc^{VII}O_4-$ in presence of stannous ions (complexed by propylene diaminotetraacetic acid) and a nitrido donating ligand such as S methyl dithiocarbazate by heating at 100°C during 15 minutes. This method has been developped since 1988[3, 5, 6, 9].

VII   (PDTA)   V

$$TcO_4^- + Sn^{2+} + = N - N = \ ---> \ (Tc \equiv N)^{2+}$$

reducing   nitro-donating
agent   ligand

Finally the TcN-NOET is obtained by exchange of ligands at room temperature according the reaction :

$$2 \quad \begin{array}{c} OC_2H_5 \\ \diagdown \\ \diagup \\ C_2H_5 \end{array} NC \diagup^{S}_{S-Na} \quad + \ (TC \equiv N)^{2+} \ int \ --->$$

The complex is neutral and displays a square pyramidal geometry with $Tc^V \equiv N$ in apical position.

The radiochemical purity of the complex is superior to 95 %.

II - Labeling of Granulocytes with TcN-NOET

The "pure granulocytes" are isolated according an usual method[4]. From a blood sample on ACD-A and after sedimentation of red blood cells (RBC), the pellet of granulocytes is obtained by floatation and resuspended in 10 ml of RPMI or plasma poor in cells (PPC).

Labeling procedures were performed with isolated granulocytes and in whole blood. Blood cells are labeled with 200 MBq of a solution of TcN-NOET at pH 8 during 10 minutes at room temperature. After washing with RPMI, labeling efficiency is calculated. The percentage of radioactivity linked to granulocytes is evaluated after separation of labeled cells on polymorphprep gradient.

Different parameters influencing labeling efficiency were studied (pH, cells number, incubation time and radioactivity range). The viability of labeled cells was controled by Trypan blue exclusion tests, chemiotactic and chimioluminescence tests.

RESULTS

With a range of 2.10^7 to 10^8 of "pure granulocytes" (PMNs), labeling efficiency averaged 90 %, varying from 40 % for 10^6 PMNs to 95 % for 5.10^8 PMNs (fig 1). The curve of labeling efficiency according the number of cells is close to the curve obtained by labeling PMNs with 111In oxinate. Labeling efficiency of PMNs labeled with 99mTc HMPAO is significantly lower.

Incubating 10 minutes 2.10^7 to 10^8 PMNs with 200 MBq of TcN-NOET, at pH 8 and room temperature, labeling efficiency averaged 92 % ± 5 % (n = 10 experiments). The elution of the radiotracer from PMNs is relatively reduced : 5 % at the first hour, 10 % at the third hour (mean of 4 experiments).

When the pH of a solution of TcN-NOET is superior to 8,5 , the labeling efficiency is reduced to 30 % ; the maximum yields are obtained between 7,5 and 8,5.

Duration of incubation does not affect labeling efficiency : it raised 90 % after 5 to 10 minutes.

Labeling efficiency decreases when the amount of radioactivity is superior to 400 MBq for 3.10^7 PMNs in solution.

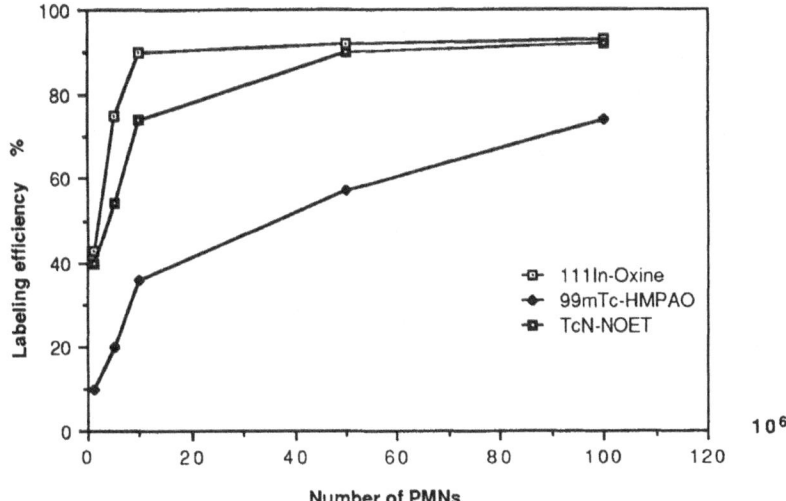

Figure 1. Labeling efficiency according to the number of PMNs.

Trypan blue exclusion tests were carried out for each experiment. The viability of labeled cells have been evaluated also by spontaneous migration and chemotaxis measurements of PMNs incubated with TcN-NOET in various conditions (Table 1).

Two tests of superoxid generation by stimulated granulocytes were evaluated. Stimulation either by PMA or zymosan was performed. The results confirmed the previous chemotaxis tests.

Some experiments were carried out in small volumes (3 ml) of whole blood. In whole blood total radioactivity bound by cells average 80 %. Cell distribution of radioactivity is evaluated with a polymorphprep gradient. The results are as follow: 42% in leucocytes ring, 35 % in RBC pellet (contaminated by leucocytes), only 6 % in plasma.

Two experiments of labeling granulocytes in whole blood were performed from 30 ml of blood. Granulocytes, lymphocytes were separated by floatation, platelets and RBC were also isolated as well as possible in each fraction. The percentage of radioactivity is estimated to be about 75 % in PNMs, 13 % in lymphocytes, very low in platelets (4 %) and red blood cells (8 %).

Table 1

SPONTANEOUS MIGRATION AND CHEMOTAXIS MEASUREMENTS OF LABELED PMNS WITH TcN-NOET

$3\,10^7$ PMNs incubated with		Chemotaxis stimulation*			
		FMLP		Serum	
		A mm/2 h	B mm/2 h	A mm/2 h	B mm/2 h
	culture medium	2,1	0,7	2,5	0,8
pH 8	200 MBq TcN-NOET	2,0	0,8	2,1	1
	300 MBq TcN-NOET	1,8	0,6	2,05	0,8
	500 MBq TcN-NOET	1,3	0,3	1,6	0,55
pH 9,5	200 MBq TcN-NOET	1,5	0,5	1,9	0,5

A   chemotaxis against an attractant (FMLP or serum)
B   spontaneous migration
*   mean of 2 experiments

CONCLUSION

TcN-NOET is a new lipophilic and neutral technetium (V) complex containing a Tc $\equiv$ N multiple bound. It is able to label isolated granulocytes with high efficiency without alteration of cell viability.

TcN-NOET gives good labeling efficiency of PNMs in whole blood compared to lymphocytes, platelets and RBC.

TcN-NOET seems to bind leucocytes with higher affinity than other well known complexes used to label white blood cells such as 111In oxine or tropolone, or 99mTc HMPAO.

These are in vitro preliminary results and need to be confirmed by in vivo biodistribution.

REFERENCES

1. Abram S, Beyer R. Blood cell labelling experiments with lipophilic technetium complexes. *Isotopenpraxis* 26, 3, 107-108, (1990).
2. Baldas J and Bonnyman J. *Int J Appl Radiat Isot*, 36, 133 : 919 (1985).
3. Duatti A, Marchi A, Pasqualini R. Formation of the Tc=N multiple bond from the reaction of ammonium pertechnetate with S-methyl-dithiocarbazate and its application to the preparation of technetium-99m radiopharmaceuticals. *J Chem Soc Dalton Trans*, 3729-3733 (1990)

4. Herry JY, Moisan A, Le Cloirec J, Bretagne JF, Darnault P, Cardin JL, Martin A. 111In autologous granulocytes in the diagnosis of abscess in the assessment of inflammatory bowel disease. *Nucl Med Biol*, 13 183-190 (1986).

5. Marchi A, Duatti A, Rossi R, Magon L. Technetium (V)-nitrido complexes of dithiocarbazic acid derivatives. Reactivity of $[Tc=N]^{2+}$ core towards schiff bases derived from S-Methyl dithiocarbazate. Chrystal structures of [S-Methyl 3-(2-hydroxyphenylmethylene) dithiocarbazato] nitrido (triphenylphosphine) technetium (V) and bis (S-methyl 3-isopropylidenedithiocarbazato) nitridotechnetium (V). *J Chem Soc Dalton Trans*, 1743-1747 (1988).

6. Pasqualini R, Bellande E, Comazzi V, Duatti A. Improved synthesis of Tc-99m nitrido dithiocabamate. *SNM, Los Angeles, 39th Annual Meeeting, JNM, abstract*, 33, 5 (1992).

7. Pasqualini R, Bellande E, Comazzi V, Fagret D, Mathieu JP, Comet M. Effect of side chain modifications of bis (dithiocarmato) nitrido technetium (V) on myocardial uptake in dogs. *SNM, Los Angeles, 39th Annual Meeeting, JNM, abstract*, 33, 5, (1992).

8. Pasqualini R, Comazzi V, Bellande E, Brucato V, Lamy M, Hoffschir D, Mathieu JP, Fagret D, Comet M, Duatti A. Préparation et biodistribution chez différentes espèces animales de complexes nitrurobis dithiocarmato technetium (99mTc) : Une nouvelle classe de composés neutres pour l'imagerie du myocarde. *J Med Nuc et Biophys* 16, 3 : 295-296 (1992).

9. Pasqualini R, Comazzi V, Bellande E, Duatti A, Marchi A. A new efficient method for the preparation of [99mTc]-radiopharmaceuticals containing the Tc=N multiple bond. *Appl Radiat Isot* 43, 11 : 1329-1333 (1992).

10. Zhang Z, Maublant J, Ollier M, Papon J, Michelot J, Bellande E, Comazzi V, Pasqualini R, Veyre A. Etude comparative sur cultures de cellules entre le Tc-99m-NOET, le TL-201, le Tc-99m-Sestamibi et le Tc-99m-Teboroxime. *J Med Nuc et Biophys* 16, 3, 335 (1992).

ARTERIOSCLEROSIS AND MONOCYTE-ADHESION *IN VIVO*

I. Virgolini, S. Li, Y. Qiong, P. Fitscha, J.R. Gerrity and H. Sinzinger

Department of Nuclear Medicine
University of Vienna
A-1090 Vienna, Austria

INTRODUCTION

The pathogenesis of arteriosclerosis appears to involve a sequence of critical events that are based on the interaction of cellular (platelets, monocyte-macrophages) and noncellular (lipoproteins) blood elements with the arterial wall.

Circulating peripheral blood monocytes seem to play a very important role during the early steps of atherogenesis. Their adhesion to the endothelium, migration into the subendothelial space and transformation into foam cells has been recognized under various experimental *in vitro*-conditions[1-3], of which hypercholesterolemia seems to be the most important one. Hypercholesterolemia leads to an increased adhesion of monocytes[1,2] to the endothelium of the artery *in vitro*, and is also causatively related to the typical pathoanatomical changes seen in arteriosclerotic vessels.

On the basis of these experimental observations we aimed to explore whether hyperlipoproteinemia would influence also *in vivo* monocyte adhesion to the arteries. This goal was to be reached by developing the "monocyte scintigraphy" which uses 10^8 purified peripheral blood monocytes labeled with 0.42 MBq 111In-oxine (viability >95%).

METHODS

The study protocol was approved by the Ethics Committee of the Medical Faculty of the University of Vienna. Written informed consent was obtained from all patients.

Based on initial *in vitro* studies on labeling efficiency and cell viability, patients had to undergo lymphocytopheresis (IBM 2997 blood cell separator). The collected buffy coat was diluted 1:2 with phosphate buffered saline (PBS)/heparin (10 I.U./ml). Following centrifugation (1800 rpm, 25 minutes, 22°C) on Ficoll Hypaque (d=1.077 g/ ml), the mononuclear cell fraction was diluted 1:2 with Ca^{++} and Mg^{++} free PBS containing 2 mM EGTA (0.38 g), pH 7.4.

This study was supported by a grant of the Fonds of the **Bürgermeister der Bundeshauptstadt Wien**. The study was qualified for the International Award for Angiology and was presented at the 8th World Congress on Angiology, Paris, September 1992.

The cells were washed 2 times in elutriation medium (Ca^{++} and Mg^{++} free PBS, 0.5 mM EGTA, pH 7.4) and thereafter resuspended in 3 ml medium. Monocytes were then isolated by centrifugal elutriation using a JE6 elutriator rotor in a J6-M refrigerated centrifuge (Beckman). About 1.5×10^9 mononuclear cells were used for elutriation centrifugation. The flow rate was kept constant (15 ml/min) and the rotor speed was reduced stepwise.

Monocytes ($9.1 \pm 0.6 \times 10^7$) were labeled in a volume of 1 ml 0.9% NaCl solution by adding approximately 15 μCi (0.42 Mbq) of 111In-oxine (20 μg oxine/10^8 cells) for 10 minutes at 37°C. Monocytes were washed twice in RPMI 1640 with 10% FCS to remove unbound 111In, and resuspended in 0.9% NaCl solution.

111In-oxine-labeled autologous monocytes were i.v.-injected just after labeling. All patients were placed in a supine position under a large field-of-view gamma camera (Searle, Inc., NL) connected to a data processor (PDP11/34, Digital Equipment Int. Ltd., Galway, Ireland). The gamma camera was equipped with a high-sensitivity collimator; the lower energy peak of 111In (173 keV) was selected as the energy window.

In all patients sequential images were recorded during the first 30 minutes after reinjection (1 frame/minute) with the collimator placed over thigh or lower leg arteries. Late planar images for 10 minutes each were taken at different time intervals after reinjection.

If a patient showed monocyte uptake appearing as a visible "hot spot", regions of interest (ROI) were inserted and the monocyte uptake ratio (MUR) was calculated. MUR was determined after (non-vascular) background subtraction by the cpm measured in the ROI over the lesion site in relation to the cpm measured in a ROI of same size inserted over a contralateral area without visible monocyte uptake.

RESULTS AND DISCUSSION

As already reported previously[4-7] the spleen was the major organ of monocyte uptake in human in vivo. "Hot spots" over the vascular bed became visible within 1 to 8 hours after reinjection.

In normolipemic patients, 50% of angiographically positive arteriosclerotic lesions (defined as a 30-60% luminal stenosis) and 40% of angiographically negative lesions showed monocyte accumulation. However, all FH patients with positive angiography also showed "hot spots" over at least one investigated area ($p < 0.001$).

The fact that hot spots of even comparable density can be found in lesions that are angiographically positive and negative fits well into the concept that radiosensitive techniques do allow the monitoring of the functional stages of arteriosclerosis rather than its extent which is obtained by angiography.

The MUR was calculated for an area whenever a "hot spot" had become evident. In such areas the time course of appearance of monocytes was studied from the image taken at 30 minutes (last sequential image) to the last control image at 48 hours. The MUR was significantly ($p < 0.001$) higher in FH patients as compared with controls, in both groups, those with positive and those with negative angiography (Fig.1).

With respect to monocyte accumulation in terms of appearance of "hot spots" and MUR, smoking patients with FH who had a positive angiography were not different from nonsmoking patients with FH with a positive angiography. There was also no statistical difference between smokers in the normolipemic group with positive or negative angiography. Furthermore, no effect of hypertension on monocyte accumulation could be found. Also the presence of multiple risk factors did not further contribute to an enhanced monocyte adhesion in human in vivo.

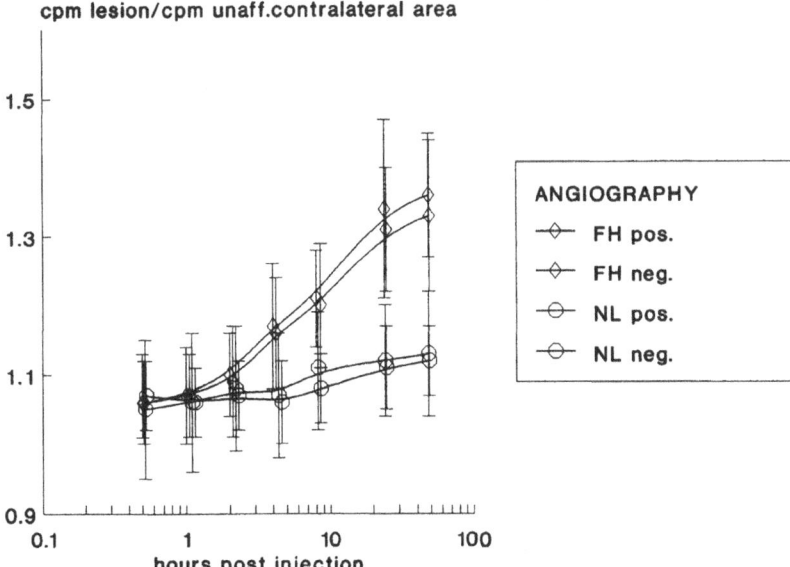

Fig.1. Time course of appearance of monocytes (expressed as monocyte uptake ratio; MUR) in arteriosclerotic lesions. In patients with familial hypercholesterolemia (FH) independent from angiographical results a significantly ($p < 0.001$) higher uptake of monocytes was found as compared with normolipemic patients. The MUR was calculated for lesions which were identified as single "hot spots" of either thigh or lower leg arteries.

In FH patients undergoing LDL-apheresis and/or hypolipemic drug therapy, the monocyte scintigraphy was repeated 2 months after the onset of therapeutic intervention. Whereas there was no difference in the appearance of "hot spots", successful intervention led to a significantly decreased MUR (1.35 ± 0.07 vs 1.19 ± 0.08; $p < 0.001$).

Our imaging results show that while in normolipemics the incidence of monocyte uptake into the vascular area is low, almost all patients with (heterozygous) FH do have *in vivo* monocyte adhesion onto at least one of the possible lesion sites studied. The presence of monocytes in the vessel wall with negative angiography raises important fundamental questions and opens a new research area.

Monocyte-macrophages are precursors of the foam cells, that contain most of the lipid material in the atherosclerotic plaque[2,3]. Many factors may increase their adhesion to the endothelium *in vitro*[2,3], - an early key event in atherogenesis. Radiolabeling of monocytes and external imaging with a gamma camera might offer new interesting means of taking advantage of the metabolic activity of developing atherosclerotic lesions in order to noninvasively detect early atherosclerosis as well as for a look at the pathogenesis of the disease.

REFERENCES

1. Gerrity RG: The role of the monocyte in atherosclerosis. I. Transition of blood-borne monocytes into foam cells in fatty lesions. *Am J Pathol*; 103: 181-190 (1981).
2. Bylock A, Gerrity RG: FITC-labeling of leukocytes for tracing monocyte recruitment into atherosclerotic arteries. *Atherosclerosis*; 71: 17-25 (1988).
3. Gerrity RG, Ross JA, Soby LM: Control of monocyte recruitment by chemotactic factor(s) in lesion-prone areas of swine aorta. *Arteriosclerosis*; 5: 55-56 (1985).

4. Virgolini I, Müller C, Fitscha P, Chiba P, Sinzinger H: Radiolabeling autologous monocytes with 111In-oxine for reinjection in patients with atherosclerosis. In: Sinzinger H, Thakur ML (Eds). Radiolabeled Blood Elements. Wiley Liss Inc. NY, 1990; 271-280.
5. Müller C, Zielinski C, Linkesch W, Sinzinger H: *In vivo* tracing of indium-111 oxine-labeled human peripheral blood mononuclear cells in patients with lymphatic malignancies. *J Nucl Med*; 3: 1005-1011 (1989).
6. Heyns A Du P, Pieters H, Steyn AC: Isolation and labeling with In-111 of a viable population of blood monocytes. In: Sinzinger H, Thakur ML. (Eds.). Radiolabeled Blood Elements. Wiley Liss Inc. N.Y. 1990; 265-270.
7. Sinzinger H, Virgolini I: Nuclear Medicine and atherosclerosis. *Eur J Nucl Med*; 17: 160-178(1990).

STABILIZATION OF EXAMETAZIME FOR LEUCOCYTE LABELLING: A NEW APPROACH USING TIN ENHANCEMENT

C. Solanki, D.J. Li, A. Wong and C. Sampson

Department of Nuclear Medicine
Addenbrookes Hospital
Cambridge, U.K.

SUMMARY

We have examined the effect of the addition of two different stannous chloride formulations on the levels of primary lipophilic 99mTc exametazime. In the first study a solution containing 20 μg $SnCl_2$ $2H_2O$ was prepared ("in house" method) and used over a two week period. The mean level of radiochemical purity was 41% (range 11%-60%, n=6). In the second study a kit formulation containing 6.6 μg of $SnCl_2$ $2H_2O$/ml was prepared freshly each day. The mean radiochemical purity of 99mTc exametazime was 87% (range 68%-93%, n=5).

"Mixed" leucocytes were labelled with 99mTc exametazime which had been prepared with each of the two stannous preparations. The mean labelling efficiency (LE) of 99mTc exametazime labelled leucocytes using the in-house stannous preparation was 54% (range 18%-55%, n=130) and that for leucocytes labelled using the kit stannous solution was 67% (range 43%-96%, n=69). Clinical scintigrams of patients injected with 99mTc labelled leucocytes prepared using the two methods were examined.

INTRODUCTION

99mTc exametazime labelled leucocytes have now become widely used for the detection of sites of local infection[1], abdominal abscess[2], inflammatory bowel disease[3, 4], osteomyelitis[5], sepsis[6], pyrexia of unknown origin[7] and osteoarthritis[8].

Howewer, exametazime is relatively expensive and its efficient use for cell labelling is limited by the instability of the reconstituted freeze dried material.

The marked instability of reconstituted exametazime is due to the rapid oxidation of the small amount (7.6 μg) of stannous chloride present in the kit. This level of tin is critical for the kit. This level of tin is critical for the succesful labelling of exametazime. Excess amount of stannous ion will enhance the formation of the secondary non-lipophilic complex and too little will be insufficient to fulfill its role as a reducing agent (verbal discussion with Amersham plc).

Radiolabeled Blood Elements, Edited by J. Martin-Comin
Plenum Press, New York, 1994

The problem of improving the stability of 99mTc exametazime has been investigated by several workers. Sampson et al (1986, unpublished work) used citric acid and EDTA to maintain radiochemical purity for 6 hours, but large levels of free pertechnetate also remained. Hung et al[9] used gentisic acid to increase the levels of primary complex tp 85% for up to 6 hours post preparation, and Lan et al[10] used a weak chelating agent, and low volumes in a nitrogen environment to increase the primary complex to 92% for 2 hours after preparation.

However the value of these manipulations is limited since they have to be made after the addition of sodium pertechnetate to theKit. By reconstituting a vial of exametazime with saline and storing in the freezer at - 10°C, Sampson et al (1987 unpulished work), maintained radiochemical purity for 3 days. Ballinger[11] extended the useful life of reconstituted exametazime for 6 days by subdividing a vial and storing at - 10°C under nitrogen, and Hawkins[12] subdivided a vial of exametazime and stored the fractions at - 60°C. The level of the primary complex was maintained at 55% using exametazime which had been reconstituted 24 days previously.

In order to improve the long term stability of reconstituted exametazime we have used a novel approach based on the premise that tin lost through oxidation should be replaced by further amounts of tin to maintain the stoichimetric balance. In the first study, a stock solution of stannous chloride was prepared containing 20 μg/ml. Small aliquots were used to prepare 99mTc exametazime. In the second study aliquots were used from a commercial kit preparation containing 6,6 μg/ml stannous chloride.

METHODS

PREPARATION OF STANNOUS CHLORIDE SOLUTIONS

1. In-house Method

A stock solution of stannous chloride was prepared by dissolving 20 mg stannous chloride dihydrate in 1 litre of Sodium Chloride Infusion BP to produce a concentration of 20 μg/ml. 10 ml aliquots were transfered to sterile nitrogen filled vials and stored in the freezer (-10°C). 0.1 ml (2 μg stannous chloride) was used for each cell labelling procedure.

2. Kit Method

A kit solution of stannous chloride was prepared by reconstituting a vial of stannous medronate ("Amerscan", Amersham plc), containing 4 mg of stannous chloride dihydrate with 6 ml Sodium Chloride Injection BP. 0.1 ml of this solution was made up to 10 ml with Sodium Chloride Injection BP to give a final concentration of 6,6 μg stannous chloride) were used for each cell labelling procedure. A fresh solution was prepared on a daily basis (usually from the MUGA material already prepared for the department) at no further cost.

DETERMINATION OF THE EFFECT OF ADDITION OF TIN TO RECONSTITUTED EXAMETAZIME

A preliminary set of experiments was performed to confirm that the addition of tin using the two formulations was able to maintain satisfactory levels of radiochemical purity of the 99mTc exametazime. A vial of exametazime was reconstituted with 6 ml of Sodium Chloride Injection BP. 0.3ml aliquots were mixed with 0.1 ml of each of the stannous chloride solutions, and 400-500 MBq of freshly eluted sodium pertechnetate added. For determinations using the in-house stannous solutions, exametazime was used which had been reconstituted up to 55 days previously (n=6). For each reading a control was prepared containing saline instead of stannous chloride. Similar readings were taken using the kit solution of stannous chloride using exametazime which had been reconstituted up to 150 days previously (n=5). Determination of the level of primary lipophilic complex (PC) and free pertechnetate were carried out using thin-layer chromatography according to the manufacturer's recommended method[13].

RADIOLABELLING OF MIXED LEUCOCYTES

Mixed leucocytes from 50 ml of blood were obtained from a wide variety of patients by sedimentation and centrifugation. 99mTc exametazime was prepared as described and incubated with the plug of leucocytes for 10 minutes. Radiactivity not associated with the cells was washed off with cell free plasma, and the labelling efficiency (LE) determined.

RESULTS

The mean levels of radiochemical purity of the 99mTc exametazime prepared with the in-house stock solution of stannous chloride was 41% (range 11%-60%, n=6). The control experiment showed no primary lipophilic complex (Table 1). The mean levels of radiochemical purity of the 99mTc exametazime prepared with the kit solution of stannous chloride was 87% (range 68%-93%, n=5) (Table 2). The mean labelling efficiency using the in-house stannous solution was 54% (SD=15%, n=130), see Figure 1. The exametazime used had been reconstituted up to 8 months previously. The mean labelling efficiency obtained using the kit solution of stannous chloride was 67% (SD=19%, n=60), see Figure 2. The exametazime used had been reconstituted up to 5 months previously.

Table 1. Results of Radiochemical Purity tests with and without the addition of in-house tin solution.

Days after reconstitution	% primary complex	
	in-house solution (2 μg stannous chloride)	control solution (saline)
3	57	1
22	16	0
29	11	0
33	60	0
54	57	0
55	43	0

Table 2. Results of Radiochemical Purity tests with and without the addition of kit tin solution.

Days after reconstitution	% primary complex	
	Kit solution (0,66 μg stannous chloride)	control solution (saline)
14	93	0
15	98	0
19	90	0
146	87	0
150	68	0

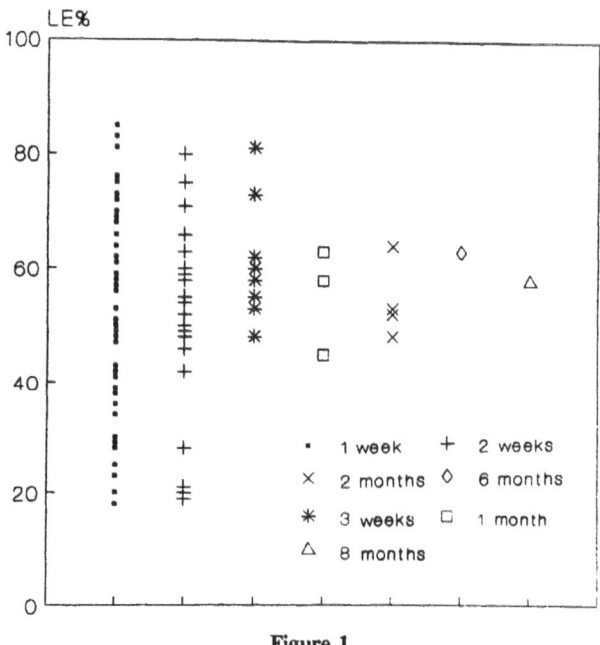

Figure 1

DISCUSSION

The preparation of the in-house stock solution of stannous chloride was time consuming , since the stannous chloride dihydrate dissolves in saline with difficulty . We did not resort to adding hydrochloric acid to enhance the solubility of the stannous chloride, since this would have affected the pH of the final preparation. Because the dissolution of the stannouschloride was not carried out under nitrogen it was prone to oxidation so that the final solution may have been of a concentration less than 20 μg/ml. Also during cold storage of the stock solutions oxidation may have occured since the saline used was not nitrogen purged.

The kit solution of stannous chloride was convenient to prepare and had an accurate amount of stannous chloride. Since the solution was freshly prepared on a daily basis it was not prone to oxidation.

Satisfactory levels of radiochemical purity were maintained with both preparations of tin, but the primary lipophilic content was higher when the kit solution was used. Labelling efficiencies were also higher using the kit solution of tin.

Scans of patients injected with 99mTc exametazime labelled mixed leucocytes prepared with the in-house stock tin, the kit tin and without tin were compared. There were no unusual bio-distribution as a result of using the different tin formulations.

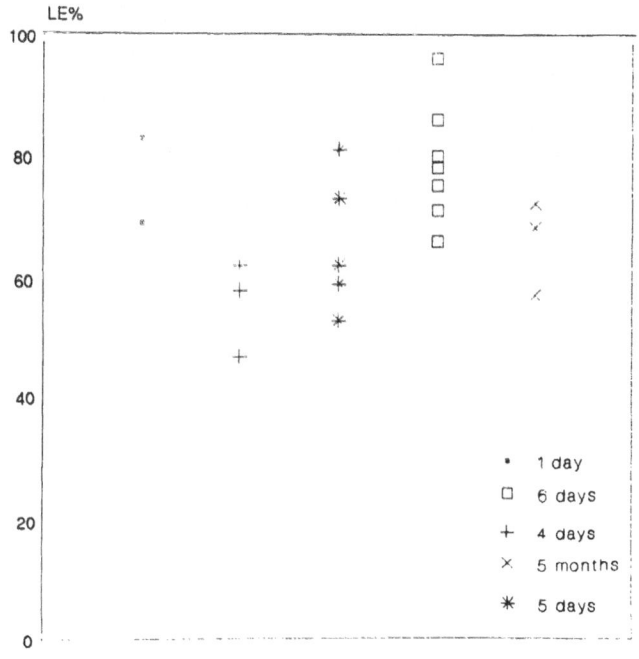

Figure 2

CONCLUSION

Long term stability of exametazime reconstituted with saline can be achieved by addition of tin to replace that lost through oxidation. We have demonstrated that high levels of radiochemical purity of 99mTc exametazime were retained following the addition of sodium pertechnetate to exametazime stabilised with tin. Fresh stannous chloride is more convenient to prepare and labelling efficiencies are higher using fresh tin. By using small volumes of exametazime, we have established a protocol for cell labelling that allows 15-18 patient doses to be removed from one vial of exametazime.

REFERENCES

1. Roddie ME, Peters AM, Danpure H et al. Imaging with Tc-99m HM-PAO lablled leucocytes. *Radiology*; 166: 767-72 (1988).
2. Mortelmans L. Clinical uselfulness of Tc-99m HM-PAO labelled white blood cell imaging in abscesses. *Clin Nucl Med*; 14: 127-30 (1989).
3. Becker W. Radiolabelled granulocytes in inflamatory bowel disease: diagnostic possibilities and clinical indications. *Ncl Med Commun*; 9:693-6 (1988).
4. Scholmerich J, Schmidt E, Schichen C et al. Scintigraphic assessment of bowel involvement and disease activity in Crohn's disease using Tc-99m Hm.PAO as a leucocyte label. *Gastroenterology*; 95: 1287-93 (1988).
5. Roddie ME, Peters AM, Osma S et al. Osteomyelitis. *Nucl Med Commun*; 9: 713-18 (1988).
6. Peters AM. Sepsis. *Nucl Med Commun*; 9: 719-23 (1988).
7. Reynolds JH, Graham D, Smith FW. Imaging inflammation with Tc-99m Hm-PAO labelled leucocytes. *Clin Radiol*; 42:195-8 (1990).
8. Al Janabi MA, Solanki K, Critchley M et al. Radioleucoscintigraphy in osteoarthritis. Is there an inflammatory component?. *Nucl Med Comm*; 13: 706-712 (1992).
9. Hung JC, Volkert WA, Holmens RA. Stabilization of Tc-99m-D, L-HMPAO using gentisic acid. *Nucl Med Biol*; 16: 675-80 (1989).
10. Lang J, Barbarics E, Lazar J at al. Effects of labelling conditions and formulations of kit on in vitro stability of Tc-99m-D, L-HMPAO. *Eur J Nucl Med*; 15:424 (1989).
11. Ballinger J. Preparation of Tc-99m HMPAO. *J Nucl Med* 31: 1892 (1990).
12. Hawkins T, Reeder A, Keavey PM et al. The long term stability reconstituted exametazime: a clinical and laboratory evaluation. *Nucl Med Commun*; 12: 1045-1055 (1991).
13. Amersham international plc: ceretec package insert.

99mTc LABELLING OF INTERLEUKIN-2 FOR IN VIVO TARGETING OF ACTIVATED T-LYMPHOCYTES

M. Chianelli[1,2], A. Signore[2], G. Ronga[2], P. Pozzilli[3], A. Fritzberg[4] and S.J. Mather[1]

[1]Dept. of Nucl. Medicine Research, St. Bartholomew's Hospital, London
[2]Nu. M.E.D. Group, Servizio Speciale, Medicina Nucleare and
[3]Endocrinologia, Clinica Medica II, University of Rome "La Sapienza"
[4]NeoRx corp. Seattle, USA

INTRODUCTION

We have recently reported that interleukin-2 (IL2) labelled with iodine-123 (123I) can be successfully used for the in vivo detection of areas of lymphocytic infiltration[1]. IL2 is a lymphocyte growth factor (M.W.:15.5kD) that binds to its specific receptor expressed on the surface membrane of activated T lymphocytes[2]. 123I is a suitable isotope for in vivo studies and for protein labelling. However, it has some disadvantages such as the poor availability, the elevated cost and the low labelling efficiency.

These aspects encourage the labelling of IL2 with 99mTc. This is always easily available, is inexpensive and has a shorter physical half life (6 hrs) that allows the injection of greater activity compared to 123I. However, most techniques available for the 99mTc labelling of proteins are too harsh for an effective labelling of a small and delicate protein such as IL2 and may result in protein damage and loss of receptor binding capacity[3].

The aim of this study is the development of a new technique for the effective labelling of IL2 with 99mTc with high specific activity (S.A.) and retained receptor binding capacity for the in vivo detection of pathological lymphocytic infiltration.

MATERIALS AND METHODS

In order to minimize the possible radiolabelling damages to IL2 and to inject low amounts of the protein we have optimised the reaction in order to achieve the labelling of the ligand with the maximum S.A. thus using only very small amounts of the ligand.

We used for our experiments a chelate with two functional sites: an N_3S group for the coordination of 99mTc and an active ester available for the binding to proteins via the lysine residues[4].

The ligand is first labelled with 99mTc and then conjugated to proteins.

Ligand Labelling

Labelling of the ligand was obtained by reduction of 99mTc with stannous chloride and transchelation via a labile complex with glucuronic acid. All reagents/parameters influencing the reaction have been studied in order to obtain the maximum ligand labelling efficiency (L.E.).

$99mTcO_4$- (740 MBq) and the ligand (16 μg/ml) were incubated (7/15/25 mins) at 80/100°C, with different concentrations of: iso-propyl alcohol (9/18/36%), glucuronic acid (2/4/8/16 μg/ml), stannous chloride (30/60/120 μg/ml), gentisic acid (30/60/120/240 μg/ml), at different pH (2/3/4). Ligand L.E. was evaluated by RP-HPLC with a C-18 column running a gradient from 5 to 28% of acetonitrile in 0.01 MPO_4 buffer. The presence of free $99mTcO_4$- was evaluated by ITLC run with acetone and colloids formation with ITLC run with 0.1 M Tris buffer.

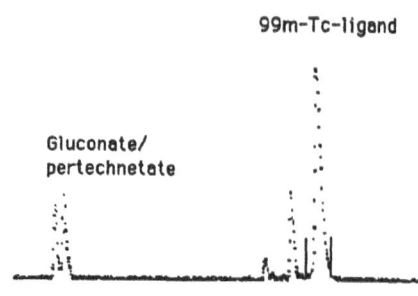

Figure 1. Ligand L.E. evaluated by RP-HPLC

IL2 Labelling and Purification

The labelling of IL2 has been studied in order to have the highest labelling efficiency with the minimum damage to the protein. All factors that could be possibly hazardous to IL2 have been studied so that the mildest conditions have been used still giving good L.E..

Labelled ligand was cooled at 4°C in a prechilled lead container to prevent heat shock of IL2 and then incubated at room temperature, at basic pH in order to promote the

Table 1. Optimal concentrations of reagents for the labelling of the ligand with high S.A.

- reagents -	- concentrations -	- effects -
iso-propyl alcohol	18%	ligand solvent
pH	2	prevent ester hydrolysis
glucuronic acid	16 μg/ml	intermediate chelate
stannous chloride	60 μg/ml	reduces 99mTc
gentisic acid	60 μg/ml	antioxidant
heating	80°C, 20 min	provides the energy for 99mTc co-ordination

reaction of the active ester with lysine residues of IL2. Different incubation times (5/15/30/60 min), pH (8/9/10), IL2 (78/150/260 μg/ml) and IPA (6/12/21%) concentrations were tested. IL2 L.E. was evaluated by ITLC run with 12 % TCA. 99mTc-IL2 was purified by a pre-packed G25M gel-filtration column (PD10, Pharmacia).

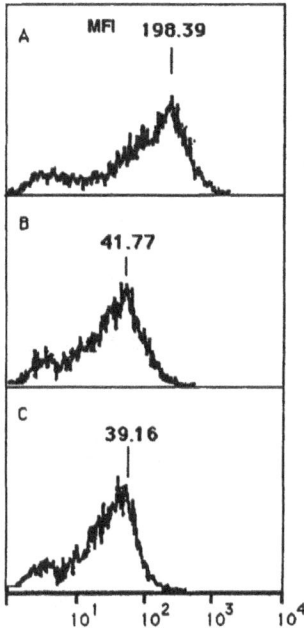

Figure 2. Histograms obtained incubating IL2R + ve cells with a fluoresceine conjugated anti-IL2R MoAb in absence of IL2 (A), in presence of unlabelled (B) and 99mTc-labelled (C) IL2. An identical decrease of mean fluorescence intensity (MFI) is obtained with 99mTc-IL2 respect to unlabelled IL2.

Characterization and In Vitro Test of Receptor Binding Capacity of 99mTc-IL2

After purification a SDS-PAGE electrophoresis was performed on 99mTc-IL2, in order to ascertain if possible alterations of the molecular structure (aggregation/fragmentation) occurred during the labelling procedure.

The capacity of 99mTc-IL2 to bind to its receptor was tested by a competitive assay based on the incubation of a fluoresceine conjugated anti-IL2R monoclonal antibody (2A3, Becton Dickinson) in presence of different concentration of IL2. Binding of IL2 is evaluated by its capacity to inhibit the binding of the fluorescinated antibody, the binding of which is directly proportional to fluorescence intensity. Receptor binding capacity of 99mTc-IL2 is determined by comparison with unlabelled IL2[5].

RESULTS

Ligand Labelling

Labelling of the ligand with high S.A. was achieved with a L.E. of about 80% (Fig.1). The labelling is obtained with a negligible formation of colloids (less than 3%)

and free 99mTcO$_4$-. Glucuronic acid played a key role for the labelling of the ligand with no colloids formation. Acid pH also was important to obtain a good L.E.. Best results are with pH no higher than 2. Also the heating time: it must be kept within 20' for the prevention of radiothermolisis products.

See table 1 for results.

IL2 Labelling and Purification

IL2 was labelled to a S.A. of about 20 mCi/mg with a L.E. of about 20%. After purification, precipitation studies with trichloracetic acid showed that greater than 98% of the 99mTc is IL2 bound.

IL2 L.E. increases with increasing IL2 concentrations and optimal incubation time was 30 minutes. Longer incubation times gives better L.E. but are likely to damage IL2. Basic pH was critical for a good conjugation of the ligand: it should be no lower than 9.

Characterization and In Vitro Test of Receptor Binding Capacity of 99mTc-IL2

Autoradiography of the gel electrophoresis of purified 99mTc-IL2 showed that radioactivity migrates according to IL2 molecular weight indicating that the labelling procedure did not affect IL2 molecular structure by molecular breakage or aggregation.

Results from binding assays showed that radiolabelled IL2 was capable of inducing the same decrease in fluorescence as unlabelled IL2, indicating that the labelling procedure, using conditions described above, has no effect on IL2 receptor binding capacity.

CONCLUSIONS

Our results indicate that the use of prelabelled ligands can be used effectively for the 99mTc labelling with high S.A. of IL2 without affecting its receptor binding capacity. This can be obtained via the labelling with high S.A. of the ligand, that is the most difficult task. The labelling is stable and is the mildest approach, to date, for labelling protein with 99mTc.

Our data are a starting point for the use of 99mTc for the labelling of small biologically active peptides and encourage the use of 99mTc-IL2 for the in vivo imaging of pathological lymphocytic infiltrations.

REFERENCES

1. A. Signore, M. Chianelli, A. Toscano, L. Monetini, G.F. Tonnarini, M. Negri, C.C. Nimmon, P. Pozzilli. A radiopharmaceutical for imaging areas of lymphocytic infiltration: 123I-interleukin-2: labelling procedure and animal studies. *Nucl. Med. Comm* 13: 713-722 (1992).
2. Morgan D.A., Ruscetti F.W., Gallo R.C. Selective in vitro growth factor of T lymphocytes from normal human marrow. *Science* 193: 1007-1008 (1976).
3. W.C. Eckelman, C.H. Paik, J. Steigman. Three approaches to radiolabelling antibodies with 99mTc. *Nucl Med Biol* 16(2): 171-76 (1989).
4. A.R. Fritzberg, P.G. Abrams, P.L. Beaumier, S. Kasina. A.C. Morgan, T.N. Rao, J.M. Reno, J.A. Sanderson, A. Srinivasan, D.S. Wilbur, J.L. Vanderheyden. Specific and stable labelling of antibodies with technetium-99m with a diamide dithiolate chelating agent. *Proc Natl Sci USA*.85: 4025-4029 (1988).
5. M. Chianelli, A. Signore, R. Hicks, E. Napoleone, P. Pozzilli, P.C.L.Beverley: Evaluation of interleukin-2 binding to its receptors by using the fluorescence activated cell sorter. 10th EFIS meeting, Edinburgh (1990). 10th EFIS meeting. S-38,2.

NITRIC OXIDE AND PROSTAGLANDIN I₂ FOR RADIOLABELLING OF HUMAN PLATELETS

I. Neumann, S. Granegger, A. Dembinska-Kiec, J. O'Grady[1], and
H. Sinzinger

Wilhelm Auerswald-Atherosclerosis Research Group (ASF) Vienna
Dept. of Nuclear Medicine, University of Vienna
Ludwig Boltzmann-Institute for Nuclear Medicine, Vienna
[1]Department of Pharmacology, University of Vienna, Austria

ABSTRACT

Both nitric oxide (NO) and prostaglandin I₂ (PGI₂) are of benefit during platelet preparation in improving platelet viability. We have examined the influence of NO and PGI₂ on in vitro and in vivo labelling parameters when using 100 μCi 111Indium-oxine. For labelling, platelets from 121 patients with clinically manifested atherosclerotic vascular disease were incubated either with PGI₂ (n=29) or NO (n=27) alone, a combination of both (n=30) or without any additive (n=35). Using platelets from 7 healthy volunteers labelling was carried out similary and the offer of the same additives examined as with the platelets derived from patients. While in the patient group no effect was seen on labelling efficiency (LE), platelet viability as reflected by recovery (REC) showed a significant improvement which was greatest with the combined use of NO an PGI₂. Platelet function (aggregation, migration) was best preserved in the presence of PGI₂ (alone or together with NO). The parallel experiments comparing all the 4 processing procedures using platelets from healthy volunteers revealed a significant benefit with PGI₂ though not with NO and the combined use produced no further benefit over that seen with PGI₂ alone. Thus, NO and PGI₂ are recommended for routine use to minimize platelet damage during extracorporal manipulations and to facilitate preservation of platelet function.

INTRODUCTION

Endothelium derived relaxing factor (EDRF) (Furchgott et al. 1980) has been shown to inhibit platelet aggregation (Moncada et al. 1988) via an elevation of intracellular cGMP. One component of EDRF has recently been discovered to be NO (Palmer et al. 1987). PGI₂ acts by increasing intracellular cAMP. PGI₂ decreases platelet trapping on reinjection set (Sinzinger et al. 1981), preserves platelets during washing (Blackwell et al. 1982; Vargas et al. 1982; Radomski et al. 1983) and inhibits platelets activation during preparation of platelet concentrates (Menitove et al. 1984) as verified by morphological studies as well (Read et al. 1985). PGI$_2$ also improved the recovery (REC) of radiolabelled platelets (Sinzinger et al. 1.984) without affecting labelling efficiency (LE) (Sinzinger et al. 1987). However, a similar property for NO has been claimed recently by Moncada's group (Radomski et al. 1988) which reported benefits during isolation and washing of platelets. PGI$_2$ and NO have been shown to synergize with each other both in vitro and in vivo (Sinzinger et al. 1991). Recently, Kotze et al.(1991) demonstrated that the labelling method is critical to the platelets in-vivo functional behaviour. Therefore, we wondered whether NO might influence the radiolabelling- and viability of human platelets and how any benefits compare to those obtained with PGI$_2$.

Finally, any synergistic effects on labelling parameters were examined.

MATERIAL AND METHODS

Volunteers and Patients

Blood from 7 healthy donors (4 males and 3 females aged 25-44 years) and 121 patients (75 males and 46 females aged 41-71a, patients data in Table 1) suffering from clinically manifest atherosclerosis was used. All the healthy donors and patients were non-smokers with normal cholesterol and lipoprotein values according to the Austrian cholesterol conference ranges (Kaliman et al. 1987). They were not taking any medication known to influence platelet function or the PG-system within two weeks of blood donation. Blood from the 7 healthy donors was processed for radiolabelling, in parallel, without any additive, with PGI$_2$ or NO alone and also in combination. In the 121 patients one of the 4 processing steps (PGI$_2$: n=29;NO : n=27; PGI$_2$ + NO : n=30; Control : n=35) were used. PGI$_2$ (3,33 μg in 100 μl [The Upjohn Company, Kalamazoo, Mi, USA]) and/or 10 mM (200 μl) NO (AGA-Edelgas GmbH, Vienna, Austria) were added once or twice, respectively, at the step of sedimentation as well as separation of platelet rich plasma (figure 1) and to the platelet pellet immediately prior to the radiolabelling procedure. NO preparation was performed as follows: 10 ml Tris-HCL-buffer (25 mM, pH = 7,4) was bubbled for 15 min with Argon gas (AGA-Edelgas GmbH, Vienna, Austria) and then for 15 min with NO-gas (AGA-Edelgas GmbH, Vienna, Austria). After the gas-bulb was sealed with a rubber stopper 1 ml was removed with a syringe and injected into another gas bulb which was filled with 9 ml with Argon bubbled (15 min) Tris-HCL-buffer. The final concentrations of NO were between 0.3 % and 0.1 %.

Table 1. Patients data

	n	f	m	a
control	35	12	23	56.9 ± 7.4
+ NO	27	12	15	60.4 ± 7.5
+ PGI$_2$	29	11	18	56.9 ± 6.6
+ NO + PGI$_2$	30	11	19	59.2 ± 6.7

f... females; m... males; a... age (years).

Platelet Labelling

Platelet labelling was performed using a simple kit (Karmed, Klosterneuburg, Austria) developed by us earlier (Jäger et al.1984). Briefly, 16 ml of blood were collected into two Monovette vials (Sarstädt, Germany) and anticoagulated using 4 ml acid citrate dextrose (ACD). Another 2 Monovettes were identically prepared to be used for the in vitro viability testing. After 10 minutes sedimentation at 22°C the vials were centrifuged for 5 minutes at 150 x g to obtain platelet rich plasma (PRP). The PRP in the supernatant was removed and by a further centrifugation step a platelet pellet was obtained. The platelet poor plasma (PPP) in the supernatant was removed and preserved in a sterile syringe. The pellet was resuspended in 1 ml freshly prepared Tyrode buffer (pH 6,2) to a final platelet concentration of 1x10E9/ml. For radiolabelling 100 μCi (100 μl) 111-indium-oxine (kindly provided by P. Angelberger PhD, Dept. of Chemistry, SGAE Seibersdorf, Austria) were added and incubated at 37°C for 5 minutes (platelet concentration 1x10E9/ml; oxine concentration 5 μg/ml) in a constantly stirred water bath. These labelling conditions have been previously described by us as being optimal (Jäger et al. 1984; Neumann et al. 1992).Thereafter, the stored autologous PPP was added to the radiolabeled platelets and the suspension was reinjected immediately. PGI₂ and/or NO were added at the various steps of the labelling procedure as indicated in Figure 1.

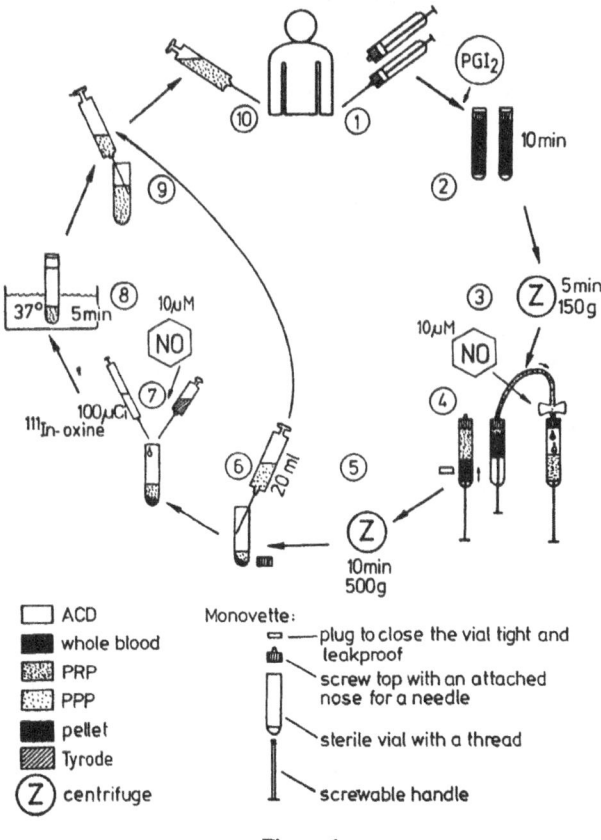

Figure 1

Labelling Efficiency

The labelling efficiency (LE) was counted from an aliquot as cell bound radioactivity (as % compared to total radioactivity); **Platelet survival** (International Committee for standardisation in Haematology 1988): 2 ml blood samples (anticoagulated by means of EDTA) were drawn at least twice daily for 10 days. The platelet bound radioactivity was counted and survival calculated using a multiple-hit-model (computer program kindly provided by Anthon du P. Heyns, Blood Transfusion Service, Johannesburg, South Africa).

In Vitro Viability Testing:

Platelet aggregation: Platelet aliquots resuspended in 600 μl PPP at a final concentration of 250 x 10E3/μl were put into a prewarmed cuvette and stirred continuously. Aggregation was induced with 10 μM (100 μl) ADP (Boehringer Mannheim, Germany). The maximal amplitude of the response curve was measured (cm) and expressed as a percentage of the theoretical maximal response.

Platelet Migration (Kaliman et al. 1983): PRP was adjusted with PPP to a final platelet count of 250 x 10E3/μl. A Petri dish was filled with 10 ml Gibco medium (Gibco, Paisley, Scotland) and a 10 cm capillary freshly filled with PRP was placed with one end at the center of the Petri dish, 100 units penicillin and 50 mg streptomycin were added. The system was closed and incubated for 24 h at 37°C under continuous supply of 95 % O_2 and 5 % CO_2. At the end of the incubation time the area into which the platelets had migrated was outlined by pencil and quantified using a plan compensation polarimeter (Zeiss, Jena, Germany). The migration area was expressed as the mean of two estimations made in parallel.

In Vivo Viability Testing, Recovery:

Two hours after reinjection of labelled platelets a 2 ml blood sample anticoagulated with 2 % EDTA was drawn from the patients. Counting the cell bound radioactivity after centrifugation (1000 x g, 10 minutes, 22°C), the REC was determined from the cell bound activity of the sample and the calculated activity at the injection time (from injected activity and estimated blood volume). REC was expressed as a percentage of the initial radioactivity.

Statistical Analysis

Data are presented as mean values $\pm$ SD; calculation of significance was done using stundent's t-test.

RESULTS

In blood from the healthy volunteer subjects processing in the presence of NO produced a significantly better LE (table 5). PGI_2 was similar beneficial, but the combined use of both did not further improve labelling data (Table 5).

Using the optimal labelling conditions for human platelets (Neumann et al. 1992) in the 121 patients the addition of NO apparently did not influence LE (Table 2). The LE in the presence of PGI_2 was slightly, but not significantly higher (Table 2) than incubation without any additive. The addition of both, PGI₂ and NO, did not result in a significant improvement of LE.

A more pronounced effect could be demonstrated for REC, showing the lowest viability for those platelets radiolabelled without any additive, while the addition of NO (+2,4 %), PGI₂ (+4,4 %) and the combination of both (+4,8 %) were significantly improving the value. This was reflected in the correlation between LE and REC (Table 3) which was highest without additive; both NO and PGI₂ improved REC, but not LE, resulting in a much less strong correlation ($r=0.623$). No correlation between age (calculated for both sexes separately) and LE, REC or platelet survival was found.

In-vitro platelet function tested by ADP-induced platelet aggregation, as well as migration, showed a small difference in response after as compared to before the radiolabelling procedure. This difference, however, was comparable in all the four examined groups for the aggregation response, while in the presence of PGI₂ (alone as well as together with NO) a significantly ($p < 0,01$) smaller difference indicating the artificial damage was detected (Table 4). Comparable platelet function data were obtained in the healthy volunteers samples (Table 5).

Table 2. Influence of PGI₂ and NO on platelet labelling

	LE (%)	REC (%)	SUR (hrs)	a
Control (n=35)	84.9 ± 5.7	61.3 ± 6.0	168.5 ± 20.8	56.9 ± 7.9
+ NO (n=27)	85.6 ± 3.5	63.7 ± 4.4	170.4 ± 21.9	60.4 ± 7.5
+ PGI₂ (n=29)	86.4 ± 3.9	65.7 ± 3.8	167.9 ± 16.3	56.9 ± 6.6
+ NO + PGI₂ (n=30)	86.4 ± 3.3	66.1 ± 3.7*	172.9 ± 16.5*	59.2 ± 6.7

$\overline{X}$ ± SD; *) $p < 0.01$ (versus controls)

Table 3. Effect of PGI₂ and NO on correlation between LE and REC

Controls	r = 0.974 *
+ NO	r = 0.939 *
+ PGI₂	r = 0.811 *
+ NO + PGI₂	r = 0.623 *

r = corr (x,y)
* $p < 0.01$

Table 4. In-vitro platelet function testing

	n	Aggregation[1]	Migration[2]
Controls	35	20.86 ± 2.57	40.27 ± 4.16
+ NO	27	19.81 ± 3.02	37.11 ± 3.73
+ PGI₂	29	18.57 ± 2.62	31.86 ± 2.75 *
+ NO + PGI₂	30	18.83 ± 2.77	30.12 ± 2.19 *

$\overline{X}$ ± SD; * p<0.01 (versus controls)
[1] % difference in maximal amplitude before vs. after labelling
[2] difference (mmE2) in migration area before vs. after labelling

Table 5. Influence of PGI₂ and NO on LE and platelet function using blood from 7 healthy volunteers

	LE	Aggregation[1]	Migration[2]
Controls	87.56 ± 2.48	22.66 ± 1.02	40.43 ± 2.51
+ NO	88.37 ± 2.48 *	20.23 ± 0.79 *	34.70 ± 3.94 *
+ PGI₂	92.01 ± 2.76 *	19.59 ± 0.96 *	33.20 ± 3.59 *
+ NO + PGI₂	92.54 ± 2.99 * **	19.27 ± 0.77 * **	31.67 ± 3.17 * **

$\overline{X}$ ± SD; * p<0.01 (versus controls); ** p>0.01 (vs PGI₂)
[1] % difference in maximal amplitude before vs. after labelling
[2] difference (mmE2) in migration area before vs. after labelling

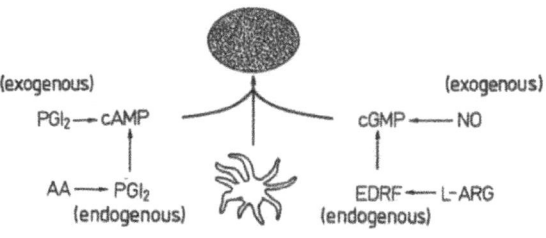

Figure 2. Mechanisms of Platelet Deactivation.

DISCUSSION

Numerous attempts were done to improve radiolabelling of platelets (Thakur et al. 1976; Heyns et al. 1979; Goedemans et al. 1982; Hawker et al. 1983; Sinzinger et al. 1984; Hill-Zobel et al. 1987; Kotze et al. 1991; Neumann et al. 1992) either by modifying the procedure or adding various pharmacological agents, such as PGE_1, PGI_2 and theophylline.

PGI_2 is a short-lived compound derived from arachidonic acid metabolism which stabilizes the platelet membrane via specific membrane receptors and subsequent elevation of intracellular cAMP (Moncada et al. 1976).

In 1981 we were the first to report that the use of PGI_2 during radiolabelling is of benefit (Sinzinger et al. 1981), not only by improving platelet recovery but also by decreasing the number of platelets trapped in the reinfusion set. It has previously been shown that PGI_2 is of significant benefit during the radiolabelling of human and experimental animal platelets (Sinzinger et al. 1989) by preventing ex-vivo activation. Our findings were later extended to the use PGI_2 for separation, washing and preparation of platelet concentrates (Radomski et al. 1983) proving the preservation of cells by morphological means (Read et al. 1985) and demonstrating a significantly enhanced viability (Kernan et al. 1985; Menitove et al. 1984). Recently, the addition of PGE_1, a compound which has a comparable mode of action to PGI_2 has been reported to improve platelet transfusion when added during platelet preparation (Kernan et al. 1985). NO shares a variety of properties (Moncada et al. 1988) with PGI_2, such as the inhibition of platelets adhesion and aggregation. Our findings show that NO improves only REC and does not influence LE significantly. Although PGI_2 and NO act via different mechanisms, PGI_2 by an increase of cAMP and NO by an increase of cGMP, and these compounds have been shown to synergize under certain conditions (Sinzinger et al.1989), no such synergism of PGI_2 and NO was apparent demonstrated under in vitro or in vivo conditions after radiolabelling.

The major difficulties in working with NO are that it is an aggresive and toxic gas which rapidly reacts with oxygen, and which in vivo is inactivated by the presence of haemoglobin. This fact, however, does not allow to add NO even in large amounts (more than 100 μM) at an earlier stage for platelet preservation during radiolabelling. Adding an NO-donor, however, would require enormous amounts of substance. Assuming a molecular weight of about 65000 for oxyhaemoglobin, of about 250 for SIN-1 (the active compound of molsidomine formed in the liver and acting as an NO-donor) and a haemoglobin concentration of 14 g% as well as a homogenous intra-and extracellular distribution 500 μg SIN-1 would be necessary to neutralize only 1 ml whole blood. Thus, in order to achieve a protective effect on platelets in whole blood about a tenfold amount, i.e. 1-5 mg SIN-1/ml would be required (personal communication, B.A.Peskar, Dept. of Pharmacology, Ruhr-University, Bochum, Germany). It may well be that only an immediate addition of the platelet function preserving agent e.g. before the first centrifugation step, is able to induce the expected beneficial result. This may account for the difference in viability results obtained in the presence of PGI_2 as compared to NO. An addition of NO at an earlier preparation step might well show the synergism known to occur under other circumstances but not confirmed by these experiments. Whether in vivo NO-donors, such as for example nitrates or molsidomine, which would be needed in enormous amounts, could solve this problem still has to be assessed.

ACKNOWLEDGEMENTS

The technical help by our technicians Judith Bednar and Ulrike Horvath is gratefully acknowledged.

REFERENCES

Blackwell GJ, Radomski M, Vargas JR, Moncada S, 1982. Prostacyclin prolongs viability of washed human platelets. *Biochim Biophys Acta* 718: 60-65.

Furchgott F, Zawadski JV,1980. The obligatory role of endothelial cells in the relaxion of arterial smooth muscle by acetylcholine. *Nature* 286: 373-377.

Goedemans WTH, 1982. Indium-111-tropolone versus oxine. *J Nucl Med* 23: 455.

Hawker RJ, Hall CE, Gunson BK, 1983. Indium-111 tropolone versus oxine. *J Nucl Med* 24: 367.

Heyns A duP, Badenhorst PN, Pieters H, Lotter MG, Minnar PC, Duyvene de Wit LJ, Van Reenen OR, Retief RJ, 1979. Preparation of a viable population of indium-111-labeled human blood platelets. *Thromb Haemost* 42: 1473-1482.

Hill-Zobel RL, Gannon S, McCandless B, Tsan MF, 1987. Effects of chelates and incubation media on platelet labelling with indium-111. *J Nucl Med* 28: 223-228.

International Committee for Standardisation in Haematology. Recomended method for indium-111 platelet survival studies, 1988. *J Nucl Med* 29: 564-566.

Jäger E, Kolbe H, Silberbauer K, Sinzinger H, Höfer R, 1984. Technik der radioaktiven Markierung autologer menschlicher Trombozyten mit 111-Indium-oxin und 111-Indium-Oxin-Sulfat und deren klinische Anwendung. *Wr Klin Wschr* 96: 106-112.

Kaliman J, Sinzinger H, Joskowicz G, 1983. Clinical value of platelet migration test in patients with peripheral vascular disease. *VASA* 12/4: 357-362.

Kaliman J, Kostner G, Kraupp O, Kunze M, Sinzinger H, Widhalm K, 1987. Richtlinien zur Prävention der Atherosklerose. *Wr Klin Wschr* 99: 589-590.

Kernan McA, Bareford D, Hesslewood SR, Harding LK, Turner VS, Hawker RJ, 1985. Does prostaglandin improve the quality of transfused platelets?. *Nucl Med Comm*: A 130.

Kotze HF, Heyns A du P, Lötter MG, Pieters H, Roodt JP, Sweetlove MA, Badenhorst PN, 1991. Comparison of oxine and tropolone methods for labelling human platelets with indium-111.*J Nucl Med* 32: 62-66.

Menitove JE, Frenzke M, Aster RH, 1984. Use of prostacyclin to inhibit activation of platelets during preparation of platelet concentrates, *Transfusion* 24: 528-531.

Moncada S, Radomski M, Palmer RMJ, 1988. Commentary: endothelium-derived relaxing factor identification as nitric oxide and role in the control of vascular tone and platelet function. *Biochem Pharmacol* 37: 2495-201.

Neumann I, Strobl-Jäger E, Angelberger P, O'Grady J, Sinzinger H, 1992. A comparison of 111-In-oxine with 111-In-oxine-sulphate for human platelet labelling *Thromb Haem Dis* 5: 5-10.

Palmer RMJ, Ferridge AG, Moncada S, 1987. Nitric oxide release accounts for biological activity of endothelium-derived relaxing factor. *Nature* 327: 524-526.

Radomski M, Moncada S, 1983. An improved method for washing of human platelets with prostacyclin.*Thromb Res* 30: 383-389.

Radomski M, Palmer RMJ, Rad NG, Moncada S, 1988. Isolation and washing of human platelets with nitric oxide. *Thromb Res* 50: 537-546.

Read NG, Radomski M, Goodwin DA, Moncada S, 1985. An ultrastructural study of stored human platelets after washing using prostacyclin. *Brit J Haematol* 60: 305-314.

Sinzinger H, Angelberger P, Höfer R, 1981. Platelet labelling with 111In-oxine-benefit of prostacyclin (PGI2)-addition for preparation and injection. *J Nucl Med*22: 292.

Sinzinger H, Strobl-Jäger E, Pesl H, 1984. Radiolabelling of human platelets. *Wr Klin Wschr* 96:357A.

Sinzinger H, Kolbe H, Strobl-Jäger E, Höfer R, 1984. A simple and safe technique for sterile autologous platelet labelling using "Monovette vials". *Europ J Nucl Med* 9: 320-322.

Sinzinger H, Fitscha P, Kaliman J, 1987. Prostaglandin I2 during radiolabelling improves recovery, but does not change platelet half-life and platelet uptake over active human lesion sites. *Prostaglandins* 33: 787-790.

Sinzinger H, Fitscha P, Kaliman J, 1989. Indikation und Methoden zurThrombozytenmarkierung. *Wr Klin Wschr* 101: 179A.

Thakur ML, Welch MJ, Joist LH, Coleman RE, 1976. Indium-111 labeled platelets: studies on preparation and evaluation of in vivo functions. *Thromb Res* 9:345-357.

Vargas JR, Radomski M, Moncada S, 1982. The use of prostacyclin in the separation from plasma and washing of human platelets. *Prostaglandins* 23:929-945.

111In LABELING OF HUMAN IgG USING A DTPA-IgG KIT

M. Roca, I. Carrió[1], L. Prat, J. Blasi[2], I. Ferrer[2], J. Mora and
J. Martín- Comín

Department of Nuclear Medicine and [2]Department of Histology
Ciutat Universitaria de Bellvitge
[1]Department of Nuclear Medicine, Hospital de la Sta Creu i St Pau
Barcelona, Spain

INTRODUCTION

The use of 111In-human nonspecific Immunoglobulin G has been described as an effective tool in detecting focal infection[1] and inflammation[2], as well as being useful in the detection of osteomyelitis[3] and experimental atherosclerosis[4].

There are a lot of works describing different methods of coupling bifuncional chelator agents to proteins and their labeling with 111In[5, 6, 7, 8].

The lack of a commercial source for 111In-human IgG has led us to design a two vial kit as a rapid and easy way to get this trazer.

MATERIAL AND METHODS

The first step was directed to obtaining the DTPA coupled to the IgG. The human, nonspecific, polyclonal immunoglobulin was obtained from a commercial preparation for intravenous use (Endobulin[R], IMMUNOAG) with the following composition in a liophylized form: 500 mg of human IgG, 500 mg of Glucose and 30 mg of NaCl. This was dissolved in 0.1N NaHCO3 (pH: 8.3) to a final concentration of 10 mg/ml.

We used the bicyclic anhidride DTPA (SIGMA) freshly dissolved in Dimethyl Sulfoxide (SIGMA) to a concentration of 2.1 mg/ml.

DTPA was conjugated to the IgG at a molar ratio of 5:1 by incubating both solutions at 4°C for 50'.

After that, we eliminated the DTPA not bound to the protein by means of Centricon-100 centrifugal miniconcentrators (AMICON) that had been previously coated with IgG.

This method of purification doesn't dilute the DTPA-protein conjugate, doesn't cause a loss of IgG, and prevents the possible contamination with metallic ion impurities.

Using the same device in its recovery mode, we changed the medium to phosphate buffered saline (PBS) pH: 7.2 in order to achieve a concentration of 10 mg/ml of IgG.

Radiolabeled Blood Elements, Edited by J. Martin-Comin
Plenum Press, New York, 1994

Aliquotes of 0.1 ml, containing 1 mg of IgG each, were dispensed in vacuum sealed glass vials and stored at 4°C until their use.

In a lot of these vials we added 10% of maltose as a preservative agent.

DTPA-coupled IgG was labeled with 111In by citrate transchelation: 1.0 ml of citrate buffer (pH: 5) (vial II) was added to vial I containing the protein and, after that, the 111In cloride (MEDGENIX) required was added.

The kinetics of the reaction was tested with and without the addition of maltose as a preservative agent.

The labeling efficiency was measured by mixing the labeled IgG with 0.05 DTPA volume to volume. After that, we performed a thin layer chromatography using ITLC/Silica Gel chromatographic strips with saline as solvent.

The absence of dimers and polimers of IgG, as well as other unwanted labeled forms was tested by means of Sephadex G-200 gel colum chromatography and polyacrylamide gel electrophoresis.

RESULTS AND DISCUSSION

An incubation time of 10 minutes was enough to reach the maximum labeling efficiency (Fig 1).

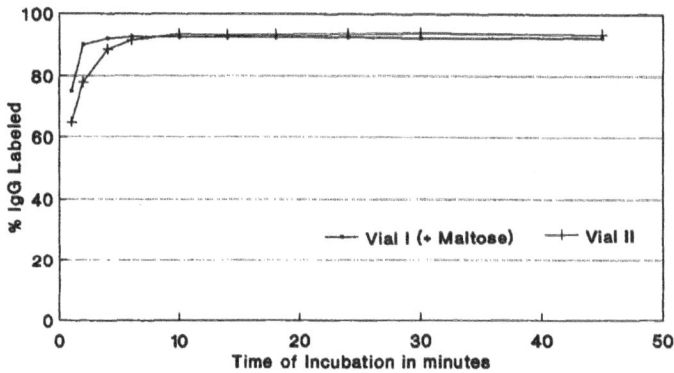

Fig. 1. Labeling kinetics of DTPA-IgG with 111In using vial A (+ Maltose) and vial B.

When the mixture was centrifuged only once, in order to eliminate the free DTPA, the labeling efficiency was guaranteed to be equal or more than 90% (n = 6). But when this step was done twice, adding more PBS, labeling efficiency grew to more than 95% (n = 6).

Labeling efficiency variation with increasing In-111 activity added from 500 to 2000 μCi is nearly inexistent.

After the labeling, the filtration of the solution through a low protein binding 0.22 μ filter is adviseable. Around 10% of the Indium activity is retained in the filter. As we show further on, this is due to unspecific binding and not to colloid formation.

The stability of the 111In-DTPA-IgG was well mantained both at 4°C and room temperature, for 7 days following the labeling (Fig. 2).

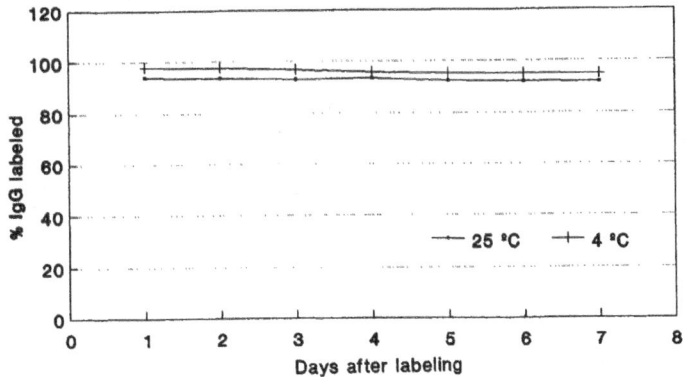

Fig. 2. Stability of 111In-DTPA-IgG.

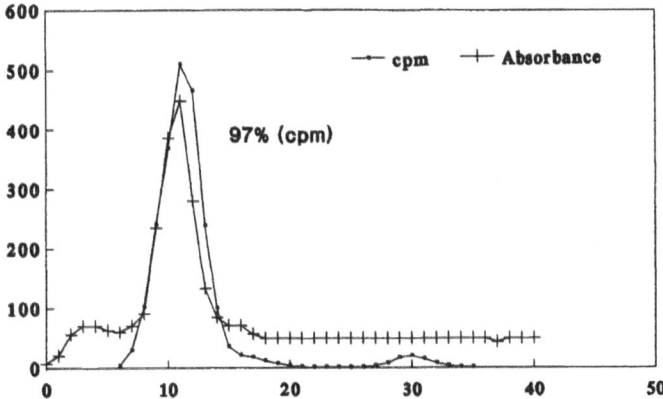

Fig. 3. Chromatogram (Sephadex G-200) and radioactivity profile of a sample of 111In-DTPA-IgG (5:1, DTPA:IgG molar ratio) 5 days after labeling.

The chromatogram and radioactivity profile show only one peak of labeled IgG form (Fig. 3).

No differences in the electrophoretic pattern could be seen between the labeled and the unlabeled intact IgG forms either at 1:1 or at 5:1 DTPA:IgG molar ratio. The autoradiography of the same sheets shows the radioactivity be present in the same areas as the dyed ones (Fig. 4).

The stability of vial I containing DTPA-IgG in the described form at 4°C is perfectly mantained up to at least 3 months with or without maltose. However, when vial I is made using a 1:1 DTPA:IgG molar ratio, the labeling efficiency falls under 90% and it decreases to under 70% 2 months after its preparation (Fig. 5).

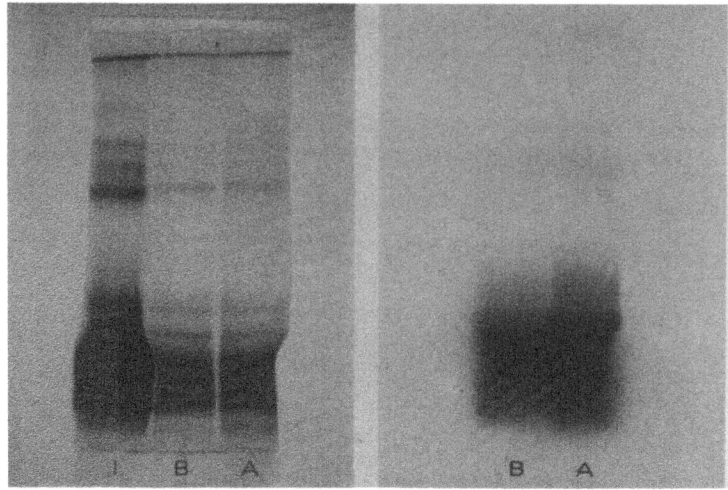

Fig. 4. Left: Electrophoretic sheets of the intact IgG (I) and the 111In-DTPA-IgG at 1:1 (B) and 5:1 (A) DTPA:IgG molar ratio. Right: Autoradiography of B and A.

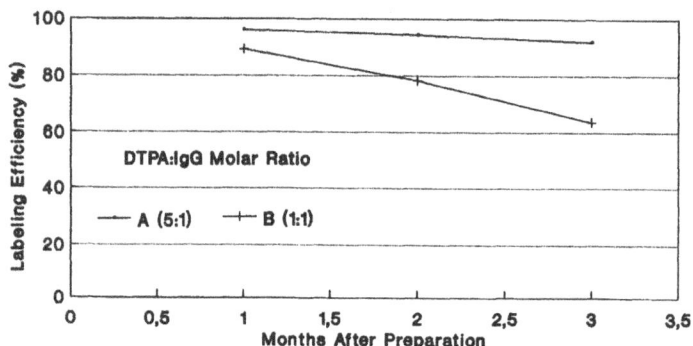

Fig. 5. Labeling efficiency of IgG using 1:1 and 5:1 DTPA:IgG molar ratio preparations after their storage at 4 °C.

CONCLUSION

The two-vial kit form here described is a sure and feasible way of obtaining 111In labeled human IgG to use for diagnostic or experimental purposes.

REFERENCES

1. Rubin RH, Fishman AJ, Callahan RJ, et al. 111In-Labeled nonspecific immunoglobulin scanning in the detection of focal infection. *N Engl J Med*; 321: 935-940 (1989).
2. Sefarini AN, Garty I, Vargas-Cuba R, et al. Clinical evaluation of a scintigraphic method for diagnosing inflammations / Infections using Indium-111-labeled nonspecific human IgG. *J Nucl Med*; 32: 2227-2232 (1991).

3. Oyen WJG, Netten PM, Lemmens AM, et al. Evaluation of infectious diabetic foot complications with Indium-111-labeled human nonspecific Immunoglobulin G. *J Nucl Med*; 33: 1330-1336 (1992).

4. Fishman AJ, Rubin RH, Khaw BA, et al. Radionuclide imaging of experimental atherosclerosis with nonspecific polyclonal Immunoglobulin G. *J Nucl Med*; 30: 1095-1100 (1989).

5. Hnatowich DJ, Childs RL, Lanteigne D and Najafi A. The preparation of DTPA-Coupled antibodies radiolabeled with metallic radionuclides: an improved method. *J Imm Meth*; 65: 147-157 (1983).

6. Paik CH, Hong JJ, Ebbert MA, Heald SC, Reba RC and Eckelman WC. Relative reactivity of DTPA immunoreactive antibody-DTPA conjugates, and nonimmunoreactive antibody-DTPA conjugates toward Indium-111. *J Nucl Med*; 26: 482-487 (1985).

7. Bhargava KK and Acharya SA. Labeling of monoclonal antibodies with radionuclides. *Semm Nucl Med*; 19 (3): 187-201 (1989).

8. Sumerdon GA, Rogers PE, Lombardo CM et al. An optimized antibody-chelator conjugate for imaging of carcinoembryonic antigen with indium-111. *Int J Rad Appl Instrum*; 17 (2): 247-254 (1990).

QUANTITATION OF PLATELET CONSUMPTION IN HEALTH AND DISEASE

M.K. Dewanjee

From the Departments of Radiology, Surgery and Biomedical Engineering
University of Miami, School of Medicine, Miami
Florida, USA

SUMMARY

The cloning of platelet receptors (glycoproteins) by recombinant-DNA technology and blocking the receptor functions by monoclonal antibodies, platelet consumption in health and diseases is being understood at a molecular level. The platelet survival times in healthy volunteers and patients were determined with three markers: 51Cr-disodium chromate in ACD-plasma, 111In-oxine in ACD-saline and 111In-tropolone in ACD-saline and ACD-plasma media. Difference found between 51Cr and 111In labels can be attributed to a variation in localization of the label on the subcellular components and renal handling of the label after release. The mean platelet survival time with 51Cr was slightly longer than 111In and showed a sex difference not seen with 111In-oxine. Protein bound plasma 51Cr was lower than plasma 111In and remained constant throughout the study. Plasma 111In increased with time and correction by subtraction of free 111In from blood radioactivity is necessary. Both In-markers gave similar survival time and biodistribution; elaborate plasma labeling with 111In-tropolone showed no measurable advantage. The contribution of platelets and clotting factors in thrombosis on cardiovascular diseases, prostheses and the effect of platelet-inhibitors, anticoagulants and plasminogen-activators on the dynamics and organization of adherent thrombus, had been evaluated with several radiolabeled tracers. The platelet consumption by the three processes, phagocytosis, thrombosis and fragmentation could be quantitatively evaluated with radiolabeling, platelet kinetics, imaging with a gamma camera, flow-cytometry and autoradiography.

The 111In radioactivity was found in the reticuloendothelial system from the early phase post-intravenous injection to late phase, probably due to retention in fenestrated vessels of RES organs, phagocytosis of intact platelets and the microparticles generated from platelets by resident macrophage. In plasma, the lipid-soluble complexes of In-oxine and In-tropolone were found to be associated with plasma lipoproteins.

Thrombus formation in vivo could be measured semiquantitatively in animal models and patients with 111indium, 99mtechnetium labeled platelets, iodine-123, iodine-131 labeled fibrinogen, and 111In and 99mTc labeled antibody to the fibrinogen-receptor on the platelet-membrane, or fibrin; however, these radiolabeled antibodies could not be used for platelet-kinetics. These radiolabels only indicate the fate of antibodies and partial association with platelets and other cells with cross-reacting adhesion receptors. Platelet labeling with 99mTc HMPAO does not fix the label to organelles and cytosolic proteins as 111In; this partial binding to small molecules results in continuous release of 99mTc at high shear rate of circulation and excreted in urine. Hence this label is not adequate for quantitation of platelet survival time, platelet adhesion and platelet-density calculations.

The platelet labeling with lipid-soluble 111In complex provided a simple, sensitive and reproducible technique for the type, amount and timely administration of the drugs on platelet-pharmacology in transient ischemic attack, atrial/ventricular thrombus, deep vein thrombosis, coronary-bypass graft, balloon-angioplasty, cardiopulmonary bypass procedure, immune thrombocytopenia, development of thromboresistant prostheses (synthetic vascular grafts, artificial heart valves and catheters). Thrombus localization by imaging with 111In labeled platelets had been possible for large thrombus on thrombogenic surface of prostheses or anastomoses of graft to vessels or ulcerating plaques of atherosclerotic artery, deendothelial surface of vein graft or vessels undergoing angioplasty or phlebitis of deep vein in the acute phase. Although labeled platelets help in the identification of the intensity and kinetics of platelet deposition on thrombogenic surface, we observed that fibrin/platelet ratio, platelet-density and size of adherent thrombus are more important for the estimation of tissue ischemia/necrosis in the distal organ bed. The lesser density of packed platelets (10^7-10^9/ml of thrombus) and fibrin/platelet ratio of 1-2 millions undergo rapid thrombolysis as we see in the studies of catheterization and cardiopulmonary bypass surgery. On the other hand, packed platelets (10^{10}-10^{12}/ml) and higher fibrin ratio of 4-6 millions in the organized thrombus in the sewing-ring adherent thrombus in the tissue valves do not undergo fragmentation after embolization and are responsible for the major thromboembolic complications. Hence, for pharmacologic studies in animal models, the estimation of these parameters rather than the intensity of platelet deposition on thrombogenic surface as measured with a computerized gamma camera, will be essential for effective evaluation of platelet-inhibitors, anticoagulants and fibrinolytic drugs. The dynamics of the process and the absolute amount of thrombus formed depend on the size of the annulus, type of prostheses and the velocity of blood flow. In addition, in vitro quantification permits platelet-, fibrin-density, and determination of the number of fibrin-monomer/platelet in the sewing ring or leaflet-adherent thrombus. The role of low-dose aspirin, aspirin-persantine, heparin, warfarin and hirudin on platelet-thrombosis in mechanical and pericardial tissue valves implanted in dogs, calves, baboon and patients had been evaluated. These studies indicate that these drugs induce only partial platelet-inhibition. These tracer techniques thus provided invaluable information about platelet-fibrin deposition, their organization, dissolution of adherent thrombus and development of less thrombogenic surface for use in cardiovascular prostheses. In addition, we observed that platelet-thrombus calcifies; the reduction of platelet-thrombosis indirectly decreases the kinetics of calcification of tissue-valves.

INTRODUCTION

To appreciate the role of platelets in primary hemostasis, it is essential to be familiar with the structure and function of the platelet membrane glycoproteins (GP). Over 30 proteins were characterized by two-dimensional gel electrophoresis of surface labeled (H-3 or I-125) platelets[18, 23]. The list of platelet receptors are shown in table 1. Many glycoproteins are noncovalently associated in the heterodimeric complexes (1:1) of α and β subunits. The functional roles of two important complexes GPIb-IX and GPIIb-IIIa, were derived from the congenital platelet abnormalities (Glanzmann's thrombasthenia and Bernard-Soulier syndrome) and monoclonal antibodies. These surface proteins mediate two important functions of adhesion and aggregation by interacting with other adhesive glycoproteins. Three heterodimer complexes, GPIIb-IIIa, GPIc-IIa, and GPIa-IIa represent prototypes of a superfamily of cell adhesion receptors; they share the structural and antigenic homologies with endothelial cells, fibroblast and lymphocyte. Other members of this superfamily include the very late activation antigens (VLA) of lymphocytes, human fibroblast collagen receptor and fibronectin receptor, human endothelial cell vitronectin receptor and other lymphocyte-associated receptors. The von Willebrand factor (vWf) links GPIb-IX complex on unstimulated platelets with the subendothelial matrix of damaged vessels. The fibrinogen receptor GPIIb-IIIa complex formed via a Ca^{2+} bridge (50,000 copies/platelet) are most abundant and represent 1-2% of the total proteins; about 50% of these complexes are present in the surface-connected canicular systems of platelets and interact with cytoskeletal proteins (actin, tubulin) in stimulated and aggregated platelets. GPIa-GPIIa, GPIc-GPIIa complexes, GPIIIb and GPV function as receptor for collagen, fibronectin, thrombospondin and thrombin respectively. A variety of cytokines transform the membrane of the endothelial cells from thromboresistant to procoagualant surface. The terminus of some cell surface glycoproteins and glycolipids contains a tetrasaccharide unit called sialyl Lewis[x]. Endothelial cells activated by cytokines produce cell- adhesion molecules called selectins (lectin: carbohydrate-binding protein). The adhesion molecule of leukocyte (LAM) interacts with endothelial selectin (E-selectin) via sialyl Lewis[x] of LAM and enhance diapedesis to the site of injury. The other two selectins (lymphocyte L- and platelet P-selectin) also recognize sialylated ligands.

Effect of Shear Rate on Ligand Binding to Platelet Receptors

The flow-chamber experiments with denuded vessel or biomaterials and anticoagulated blood with labeled or non-labeled platelets and nature of platelet spreading, adhesion, thrombus formation as observed by electron microscope or quantitation of platelet deposition revealed that the interaction of ligands (adhesive plasma proteins) and platelet receptors depend on the shear rate[16 - 23, 32 - 34]. At higher shear rate, initial contact with denuded subendothelial matrix is mediated by GPIb-IX complex, which is composed of $GPIb_{\alpha}$, $GPIb_{\beta}$ and GPIX; $GPIb_{\alpha}$, $GPIb_{\beta}$ are disulfide-linked and GPIX are non-covalently linked. These 3 subunits have been cloned from human erythrocyte leukemia (HEL) cell cDNA libraries. Each subunit has been derived from a separate gene and has cytoplasmic domains. Antibodies against vWf inhibited adhesion to subendothelium at high shear rate (> 1000 sec[-1]), but little adhesion at low shear rate of large blood vessels (> 500 sec[-1]) where the role of collagen and fibronectin binding with GPIV (GPIIIb) and GPIc-GPIIa receptors may play predominant role in platelet adhesion and thrombosis. In addition, at high shear rate the platelet adhesion was found to be independent of fibrinogen. These in vitro studies suggested that at low shear rate, fibrinogen promotes platelet adhesion and thrombus formation; on the other hand, at high shear rate, vWf mediates these processes. The conformational change of GPIIb-IIIa complex at high shear rate may promote vWf binding[21, 32 - 34, 63].

The activation process of platelets used in a vague manner, encompasses the saga of numerous different phenomena as described below:

1. platelet shape change,
2. induction of platelet GPIIb-IIIa receptor exposure or other receptors to bind soluble or matrix ligands,
3. elevation of cytosolic calcium ions,
4. induction of arachidonic acid metabolism,
5. activation of protein kinase C by generation of diacylglycerol and inositol triphosphate,
6. release of α-granule or dense granules or lysosomal contents,

7. induction of platelet coagulant activity and finally
8. initiation of platelet adhesion and aggregation.

The nature of activation also depends on the type of agonist, dose and the platelet handling procedures: platelet rich plasma, washed platelets and gel-filtered platelets.

In a normal healthy person, there is a steady state in the platelet production and consumption per day (Tables 5, 6); this steady state is disturbed when hematopoietic activity of bone marrow is depressed by disease, drugs or radiation. The platelet survival value in healthy volunteer indicates the normal value of platelet survival time and turnover rate; in atherosclerotic disease and hemorrhage this balance is disturbed and platelet consumption increases[54, 58, 59]. In addition, patients implanted with cardiovascular prostheses (valves, vascular graft, arterio-venous shunts, stents, ventricular assist devices) or undergoing cardiopulmonary bypass or hemodialysis or catheterization, have a higher level of platelet consumption. The higher level of platelet consumption in these patients is due to thrombus formation, embolization and fragmentation. Platelet consumption by fragmentation are studied by fluorescence-labeled murine monoclonal antibodies (von Willebrand factor, GP Ia or fibrinogen receptor: GP IIb-IIIa) and flow-cytometry.

Platelet consumption in normal healthy persons and patients have been dealt by mathematical methods, where survival times are calculated by linear, exponential and multi-hit models. In patients, accelerarated consumption could also be described by additional exponential factors in the exponential model[44, 48].

MATERIALS AND METHODS

The experiments reported herein were conducted according to the principles set forth in the "Guide for the Care and Use of Laboratory Animals." from the Institute of Laboratory Animal Resources, National Research Council (NIH 85-23, 1985). Human studies were carried out with informed consent from the volunteers and patients. The details of blood collection, platelet labeling with 111In tropolone and static and dynamic measurements of adherent thrombi to oxygenator and arterial filter and emboli in lung, brain, heart and kidneys by imaging with gamma camera, ionization chamber, gamma counter and Geiger probe are described in details before[7, 42, 57, 62, 63].

A. Labeling of Autologous Platelets with 111Indium Tropolone

The platelets were labeled according to the method of Dewanjee et al.[7]. Forty to sixty milliliters of whole blood were collected from patients or animals in 10 ml of modified ACD anticoagulant solution (NIH-A, Fenwal Lab.); the platelets separated by differential centrifugation were incubated with 111In tropolone (600-700 μCi) for 20 minutes and washed by centrifugation. The 111In labeled platelets were measured with an ionization chamber (Capintec CRC-5RH3) and injected via the antecubital vein in patients or ear-vein or jugular vein in animals. The platelet harvesting efficiency of typically (40-45)% and labeling efficiency of (80-95)% were obtained routinely.

B. Dynamic Measurement of Radioactivity of 111In Platelets in the Oxygenator and Arterial Filter During Cardiopulmonary Bypass Procedure

The radioactivity in the sequestering organs and components of extracorporeal circulations, e.g. hemodialyzers, oxygenator and arterial filter during CPB was measured with a lead-collimated Geiger probe detector (Ludlam Inc.). The background radioactivity was subtracted from the total radioactivity of adherent thrombus in oxygenator and trapped embolus in the arterial filter and the net radioactivity was plotted with time of CPB[62].

C. Scintiphoto of Platelet Deposition with the Gamma Camera, Ionization Chamber and Gamma-well Counter

Since the platelet consumption by devices is dynamic and regional, the components of the cardiovascular prostheses, e.g. vascular grafts, valves, arterial filter and hollow-fiber oxygenator were removed from the implanted organs and extracorporeal circuits. The intact device and components were imaged with the gamma camera (Siemens,Gammasonics V). The radioactivity in the components was measured in the ionization chamber (Capintec CRC-5R). The samples of large components and tissue samples were weighed in a microbalance and the radioactivity were determined with a gamma-well counter in the 111In channel. All the detectors were calibrated with standard sources of 111In to convert the microcurie into counts/min and calculate the percent of injected dose of 111In platelets deposited in components of device, organs and tissues.

D. Technical Problems in Platelet Labeling, Sample Collection and Correction of Non-Platelet Bound 111In Radioactivity

The technical information about the platelet harvesting, venipuncture with a 19 G needle, platelet separation and washing with ACD-saline, radiolabeling, IV injection, blood sampling time, 10-12 sampling times for a period of 8-10 days, 2 samples on day 1, first sample two-three hours after injection, second sample 6-10 hours, one sample a day, approximately, every 24 hour interval, sampling volume (5-6 ml, for separating plasma from cell-pellet), subtraction of free 111In in blood and the analyses of radioactive platelet clearance data for the estimation of survival and recovery are presented. Sufficient number of platelets, representative of the circulating platelet population in the host should be harvested [43 ml and 43,000 μlX(80,000-300,000/μl)X(0.30-0.45) platelets] and radiolabeled for an optimal study; the harvesting efficiency is 30-45%. In ITP patients 86 ml of blood is taken for labeling sufficient number of platelets in the survival and sequestration study. The descriptive data on final platelet preparations for 51Cr and 111In oxine and tropolone are shown in Table 2. The cell contaminants in the labeled platelet preparations are much lower than that of granulocytes, monocytes and lymphocytes (Table 3). Without subtraction of free 111In, the survival time will be overestimated (Figure 5).

Factors affecting platelet fragmentation are recognized. We have observed higher level of platelet-vesicles formed by immune complex, membrane attack complex, alcohol, detergent and mechanical manipulation e.g. rapid blood withdrawal and pelleting during platelet harvesting, radiolabeling and resuspending platelet-pellet in ACD-saline or plasma for washing and injection. During hemodialysis, these radiolabeled platelets also demonstrated slightly higher values of vesicle-formation than unlabeled platelets. In large volume sodium iodide crystal detector [NaI(Tl): 3 inch X 3 inch, well-type or bore perpendicular to cylindrical axis], the sum peak at 416 keV accounts for a major fraction of the gamma ray photons. We include the 171, 245 and the sum peak (416 keV) in the wide window of the spectrometer. The platelet deposition in the components of complex cardiovascular prostheses could be determined in a non-destructive way by swabbing the platelet-associated radioactivity with cotton-tip swab and measurement of radioactivity in a gamma counter[65].

Only the latter part of the platelet-radioactivity curve after equilibration time of labeled platelets with circulating platelets, should be used in estimation of half-life of platelets (Tables 6, 7). The mean survival time is the best estimate of platelet survival time. Calculations based on exponential, linear, weighted mean and multiple hit model are sufficient for the analysis of survival time. Other models e.g. Dornhorst, Meuleman, polynomial and alpha order are more sensitive to noise[42-48]. Labeling, IV injection, sample collection and data analysis are equally important for estimation of platelet survival time. Only meticulous methods and data analysis of platelet survival times and platelet deposition on lesions, and prostheses obtained with gamma camera, will contribute to the mechanism of platelet consumption in health, cardiovascular diseases, evaluation of drug treatment protocol in appropriate animal models and selected patients, selection of effective drug and development of cardiovascular prostheses with reduced thromboembolic complications.

E. Random and Cohort Survival Times and Radiolabeling of Platelets

The data for cohort survival time is more convenient to analyze than random survival time. In these studies, S-35 sulfate, S-35 or Se-75 methionine administered intravenously labels megakaryocytes; the former is incorporated in sulfated proteoglycans[1] and the latter amino acid is incorporated in newly synthesized proteins[4]. Unfortunately the megakaryocyte labeling time is long compared to mean platelet survival time and labeled platelets are not released as a bolus or spike. Due to technical difficulties of measurement and difficulty of interpretations of data, these procedures are not used clinically.

Platelet labeling with other labels was not successful due to leaching of labels during circulation and the results are not reproducible (S-35, sulfate, P-32 phosphate and I-131 iodide). Odell et al.[1] studied the survival of S-35 methionine labeled platelets in rats; life span of 4-5 days was observed. McIntyre et al.[4] studied Se-75 labeled platelets in healthy human volunteers. Since this precursor is incorporated in plasma proteins and cellular elements of blood, separation of platelets is essential for estimation of platelet survival time.

During random labeling, a sample population representing true age distribution of functional platelets is labeled with 51Cr, 99mTc, 111In radionuclides[2, 5, 6, 7]. Although random labeling can be carried out by in vitro or in vitro procedure, currently the in vitro labeling with 111In oxine or 111In tropolone is followed. In the in vivo procedure, the time to reach the original pre-aspirin level of the chemical malondialdehyde is measured. In this procedure, synthesis of thromboxane and malondialdehyde is inhibited by aspirin administration. The return to pre-aspirin level reflects time interval for new entry of platelets in circulation and hence platelet survival time. The procedure is not sensitive and needs large number of platelets[3]. In vivo random labeling was also carried by IV injection with C-14 or P-32 labeled diisopropylfluorophosphate (DFP). Since red cells and white cells are also labeled, they must be separated from platelets before measurement of radioactivity. A plateau DFP-level of 10-15% of original blood level suggests that the label is recycled. Due to technical difficulties and high radiation dose these methods are abandoned.

In the past, random labeling was carried out widely with 51Cr disodium chromate[2, 5, 45]. Poor photon abundance (10%), high energy gamma ray (320 keV), and low platelet labeling efficiency (5-8%) and requirement of 400-500 ml of blood, high cost of 51Cr and low accessibility are good reasons for abandoning this radionuclide. Neither 51Cr or 111In is eluted or recycled by other cells; less than (0.2-0.3)% of 111In was found in the urine of healthy volunteers. Only 0.4% of 111In labeled platelets crossed the placental barrier in a female dog and found in the fetus (4 pups). This is not true for the 99mTc HMPAO. About 15-25% of 99mTc from 99mTc HMPAO labeled platelets, is excreted in the urine within a period of 24 hours[63]. This radioactivity in kidneys and urine, obscures the view for thrombus imaging in the pelvis and abdomen. The d,l stereoisomer of 99mTc HMPAO, is incorporated faster than meso stereoisomer; although both transchelates the 99mTc label to cytosolic proteins and other small molecules, e.g. glutathione, at the same level at 60-90 minutes. It is not known whether the 3-D orientation of the isomers retards the permeability or the rate of intracellular transchelation. The loss of 99mTc is also found to be dependent on shear rate; at physiological shear rate, the 99mTc small molecules are lost from labeled platelets.

Currently, a few I-123, 111In and 99mTc labeled antibodies, are being evaluated for thrombus imaging. These tracers radiolabel the glycoprotein receptors, (GPIIb-IIIa, GMP-140) on the platelet membrane. The antibody level is reduced to saturable 5-10% of antigen level in the platelet pool. In spite of pre-incubation, the clearance is much faster than in vitro labeled platelets. This faster clearance may facilitate thrombus imaging. These murine antibodies also provoke human antimouse response (HAMA) preventing repeated use and possible adverse reactions.

Due the above-mentioned difficulties, in vitro labeling of platelets with 111In oxine or tropolone, is the most reliable and widely used method to evaluate platelet survival. The radionuclide has high photon abundance (%) with gamma rays of 171.3(90.5%) and 245(94.0%) keV. Although the conversion [144.6(8.4%), 168(1.3%), 218.6(5.0%), 242.1(1%)] and Auger electrons [18.57-25.44(14%), 3.0-3.7(31%), 2.5-3.5(73%), 0.51(191%)] and x-rays 23.1(68%), 26.2(14.6%) increase dose, the low energy electrons are superb for high resolution autoradiography[11]. The physical half-life of 111In 68 hours is about 68% of the mean platelet survival time. The only radionuclide contaminant (0.08-0.1%) of minor concern is 114mIn with a half-life of 49.7 days[8, 11, 48]. These two tracers provide high labeling efficiency with a high degree of reproducibility. The level of toxicity is low and there is release of 111In label (bound to vesicles, fragments of organelles and platelet proteins) as the circulating platelets are degraded. The exact chemical form is not known; but the radiolabel, is neither recycled nor excreted in urine. The high incorporation in the bone marrow at later times post-injection, indicates that the part of 111In label is incorporated in the transferrin pool; majority of 111In labeled vesicles, organelles and their fragments are phagocytosed in the resident macrophage of liver, spleen and bone marrow[13, 14, 62].

F. Mathematical Models and Calculations of Platelet Survival Times: Analysis of Platelet Radioactivity Time Curve for the Estimation of Mean Platelet Survival Time

A general discussion of the of the problem of platelet survival time was presented by Murphy and Francis[42, 43]. A range of values of platelet survival times from 1-4 days to the accepted value of less than 12 days is available in the literature. The problem arises from the lack of agreement of a mathematical model to describe platelet survival. Fitting of mathematical models to radioactivity time curve requires occasionally a handheld calculator (weighted mean survival time) or a microcomputer (multiple hit). Iterative nonlinear curve fitting techniques require initial estimate of regression constants; these values are calculated from the estimated mean platelet survival time and Y-intercept obtained by the weighted mean method. The iteration is terminated when the relative change in regression constant is less than 0.001. The summary of equations are shown in Table 5.

In all of these platelet survival and biodistribution studies, there is appreciable individual variation in the initial distribution of intravenously administered 111In labeled platelets; the disappearance rates of 111In from the blood are quite similar. The blood-radioactivity curve for the first 5 days was well described by single exponential function. At later times (upto 10 days), no indication of a slower component was observed. By pooling the data and averaging the means weighted by the number of subjects, a composite mean lifetime of platelets in the blood of about 154 hours was derived.

Radioactivities measured by single-view gamma camera imaging, in the liver and spleen typically have early (first hour) values of 8% and 30% of injected activity respectively. During the next 10 days, decay-corrected radioactivity in these organs, rises asymptotically to about 25% in the liver and 40% in the spleen. At 1 hour post-injection, 98% of injected 111In platelets, is accounted for in the blood, liver and spleen. At 200 hours, only 65% was found in these organs; other 35% was diffusely distributed in the bone marrow and remainder of the body. In dosimetry study, 19% was assumed to be present in the bone marrow. The liver and spleen data for each subject were fitted by the following exponential equation:

$$A = \alpha_1 e^{-\lambda_1 \cdot t} + \alpha_2,$$

where A is the radioactivity, α_n is the Y-axis intercept of the nth component, λ_1 is the biological disappearance constant and t is the time post-injection. The averaged results and the residence times, which are calculated from the biological parameters are shown in Table 7. The residence times calculated by ICRP were listed (Table 7) assuming that fractions of 0.3 and 0.1 are immediately deposited in the spleen and liver respectively and the remaining fraction (0.6) is cleared from the blood with a half-life of 4 days. These assumptions yield the following dose estimates as shown in Table 7. These dose estimates assumed that radioactivity distributed uniformly in all organs and connective tissues; autoradiography of bone, marrow, kidneys in animal models definitely indicated that these assumptions are not valid.

G. Algebraic Equations for Normal and Abnormal Platelet Consumption and Platelet-survival Time and Platelet Turn-over Rate: Multiple hit, Linear and Exponential Models for Platelet Survival Study

This model assumes that platelets are removed from the circulation after sustaining a number of hits or insults. If platelets are removed after a single hit, it reperesents a random removal from circulation and plotting of platelet radioactivity with time will result in a exponential curve. Removal of platelets after an infinite number of hits, will theoretically result in a linear clearance of radioactive platelets with time and linear survival time will be more appropriate. The multiple hit model has been recommended by the International Committee of Standardization in Hematology (ICSH) and has been widely used for platelet survival studies in health and diseases[9]. We used the MH model to determine the effect of omitting the sampling values less than 2.5 hours on platelet survival time. It reduced the mean survival time from 10.4 days with all sampling points included to 8.9 days. When all data points are included in the statistical analysis, the number of hits was nine or more for all 8 subjects. When first 2 samples are excluded, 5 of 8 subjects had 5 or fewer hits (Table 6).

The exponential model was very sensitive to the deletion of the first sampling point after injection, whereas the estimate based on a linear regression was not. When the first sampling point was excluded, the average difference in MPST between linear and exponential estimates continued to be large (3.7 days); linear estimate yielded the highest MPST. All 3 groups had a gaussian distribution of calculated MPST values regardless of the model used.

No significant correlation was detected between mean platelet survival times and age, height, weight or body surface area of the subjects studied. The MPST for both In-oxine and tropolone markers was shorter than that obtained with 51Cr marker (Tables 4 and 6). The men had a shorter MPST than women with 51Cr marker but not when 111In oxine was used[45].

For random (non-cohort) or population labeling of platelets, Murphy and Francis developed the general mathematical principles for platelet survival and the multiple hit (MH) model. This model assumes that platelets are removed from the circulation after sustaining a number of insults or hits. If platelets are removed after a single hit, it reflects random removal and exponential radioactivity-time curve will result. On the other hand, platelet-removal after an infinite number of hits wil result in a linear radioactivity-time curve. The MH model thus encompasses both the features of exponential (one hit) and linear (multiple hits >5-50) platelet survival curves. The biochemical implication of "hit" at molecular level is still under investigation in a variety of pathology (radiation-induced cell-death, apoptosis or loss of cellular organization e.g. equilibrium for polymerization of tubulin shifted to depolymerization, due to energy depletion).

The radioactivity (Y_{MH}, proportional to the no. of platelets), in the ordinate of the radioactivity-time curve at any time t, is given by the following equation:

$$Y_{MH} = \frac{c}{n} \sum_{i=0}^{n-1} e^{-at} (at)^i \frac{(n-1)}{i!}$$

The mean platelet-survival time ($MPST_{MH}$) is given by the equation:

$$(MPST)_{MH} = \frac{n}{a}$$

The radioactivity-time curve for the linear platelet-survival (Y_{Lin}) value is described by the following equation:

$$Y_{Lin} = A + Bt$$

The mean platelet-survival time ($MPST_{Lin}$) is given by the equation:

$$(MPST)_{Lin} = -\frac{A}{B}$$

The radioactivity-time curve (Y_{Exp}) for the exponential platelet-survival value is described by the following equation:

$$Y_{Exp} = \alpha e^{\beta t}$$

The mean platelet-survival time ($MPST_{Exp}$) is given by the equation:

$$(MPST)_{Exp} = -\frac{1}{\beta}$$

where A, B, α and ß are parameters to be estimated from the blood-clearance data; e denotes the base of natural logarithms, 2.7183.

H. Weighted Mean Method (Empirical Model)

The linear and logarithmic functions can be fitted to radioactivity time curve by the standard linear least square method. The weighted mean survival time (T_w), as proposed by ICSH is given by the following equation:

$$T_w = (S_e * T_1 + S_1 * T_e) / (S_e + S_1)$$

where T_1 is the linear survival time, T_e is the exponential survival time, S_1 is the linear variance and S_e is the exponential variance. When the survival curve is linear, $S_e > S_1$ and $T_w = T_1$. For predominantly exponential curve, $T_w = T_e$.

A weighted mean regression curve at any time t, is formulated from the following equation:

$$M_w (t) = (S_e * M_1 (t) + S_1 * M_e (t)) / (S_e + S_1)$$

where $M_1(t)$ and $M_e(t)$ represent the calculated linear and exponential regression curve mean values at time t, respectively. The "goodness of fit" of the radioactivity time curve could be calculated from the generated weighted mean regression curve.

I. Abnormal Platelet Consumption and Platelet-survival Time and Platelet Turn-over Rate

The normal values of platelet survival time in animal models and patients and shortened values in a variety of thromboembolic disorders are described by multiple hit model, linear or exponenetial equations.

The normal consumption of single platelet will be accelerated by consumptive process of platelet adhesion, aggregation and platelet-fragmentation during CPB. The disappearance of single platelets and platelet-aggregates is described by the following equations:

$$D_{Sp} = N_{Sp}\lambda_{Sp}$$
$$\frac{dN_{Pa}}{dt} = \lambda_{Sp}N_{Sp} - \lambda_{Pa}N_{Pa}$$

$$(D_{Pa})_t = \lambda_{Pa}N_{Pa}$$
$$= \frac{\lambda_{Pa}(D_{Pa})_o(e^{-\lambda_{Sp}t} - e^{-\lambda_{Pa}t})}{(\lambda_{Pa} - \lambda_{Sp})}$$

J. Platelet Survival Time in ITP Patients

In idiopathic thrombocytopenic purpura (ITP), the radioactive platelet clearance curve is very rapid and biexponential[30, 44]. This may result from pooling of platelets in the spleen and rapid destruction of antibody-coated platelets; the latter process may decrease the level of platelet-bound radioactivity from 95% to 80-70% within a short time after injection. These platelet-bound radioactivity also decreases from 95% to 80%, in the latter part of blood collection in the healthy human volunteer for both 111In oxine and 111In tropolone (Figure 5). Subtraction of free 111In is essential for calculation of accurate platelet survival time[45]. Flow-cytometry with fluorescent conjugated monoclonal antibodies is becoming an essential tool for the estimation of the microparticles generated by autoimmune diseases[35, 36].

Hemorrhage occurs in the gastrointestinal, urinary tract and cranium in neonatal alloimmune thrombocytopenia (NATP) induced by placental transfer of alloantibodies from mother to fetus following sensitization to fetal platelet antigens during pregnancy. The hemorrhage (blood) in urine and feces could be easily detected than RES systems. Since these fenestrated organs, accumulate (spleen 35%, liver 20%, bone marrow 15%) about 70% of total platelets and the platelet residence times in these organs (spleen 33 h, liver 15 h and red marrow 8 h) are considerably higher than other organs, at low platelet concentration, platelets are used in these fenestrated vessels to prevent hemorrhage and protein-leakage in these organs. At low platelet concentartion (50,000/μl), there should be hemorrhage in these organs, although difficult to detect. When we sacrificed animals with saturated potassium chloride and exsanguination, we observed lower values of organ radioactivity (spleen, liver); but this radioactivity only decreased by 30-40%, again suggesting a fraction of platelets are retained by the fenestrated organs for maintaining integrity of fenestrated vessels. Biopsy of these organs also could increase hemorrhagic risks. Autoradiography with large amount of 111In labeled autologous platelets in a smaller animal will provide the answer about the location of these platelets in fenestrated organs. The methodological advances indicated that platelet destruction can be induced by alloantibodies [10 platelet membrane antigens: Pl^{A1}, Pl^{A2}, Ko^a, Ko^b, Pl^{E1}, Pl^{E2}, Bak^a, Bak^b, $Pen^a(Yuk^b)$, $Pen^a(Yuk^b)$], drug-dependent alloantibodies, autoantibodies and immune complexes. Complement-dependent 51Cr or 111In release assays are used for the detection of relevant antibodies[30, 31, 63]. Only 0.2-0.4% of total 111In labeled platelets was found in the fetus at 24 hours after injection in a female dog during CPB; this accumulation may represent accumulation of platelet-microparticles formed by high shear rate[60, 61].

K. Complement System and Membrane Attack Complex in Platelet Fragmentation

The contact-activation system in blood and hemolymph evolved to serve two primary functions of hemostatic and fibrinolytic functions to maintain vascular integrity, i.e. to plug injured vessel wall while maintaining patency to flow and an immune recognition and clearance function required to resist colonization by microorganisms[31]. The abnormal platelet function observed in patients with immune complex disease and patients with chronic ITP, suggests in vivo activation of platelets and leukocytes by immune complex systems and components of the complement systems. The complement system includes more than 20 plasma proteins that interact through two interlinked enzymatic pathways (classical and alternative) to initiate the controlled production of activated molecular species with distinct immunoregulatory, opsonic and inflammatory activities. The complement system interacts with a variety of the receptor proteins present on the plasma membrane of several types; these complement receptors serve in adhesion and regulatory functions to mediate the stimulus-response transduction to initiate the cell activation. The deposition of the membrane attack complex (MAC) leads to rupture of the plasma membrane and collapse of the electrochemical gradients. The actual pore exclusion size of the membrane lesions by the C5b-9 complex proteins depends on the density and stoichiometry of the bound C5b-9 proteins, as well as the species homology of the target membrane. The interplay between hemostatic and inflammatory mechanisms is mediated through complement-platelet interactions[31].

L. Platelet Consumption by Phagocytosis of Intact Radiolabeled Platelets and Fragments

From the previous platelet kinetic studies, in healthy volunteers, and in patients (ITP, CPB), and patients with cardiovascular prostheses (mechanical valves, thrombotic thromcytopenic purpura: TTP), we could conclude that platelets are consumed by three principal mechanisms (phagocytosis, thrombosis and fragmentation of platelets into microparticles or vesicles):

I. Platelet consumption in healthy volunteer by phagocytosis and fragmentation post-sealing of fenestrated vessels in RES organs. The platelet microparticle formation by i) calpain (Ca^{2+}-protease) induced destruction of platelet skeleton (actin, myosin, tubulin etc.), ii) change of membrane fluidity or iii) loss of ATP during exocytosis and less energy generated by platelet mitochondria resulting in the presumed depolymerization of structural proteins, is under intense investigation[35, 38, 63]. In general, all cells in the host, dye (necrosis) by nutritional deficiency, toxic cytokines, free radicals or they undergo programmed cell death (apoptosis) induced by exposure of specific phospholipid[37], antigen exposure by shear and antibody binding[36] and dissolution of microtubule or other cytoskeletons[35]. Although the platelets are consumed at the site of vessel injury, some of these platelets come back in circulation in the case of unorganized thrombi or reversible injury during radiolabeling or storage. Shear- and IgG-induced fragmentation may fall under apoptosis.

II. Thrombosis/embolization and wedging in smaller vessels, fragmentation of emboli followed by phagocytosis of radioactive platelet fragments in patients. The patients in these groups may have focal or diffuse vascular diseases or cardiovascular prostheses and

III. Phagocytosis of opsonized (antibody and/or complement-mediated) platelets, in ITP and other autoimmune diseases.

The platelets in healthy volunteer are used to seal fenestrated vessels and stored for future consumption in RES organs. At the end of their lifespan, these platelets undergo fragmentation and these intact platelets or fragments are consumed or sequestered by resident macrophage post fragmentation. Platelets are formed from megakaryocytes by fragmentation; it will not be surprising to suggest that they may disappear (sequestered by resident macrophage) post fragmentation in RES organs. In ITP and other types of autoimmune diseases, opsonized intact platelets may be phagocytized, even in these patients, we observe higher rate of formation of platelet vesicles and higher level of circulating vesicles (5-10 fold) in blood. In a healthy individual, the vesicle concentration is low (4-5)%; on the other hand these number increases during shear-induced platelet activation during hemodialysis (10-15)% and cardiopulmonary bypass (15-30)%. Ultimately all the above-mentioned processes lead to platelet fragmentation and phagocytosis. The longer residence times of 111In radioactivity in RES organs may result from continuous phagocytosis of radioactive fragments by new generation of resident macrophage (Table 7). These vesicles are quantified by fluorescent-conjugated murine antibodies made against vWf receptor or fibrinogen receptor on platelet membrane and flow-cytometry. The radioactive vesicles (0.5 μm) could be separated by pelleting of red cells and intact platelets at 2500 g and further centrifugation of supernatant at 90,000-100,000 g value. Addition of thrombin to platelets without Ca^{2+}-chelating agents, eg. EDTA, results in higher number of microparticle formation. Sufficient ATP may be necessary to mainatin the cytoskeletal proteins in polymerized forms. It has been suggested that at the end of lifespan, certain antigens on platelets are exposed; IgG-like proteins bound to these antigens result in sequestration of these aged platelets by RES organs.

Platelet kinetics provide a suitable technique for studying platelet turnover[42 - 48], thrombus dynamics (Figure 3) on highly thrombogenic prostheses, regional platelet deposition (Figures 4A and 4B) on thrombogenic surfaces, platelet lysis and platelet retention and sequestration by internal organs and platelet dosimetry[41]; however, the large variation in platelet survival time representing global platelet consumption (10-12%/day) and small change observed by cardiovascular prostheses and platelet-inhibitors are the limitations of this method. Imaging platelet deposition at the site of thrombus formation with gamma camera do provide semi-quantitative information. Quantitative data could only be obtained by measurement of platelet density on components of harvested prostheses from suitable animal models (dog, pig, baboon). Considering the large variation of platelet reactivity and fibrinolytic activity in different species of animals, further consideration should be given for extrapolating these results to human patients[57].

M. Theory of Embolization and Calculation of Rate Constant of Embolization from Oxygenator During Cardiopulmonary Bypass Perocedure

The disappearance rate constant of single platelet, λ_{Sp}, is described by the following equation:

$dN_{Sp}/dt = D_{Sp} = - \lambda_{Sp}*N_{Sp}$; T½ (Single platelet for human and pig: 4-5 and 3 days); disappearance rate (D_{Sp}) is proportional to the number of single platelet (N) and λ is the rate constant.

The disappearance rate constant of platelet-aggregates, λ_{Pa}, is described by the following equation:

$$dN_{Pa}/dt = - \lambda_{Pa}*N_{Pa}$$

The net disappearance rate, λ_{Pa}, is the summation of the three embolization rates of three average size of large, medium and small emboli:

$$\lambda_{Pa} = \lambda_{Pa(S)} + \lambda_{Pa(M)} + \lambda_{Pa(L)}$$

N. Analysis of Radioactivity-time Curve by Curve-stripping Technique for Estimation of Half-life and Determination of Rate Constants of Embolization

The assumptions we have made for modeling the process of platelet-thrombosis and embolization from a device are:

(1) Single platelet disappears from blood at a fixed rate with a fixed half-life and the disappearance rate (D_{Sp}) is proportional to the number of platelets.
(2) The disappearance rate of platelet-aggregate of a group in a specific size range (D_{Pa}) from a device is also proportional to the number of platelet-aggregates in the specific size range and
(3) The net disappearance rate constant for platelet-aggregates of three size range (small, medium and large) from a device is a additive process.

The normalized radioactivity-time curve [counts per min/injected 111In radioactivity (μCi)] of embolization, (the latter part of radioactivity-time curve after the peak value), can be represented by the sum of three exponential terms for 3 size of emboli and a constant A representing the level of single platelets in circulation. The net activity A(t) at time t is described by

$$A(t) = A + A_S*e^{-t*\lambda(S)} + A_M*e^{-t*\lambda(M)} + A_L*e^{-t*\lambda(L)}$$

where A_S, A_M and A_L are intercepts on the Y-axis, indicating the abundance of emboli of three average size (large:L, medium:M and small:S), A is the level of circulating single

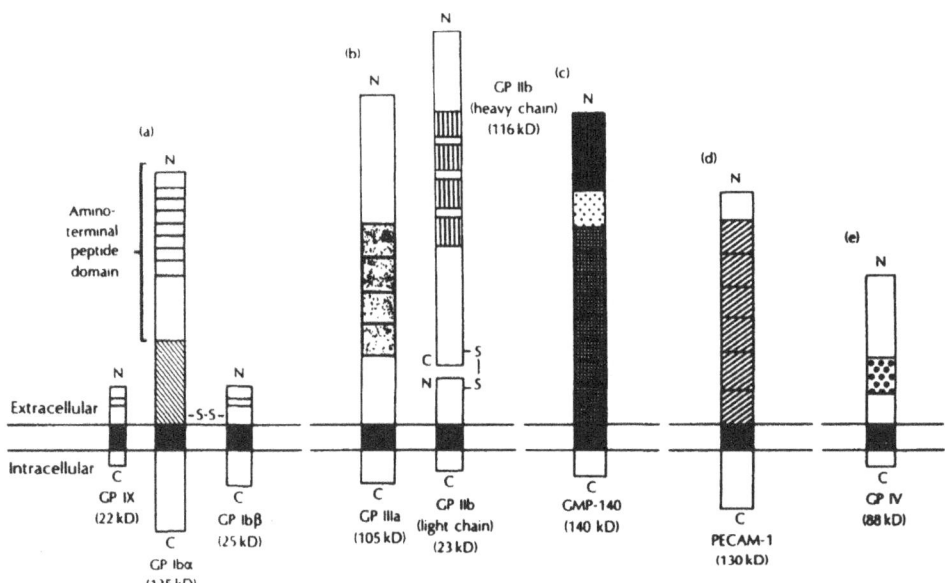

Figure 1. Platelet adhesion receptors: **(a)** glycoprotein (GP), GPIb-GPIX complex; ▦, leucine-rich domain, ▨ , macroglycopeptide. **(b)** GPIIb-GPIIIa (αIIbβ3), the major integrin receptor on platelets; ▦, cysteine-rich domain; ▥ , Ca²⁺-binding domain. Other integrins on platelets are the collagen receptor, GPIa-GPIIa (α2β1); fibronectin receptor, GPIc-GPIIa (α5β1); laminin receptor (α6β1); vitronectin receptor (α5β3). **(c)** Selectin family, Granule membrane protein GMP-140; ▧, lectin-like domain; ▨, epidermal growth factor (EGF)-like domain, ■, complement regulatory binding protein (CRB)-like domain. **(d)** PECAM-1, a member of the immunoglobin (Ig) superfamily; ▨, Ig-like domain. **(e)** GPIV; ▨, Cysteine-containing region. C, carboxy terminus, N, amino terminus; ■, transmembrane domain of the receptors (Courtesy of RK Andrews and JEB Fox).

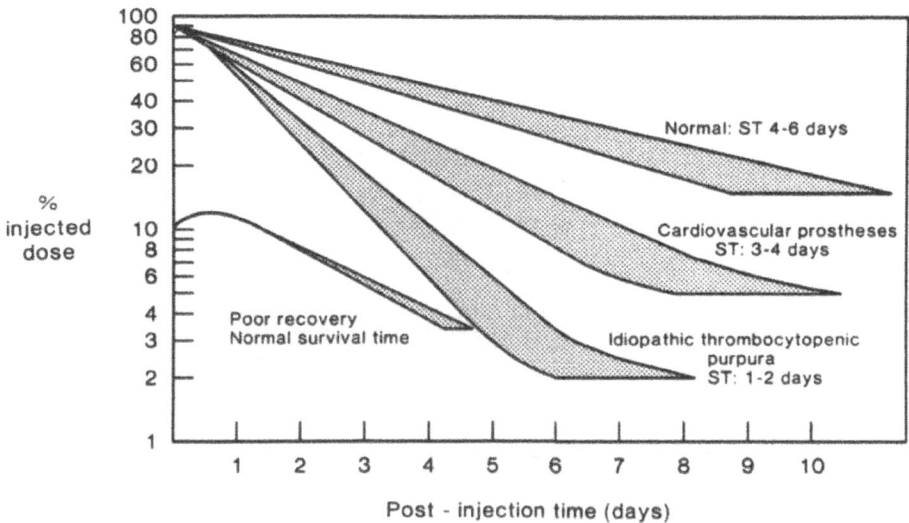

Figure 2 Platelet survival times (exponential value) in healthy volunteer and patients implanted with cardiovascular prostheses (mechanical valves) and idiopathic thrombocytopenic purpura. If platelets are poorly handled, during platelet-labeling procedures, platelet-recovery is drastically reduced.

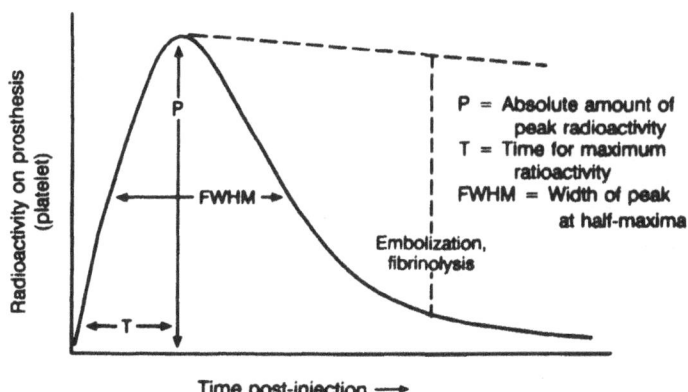

Figure 3. Thrombus formation and embolization on CV prosthesis. Thrombus dynamics on cardiovascular prostheses as measured with 111In labeled platelets. The amount of platelets involved, that could be measured with a gamma camera in a live animal or patients, varied from 0.1-10% of injected platelets.

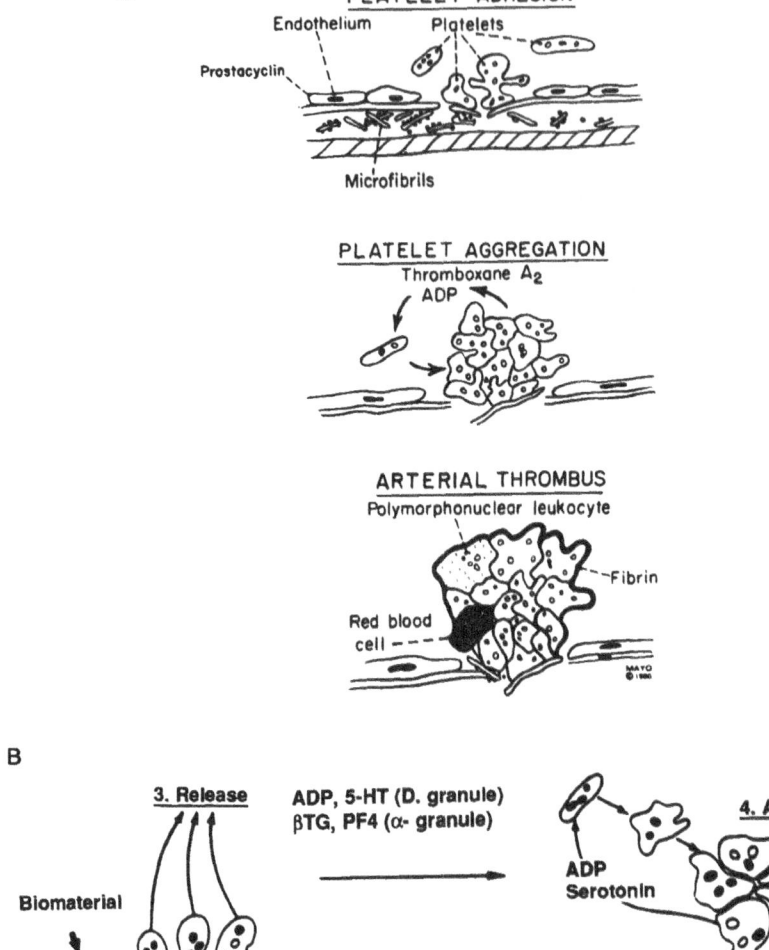

A

PLATELET ADHESION

Endothelium   Platelets

Prostacyclin

Microfibrils

PLATELET AGGREGATION
Thromboxane A$_2$
ADP

ARTERIAL THROMBUS
Polymorphonuclear leukocyte

Fibrin

Red blood
cell

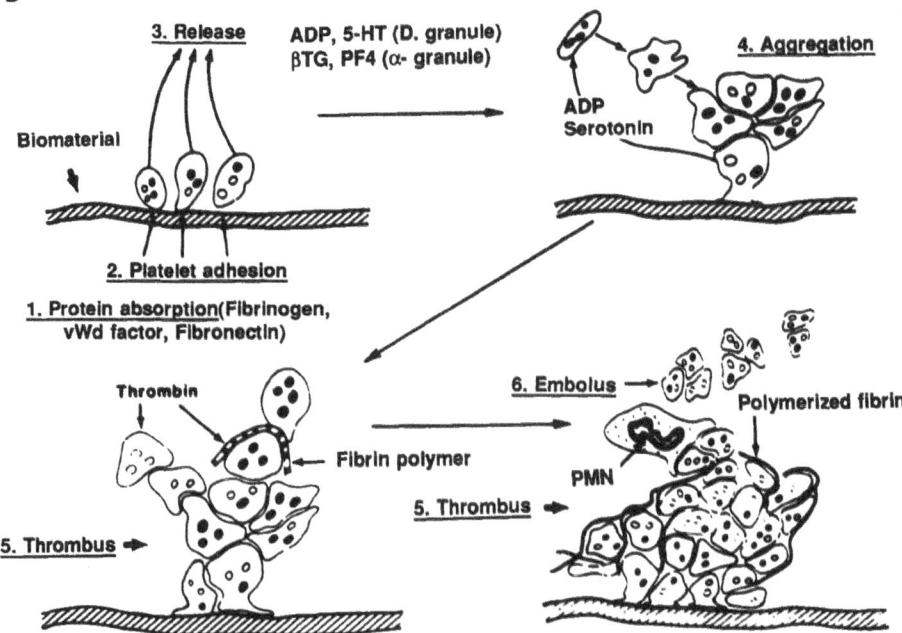

B

3. Release   ADP, 5-HT (D. granule)
βTG, PF4 (α- granule)   4. Aggregation

Biomaterial   ADP
                                         Serotonin

2. Platelet adhesion

1. Protein absorption(Fibrinogen,
vWd factor, Fibronectin)

Thrombin   6. Embolus
                                                    Polymerized fibrin
                    Fibrin polymer
                                         PMN
                                         5. Thrombus
5. Thrombus

Figure 4. Platelet consumption in deendothelialized vessel and surfaces of cardiovascular prostheses; although the initial phases of activation and adhesion in these two processes are different, the final phases of thrombus buildup and embolization is similar with the exception that consumption occurs at a much higher level in most prostheses (5-10 times) and higher level of drugs are necessary to inhibit thrombosis.

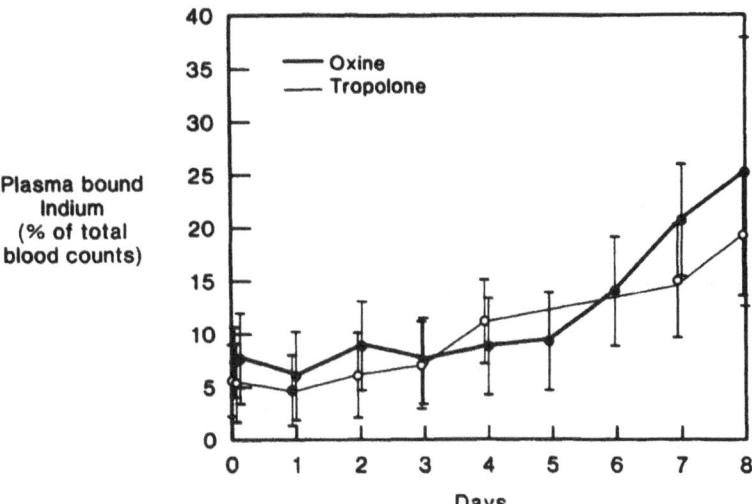

Figure 5. The amount of free 111In in both 111In oxine and tropolone labeled platelets in healthy volunteers.

Table 1. Classification of platelet adhesion receptors and their role in the adhesion with endothelial cells, platelets, other cellular elements of blood resulting in activation and thrombosis

---

A. Leucine-rich family contact activation
    at high shear > 500 sec^{-1}
  GP Ib-IX (GPIb$_a$/GPIb$_b$::1:1), (170+20): vWf, P
    Human erythroleukemia cDNA clone

B. Integrin family (adhesion receptor family: α,β subunit)

  VLA-1(α1β1), (200): very late activation antigen, L
  GPIa-IIa(α2β1), (155+130): collagen, laminin, P, E, N, M, L
  VLA-3(α3β1), (135+25): fbg, collagen, laminin, E, M, L
  VLA-4(α4β1), (150): fibronectin, M, L
  GPIc-IIa(α5β1), (150+130): fibronectin, P, E, M, L
  VLA-6(α6β1): very late act. antigen, fn, laminin, P, E, M, L
  LFA-1(αLβ2), (180): lymphocyte func.-assoc. antigen, N, M, L
  Mac-1(αMβ2), (170): leukocyte adhesion receptor, N, M
  p150/90(αXβ2), (150): leukocyte adhesion receptor, N, M
  GPIIb-IIIa(αIIbβ3), (125+25, 115): fbg, vWf, fn,
    vn, thrombospondin, cDNA transfected COS cells, P
  VNR(αvβ3), (125+25, 115): vitronection, P, E, N, M. L
    (αvβ5), E

    GP IV(GPIIIb), (95): collagen, thrombospondin, P, E, M
    GP VI, collagen, P

C. Selectin family (sugar-binding protein:lectin)

  GMP-140, (146): α-granule membrane protein, P, E
  ELAM-1, end. cell.-plt.-neut.-adhesion molecule, E
  LAM-1, lymphocyte adhesion molecule (homing), N, M, L

D. Immunoglobulin-like family, E

  VCAM-1, vascular cell adhesion molecule, P, E, N, M
  PECAM-1, platelet-endothelial cell adhesion molecule, E
  ICAM-1, E
  ICAM-2, E

E. Adhesive ligands (multi-subunit)

  i) Soluble ligands
  Fibrinogen: fbg
  Fibronectin: fn
  von Willebrand factor: vWf
  Vitronectin: vn

  ii) Matrix ligands: Collagen, laminin
  Common cell-binding domain (Arg-Gly-Asp-Ser:RGDS)

Endothelial cells (E), Monocytes (M), Platelets (P), Neutrophils (N), Lymphocytes (L) share some cell-associated receptor ligands. The molecular weight of the association complex and their subunits within parenthesis is in kilodaltons.

Table 2. Descriptive data* on Final Platelet Preparation for three Platelet Markers

Factor	51Cr-Chromate (n = 28)	111In-oxine (N = 28)	111In-tropolone (N = 28)
Volume (ml)	20.00 ± 2.10	5.00 ± 0.71	4.03 ± 1.28
Total cells injected x 10^9	47.60 ± 17.10	2.12 ± 2.65	2.80 ± 1.82
Labeling efficiency	7.80 ± 2.53	72.80 ± 7.10	76.41 ± 11.80
Plasma label (%)+	4 ± 2	-----	3.15 ± 1.12
Injected activity (μCi)	33.3 ± 14.2	178.8 ± 114.4	194.4 ± 14.4

*Shown as mean ± 1 SD.
+ Calculated at 10 minutes after injection.

Table 3. Blood Cell Contaminants in the Platelet Preparations for the three Difeerent Platelet Markers*

Cell type	51Cr-Chromate (n = 28)	111In-oxine (N = 28)	111In-tropolone (N = 28)
Plateletsl)	99.42 ± 2.33	96.30 ± 2.02	98.11 ± 1.80
Erythrocytes	0.54 ± 0.43	3.50 ± 3.80	1.81 ± 1.71
Leukocytes	0.03 ± 0.02	0.07 ± 0.15	0.07 ± 0.12

*Shown as percent of total cells (mean ± 1 SD).

Table 4. Mean Platelet Survival Times* After Injection of Platelets With Three Different Markers

Mathematical model	Group	Platelet survival time (days)	
		All sampling time included	< 21/2 hours excluded
[51Cr]Disodium chromate (N=28)			
Linear	Total	10.0 ± 0.9	10.1 ± 0.9
Exponential	Total	6.9 ± 1.0	6.8 ± 0.9
Multiple hit	Men	8.8 ± 1.6	9.1 ± 1.1
	Women	9.7 ± 1.6	9.8 ± 1.6
111In-oxine (N=28)			
Linear	Total	9.0 ± 0.6	8.8 ± 0.6
Exponential	Total	5.8 ± 0.6	5.1 ± 0.6
Multiple hit	Men	8.2 ± 0.8	7.7 ± 0.9
	Women	8.6 ± 0.8	8.1 ± 1.2
111In-tropolone (N=8)			
Linear	Men	10.6 ± 0.8	10.2 ± 0.7
Exponential	Men	6.8 ± 0.9	5.4 ± 0.7
Multiple hit	Men	10.4 ± 1.0	8.9 ± 1.4

*Data shown as mean ± 1 SD

Table 5. Mathematical Models Used for Calculation of Platelet Survival Times*

Model	Formula	Estimate of mean platelet survival
Linear	$Y = A + BX$	$-A/B$
Exponential	$Y = \alpha e^{\beta X}$	$-1/\beta$
Multiple hit	$Y = \dfrac{a^n}{(n-1)!} X^{n-1} e^{-aX}$	n/a

*A, B, α, β, and a = variables to be estimated from the data; e = base (2.718); n = integer number of hits (specified in advance); Y = percentage of injected dose remaining at time X.

Table 6. Comparison of Platelet Survival Times With Use of 111In-Oxine and 111In-Tropolone as Platelet Markers in Eight Male Volunteers and Results of Analyses by Multiple-Hit Mathematical Model

	111In-oxine (n=8)		111In-tropolone (N=8)	
	Sampling times included		Sampling times included	
	All	>2 hours	All	>2 hours
Platelet survival time (days)				
Mean ± SD	9.5 ± 1.3	8.9 ± 2.4	10.4 ± 1.0	8.9 ± 1.4
Range	7.1 - 11.6	5.7 - 13.5	9.1 - 12.3	7.5 ± 10.3
Median	8.9	8.1	10.2	9.0
N°. of hits*				
1	0	0	0	0
2-10	2	4	1	5
11-49	3	2	3	3
50	3	2	4	0

* Shown as number of patients with this number of hits.

platelet and lambda-values ($\lambda(S)$, $\lambda(M)$ and $\lambda(L)$) are the corresponding rate constants of embolization. This stripping technique was applied to the embolization curve generated from oxygenator-radioactivity during CPB[62].

The dynamic process of thrombosis and embolization on oxygenator during 3 hour CPB in a pig model provided enough emboli for using exponential equations for calculation of rate constant of embolization[62]. This dynamic embolization from oxygenator could only be observed by continuous monitoring. These significant findings suggest that at 30-40 minutes post-CPB, the arterial filter sheds emboli at the same rate of trapping, supporting preliminary data of increased screen-filter pressure[62] at similar time frame. The half-life of thrombus relates to the time of build-up and adhesivity via the platelet-receptors and fibrinogen and the adsorbed adhesive proteins on the surface of polypropylene and polyester net-work; the final retention-time may be dependent on the extra-platelet organization, fibrinolytic activity and platelet-cytoskeleton.

The principles of computational fluid mechanics helped us in identifying the transport of cellular elements of blood, differential distribution i.e. near-wall excess of platelets and areas of disturbed flow in cardiovascular systems (bifurcation, stenosis or aneurysm) or prostheses[49, 50]. But it failed to account for the interaction of activated clotting factors adsorbed on damaged vessel wall or cardiovascular prostheses and cellular elements of blood resulting in thrombus formation and embolization[54 - 63]. The interpretation of the kinetics of platelet aggregation and embolization remains tentative in the absence of rational formulations of these two aspects of dynamic pathology. We describe a kinetic scheme to derive rate equations for platelet-emboli; the process of aggregation was originally described by Jamaluddin and Krishnan[51]. The dynamic nature of thrombosis and embolization on cardiovascular prostheses was investigated with 111In labeled platelets by several investigators[52 - 62]. The normal values of platelet survival time and platelet turn-over rate were studied by several investigator[42 - 48].

Assuming the random probability of thrombosis and their embolization from oxygenator and arterial filter, we developed a mathematical model and defined equations to calculate the half-life and rate constant of embolization (RCE) from oxygenator and arterial filter with 111In labeled platelets, during CPB in pig model[62]. For regional platelet consumption, platelet density is an independent parameter; emboli trapping in brain or other organ could be estimated by absolute uptake and regional quantitative autoradiography for estimation of size and distribution in subsets of neuronal cells; regional amount of emboli and their residence time[64] are essential parameters for interventional studies. Radiolabeled platelets provide essential information about platelet consumption, thrombi and emboli that could not be obtained by any other technique.

ACKNOWLEDGEMENTS

The supports of NHLBI (HL47201, Shannon Award), Baxter Healthcare Corporation, Department of Energy grant DE-FG05-88ER60728 and Florida High Technology and Industry Council are gratefully acknowledged. The expertise of James S. Robertson, M.D.,Ph.D. and the members of the MIRD committee, in the platelet modeling calculations was highly appreciated. The author appreciates the assistance of Messers. Zulfiker Jessa in painless blood withdrawal from myself, other healthy voulnteers and Robert R. Burke and Kennneth R. Kitchens in making the photographs. The detection of the microparticles formed by variable shear rate on platelets, was carried out with the Coulter flow-cytometer (EPIC V) in Dr. Y. Ahn's laboratory. This review article is dedicated in memory of Dr. William J. Harrington.

Table 7. The radiation absorbed dose (rad/mCi), (mGy/MBq), residence times (τ) and [constants α_1, α_2 and λ_1 (h^{-1})] of 111In labeled platelets administered to healthy human volunteer to blood, viscera and connective tissue.

	Dose(rad/mCi)	Dose(mGy/MBq)	Res. time τ(h)[α_1, α_2, λ_1]
Blood	0.52	0.14	35.0[0.60, 0.0, 0.0069]
Vena cava wall	0.54	0.15	--
Aorta wall	0.46	0.12	--
Kidneys	1.4	0.38	--
Red Marrrow	1.1	0.29	8.1[-0.18, 0.19, 0.0069]
Liver	2.1	0.56	14.5[-0.17, 0.25, 0.0069]
Spleen	30.0	8.0	33.4[-0.10, 0.40, 0.0069]
Ovaries	0.46	0.12	--
Testes	0.25	0.067	--
Remainder of body	0.58	0.16	6.9[-0.15, 0.16, 0.0069]

$$\tau = \alpha_1 / (\lambda_1 + \lambda) + \alpha_2 / \lambda$$

(MIRD-Dose Estimate:15, ref. 35)

REFERENCES

1. Odell TT, Tausche FG, Furth J. Platelet life span as measured by transfusion of isotopically labeled platelets into rats. *Acta Haematol* 13: 45 (1955).
2. Morgan MC, Keating RP, Reinser EH. Survival of radiochromium labeled platelets in rabbits. *J Lab Clin Med* 46: 521 (1955).
3. Leeksma CHW, Cohen JA. Determination of life of human blood platelets using labeled di-isopropylfluorophosphonate. *Nature* 175: 552 (1955).
4. McIntyre PA, Evatt B, Hodkinson BA. Selenium-75, selenomethione as label for erythrocytes, leukocytes and platelets in man. *J Lab Clin Med* 75: 472 (1970).
5. Uchida T, Tasunuga K, Karione S, Waksiaka G. Survival and sequestration of Cr-51 and Tc-99m labeled platelets. *J Nucl Med* 15, 801 (1974).
6. McAfee JG, Thakur ML. Survey of radioactive agents for in vitro labeling of phagocytic leukocytes. I. Soluble agents. *J Nucl Med* 17: 480 (1976).
7. Dewanjee MK, Rao SA, Didisheim P: Indium-111 tropolone, a new high affinity platelet label: Preparation and evaluation of labeling parameters. *J Nucl Med* 22:981-987 (1981).
8. Weber DA, Eckerman KF, Dillman LT, Ryman JC. MIRD radionuclide data and decay schemes. Society of Nuclear Medicine, New York, 1989, pp 196-197 (In-111), pp 178-179 (Tc-99m).
9. International Committee for standardization in hematology panel on diagnostic applications of radionuclides (ICSH). *J Nucl Med* 29:564-566 (1988).
10. ICRP. Radiation dose to patients from radiopharmaceuticals. ICRP publication 53. New York, Pergamon Press, 1988.
11. Jonsson B-A, Strand S-E, Larsson BS. A quantitative autoradiographic study of the heterogenous activity distribution of different 111In-labeled radiopharmaceuticals in rat tissues. *J Nucl Med* 33: 1825-1835 (1992).
12. Rand ML, Packham MA, Mustard JF. Survival of density subpopulation of rabbit platelets: use of Cr-51 and In-111 labeled platelets to measure survival of least dense and most dense platelets concurrently. *Blood* 61: 362, (1983).
13. Steiner M, Baldini MG. Subcellular distribution of Cr-51 and characterization of its binding sites in human platelets. *Blood* 35: 727 (1970).
14. Hudson EM, Ramsey RB, Evatt BL. Subcellular localization of indium-111 in indium-labeled platelets. *J Lab Clin Med* 97:577 (1981).
15. Dewanjee MK. Indium-111 trolpolone versus oxine. *J Nucl Med* 23: 455-456 (1982).
16. Hynes RO. Integrins: A family of cell surface receptors. *Cell* 48:549 (1987).
17. Peerschke EIB. The platelet fibrinogen receptor. *Semin Hematol* 22:241 (1985).

18. Andrews RK, Fox JEB. Platelet receptors in hemostasis. *Current Opinion in Cell Biology*. 2: 894-901 (1990).
19. Bornstein P. Thrombospondins: structure and regulation of expression. FASEB J 6: 3290-3299 (1992).
20. Pober JS, Cotran R. Cytokines and endothelial cell biology. *Physiol Rev* 70: 427 (1990).
21. Kouns WC, Kirschhofer D, Hadvary P, Endenhofer A, Baumgartner HR, Steiner B. Reversible conformational changes induced in glycoprotein IIb-IIIa by a potent and selective peptidomimetic inhibitor. *Blood* 80: 2539-2547 (1992).
22. Winiarski J, Holm G. Platelet associated immunoglobins and complement in idiopathic thrombocytopenic purpura. *Clin Exp Immunol* 53:201 (1986).
23. Fitzgerald LA, Phillips DR. Structure and function of platelet membrane glycoproteins. Chap 2, In Platelet Immunobiology, Molecular and Clinical Aspects. Eds, Kunicki TJ, George JN. JB Lippincott Co., Philadelphia, 1989, pp 9-30.
24. Coller BS, Beer JH, Scudder LE, Steinberg MH. Collagen-platelet interactions: Evidence for a direct interaction of collagen with platelet GPIa/IIA and an indirect interaction with platelet IIb/IIa mediated by adhesion proteins. *Blood* 74:182-192 (1989).
25. Staatz WD, Rajpara SM, Wayner EA, Carter WG, Santoro SA. The membrane glycoprotein Ia-IIa (VLA-2) complex mediates the Mg^{++}-dependent adhesion of platelets to collagen. *J Cell Biol* 108: 1917-1924 (1989).
26. Parise LV, Criss AB, Nannizzi L, Wardell MR. Glycoprotein IIIa is phosphorylated in intact human platelets. *Blood* 75: 2363-2368 (1990).
27. Frelinger AL III, Cohen I, Plow EF, Smith MA, Roberts J, Lam SC-T, Ginsberg MH. Selective inhibition of integrin function by antibodies specific for ligand-occupied receptor conformers. *J Biol Chem* 265: 6346-6352 (1990).
28. Johnston GI, Cook RG, McEver RP. Cloning of GMP-140, a granule membrane protein of platelets and endothelium: sequence similarity to proteins involved in cell adhesion and inflammation. *Cell 56*: 1033-1044 (1989).
29. Newman PJ, Berndt MC, Gorski J, White GC, Lyman S, Paddock C, Muller WA. PECAM-1 (CD31) cloning and relation to adhesion molecules of the immunoglobulin gene superfamily. *Science* 247: 1219-1222, (1990).
30. Aster RH. The immune thrombocytopenias. Chap 19, In Platelet Immunobiology, Molecular and Clinical Aspects. Eds, Kunicki TJ, George JN. JB Lippincott Co., Philadelphia, 1989, pp 387-435.
31. Sims PJ. Interaction of human platelets with the complement systems. Chap 18, In Platelet Immunobiology, Molecular and Clinical Aspects. Eds, Kunicki TJ, George JN. JB Lippincott Co., Philadelphia, 1989, pp 354-383.
32. Weiss HJ, Hawiger J, Ruggeri ZM, Turitto VT, Thiagarajan P, Hoffman T. Fibrinogen-independent platelet adhesion and thrombus formation on subendothelium mediated by glycoprotein IIb-IIIa complex at high shear rate. *J Clin Inv* 83: 288-297 (1989).
33. Du X, Beutler L, Ruan C, Castaldi PA, Berndt MC. Glycoprotein Ib and glycoprotein IX are fully complexed in the intact platelet membrane. *Blood* 9: 1524-1527 (1987).
34. Moake JL, Turner NA, Stathoupolous NA, Nolasco L, Hellums JD. Shear-induced platelet-aggregation can be mediated by vWF released from platelets, as well as by exogenous large or unusually large vWF multimers, requires adenosine diphosphate, and is resistant to aspirin. *Blood* 71: 1366-1374 (1988).
35. Jy W, Horstman LL, Arce M, Ahn YS. Clinical significance of platelet microparticles in autoimmune thrombocytopenias. *J Lab Clin Med* 119: 334-345 (1992).
36. Kelton JG, Warkenton TE, Hayward CPM, et al. Calpain activity in patients with idiopathic thrombocytopenic purpura is associated with platelet microparticles. *Blood* 80: 2246-2251 (1992).
37. Amenta JS, Baccino FM. Proteolysis and cell death. *Revis Biol Cellular* 21: 401-422 (1989).
38. Martin SJ, Cotter TJ. Disruption of microtubules induces an endogenous suicide pathway in human leukemia. *Cell Tissue Kinet*. 23: 545-559 (1990).
39. Singer JA, Jennings LK, Jackson CW, Dockter ME, Morrison M, Walker WS. Erythrocyte homeostasis: antibody-mediated recognition of senescent state by macrophages. *Proc Natl Acad Sci* 83:5498-5501 (1986).
40. Schroit AJ, Madsen JW, Tanaka Y. In vivo recognition of red blood cells containing phosphatidyl serine in their plasma membranes. *J Biol Chem* 260: 5131-5138 (1985).
41. Cohen JJ, Duke RC, Fadok VA, Sellins KS. Apoptosis and programmed cell death in immunity. *Ann Rev Immunol* 267-293 (1992).
42. Murphy EA, Francis ME. The estimation of blood platelet survival. I. General principle of the study of cell survival. *Throm Diath Haemorrh* 22: 281-295 (1969).

43. Murphy EA, Francis ME. The estimation of blood platelet survival. II. The multiple hit model. *Throm Diath Haemorrh* 25: 53-61 (1971).

44. Turpie AGG, de Boer AC, Genton E. Platelet consumption in cardiovascular disease. *Semin Thromb Hemostasis* 8: 161 (1982).

45. Dewanjee MK, Wahner HW, Dunn WL, et al. Comparison of three platelet markers for measurement of platelet survival time in healthy volunteers. *Mayo Clinic Proc* 61: 327-336 (1986).

46. Plevak DJ, Halma GA, Forstrom LA, Dewanjee MK, O'Connor MK, Moore SB, Krom RAF, Rettke SR. Thrombocytopenia following liver transplantation. *Transplantation Proc* 20 (Suppl 1, No 1): 630-633 (1988).

47. Siegel RS, Rae JL, Barth S, et al. Platelet survival and turnover: important factors in predicting response to splenectomy in immune thrombocytopenic purpura. *Am J Hemat* 30: 206-212 (1989).

48. Robertson JS, Ezekowitz MD, Dewanjee MK, Lotter MG, Watson EE. Radiation absorbed dose estimates for radioindium labeled autologous platelets (MIRD Dose Estimate No. 15). *J Nucl Med* 33: 777-780 (1991).

49. Folie BJ, McIntire LV. Mathematical analysis of mural thrombogenesis: concentration profiles of platelet-activating agents and effects of viscous shear flow. *Biophysical J.* 56: 1121-1141 (1989).

50. Bell DN, Spain S, Goldsmith HL. Adenosine diphosphate-induced aggregation of human platelets in flow through tubes. I. measurement of concentration and size of single platelets and aggregates. *Biophysical J* 56: 817-828 (1989).

51. Jamaluddin MP, Krishnan LK. A rate equation for blood platelet aggregation. *J theor Biol* 129: 257-261 (1987).

52. Rutherford E and Soddy F. The cause and nature of radioactivity. Part I. *Phil Mag* 4: 370-396 (1902).

53. Bateman H. Solution of a system of differential equations occurring in the theory of radio-active transformations. *Proc Cambridge Phil Soc* 15: 423-427 (1910).

54. Lassen NA and Perl W. Compartmental analysis, Chap. 10, in Tracer Kinetic Methods in Medical Physiology. Eds. Lassen NA and Perl W. Raven Press, N.Y., pp 137-155 (1979)

55. Dewanjee MK, Tago M, Josa M et al. Quantification of platelet retention in aortocoronary femoral vein bypass graft in dogs treated with dipyridamole and aspirin. *Circulation* 69: 350-356 (1984).

56. Dewanjee MK: Cardiac and vascular imaging with labeled platelets and leukocytes. *Sem Nucl Med XIV*: 154-187 (1984).

57. Didisheim P, Dewanjee MK, Frisk C, Kaye M, Fass D: Animal models for predicting clinical performance of biomaterials for cardiovascular use. Chapter 10, in Contemporary Biomaterials. Material and Host Response: Clinical Applications, New Technology and Legal Aspects. Boretos JW and Eden M, Editors, Noyes Publications, Parkridge, New Jersey, (1984), pp. 132-179.

58. Dewanjee MK: Methods of assessments of thrombosis in vivo. Blood in contact with natural and artificial surfaces. Vol. 516, Theme 4, Part one. Eds. Leonard EF, Vroman L, Turitto VT. New York Academy of Science, New York, N.Y. (1987), pp. 541-571.

59. Dewanjee MK. Radiolabeled platelets in the monitoring of drug-efficacy in animal models. *Thromb Haemorrh Disorders* 1/2: 37-51 (1990).

60. Dewanjee MK, Vogel SR, Peterson KA, et al. Quantitation of platelet consumption on oxygenator and stabilization of platelet membrane with prostacyclin and ibuprofen during cardiopulmonary bypass surgery in dogs. *Trans ASAIO* XXVII: 197-202 (1981).

61. Dewanjee MK, Palatianos GM, Kapadvanjwala M, et al. Increase of intraplatelet free calcium ion during extracorporeal circulation with a hollow fiber oxygenator: arterial filter and dynamics of platelet thrombosis on oxygenator and filter in a pig model. *Trans ASAIO* 36: M668-M671 (1990).

62. Dewanjee MK, Palatianos GM, Kapadvanjwala M, et al. Rate constant of embolization and quantitation of emboli from hollow-fiber oxygenator and arterial filter during cardiopulmonary bypass. *ASAIO Journal* 39: M317-M321 (1992).

63. Dewanjee MK, Kapadvanjwala M, Ruzius K, Serafini AN, Zilleruelo GE, Sfakianakis GN. Quantitation of thrombogenicity of technetium-99m and indium-111 labeled platelets in a hemodialyzer. *Int J Nucl Med Biol* 20: 579-587 (1993).

64. Dewanjee S, Dietrich WD, Prado R, Watson BD, Dewanjee MK. Direct method of quantitation of platelet-embolus and residence time in brain with radiolabeled platelets formed by photodenudation of endothelial cells of carotid artery in a rat model. ISORBE Proc 1992.

65. Schoepherster RT, Oynes F, Nunez G, Kapadvanjwala M, Dewanjee MK. Influence of flow rate on platelet deposition in an in vitro model stenosis using In-111 labeled platelets. The Proceedings of AAMI/NHLBI Conference on Cardiovascular Science and Technology, Bethesda MD, November 12-14, 1992 p 260.

PLATELET LABELING PARAMETERS ARE INFLUENCED BY LIPIDS AND LIPOPROTEINS*

S. Granegger, I. Neumann and H. Sinzinger

Wilhelm Auerswald Atherosclerosis Research Group Vienna
Department of Nuclear Medicine, University of Vienna
Ludwig Boltzmann Institute for Nuclear Medicine
Vienna, Austria

INTRODUCTION

During one of our very first applications of 111Indium-oxine platelet labeling in patients with manifested atherosclerosis more than a decade ago now[8], we discovered an extremely low labeling efficiency of only 16 % in contrast to the normal range of 80-95 %[4]. Beside discussing the problems of a technical mistake[2, 4, 10], we were looking for underlying phenomena in potential candidates being the risk factors for the development of atherosclerosis, i.e. hyperlipoproteinemia (3; HLP), smoking and eventually an interference of drugs. In fact, this particular 56 years old male patient was suffering from isolated hypercholesterolemia (type IIa) according to Fredrickson with a total cholesterol of 424 mg/dl and a LDL-cholesterol of 398 mg/dl. As LDL is known to activate platelet function[1, 5] and to alter the cellular membrane phospholipid composition, an influence onto the labeling behaviour was quite likely.

In order to assess the potential influence of lipids and lipoproteins (LP) and to clarify whether cells derived from hyperlipidemic patients or the plasma (or both) might exert an influence - if any - onto platelet labeling efficiency (LE) and recovery (REC), we were examining clinical situations associated with qualitative and quantitative changes in lipids and the LP-profile.

METHODOLOGICAL APPROACH

Platelet labeling was performed at 37°C and a 5 minutes incubation using our standardized method described earlier[2, 4, 7]. Basic requirements are > 1.10E9 cells/ml; Tyrodebuffer pH 6.2. In order to assess the influence of lipids and LP various clinical

* This study was supported in part by a grant for the "VIP"-Screening of the "Medizinisch-Wissenschaftlicher Fonds des Bürgermeisters der Bundeshauptstadt Wien".

conditions have been examined such as

A) in-vivo

1. Hypercholesterolemia (HC)
2. Hypertriglyceridemia (HT)
3. Hypo-β-lipoproteinemia
4. Hyperthyroidism
5. Hypothyroidism
6. Omega-3-fatty acid supplement

B) in-vitro

1. oxidized LDL

    Statistical analysis: Values are means $\pm$ SD; significance was assessed by Student's t-test for paired and unpaired data, respectively.

RESULTS

A) In-vivo Experiments

1. Hypercholesterolemia

    HC is associated with a decreased LE reaching values of below 20 % at total cholesterol levels above 350 mg/dl. There is a strong correlation (p<0,01) between LE and total cholesterol (r=-0.83) and even more LDL-cholesterol (r=-0.85). This association is closest in type IIa HLP (i.e. isolated HC), the association decreasing in type IIb (r=-0.80; r=-0.82) and type IV hyperlipoproteinemic patients (r=-0.74, and r=-0.77, respectively) (table 1).

Table 1. LE in normo- and HC using different tracers

	MPO	oxine	oxine-sulphate	tropolone
a)	90.3 ± 1.1	88.7 ± 3.1	90.3 ± 2.1	89.3 ± 2.0
b)	64.7 ± 6.9*	61.6 ± 5.3*	65.1 ± 4.8*	64.1 ± 5.7*
c)	39.6 ± 6.5*	38.7 ± 6.8*	42.7 ± 4.6*	41.5 ± 3.7*
d)	19.7 ± 6.3*	22.5 ± 6.3*	21.7 ± 5.8*	23.2 ± 5.8*

Cholesterol (mg/dl): a) 200-250; b) 251-300; c) 301-350; d) 351-400; values shown are X $\pm$ SD; n= 4 - 6 each; * p<0.01

2. Hypertricliceridemia

    Extreme HT apparently does not affect LE substantially. The minimal change in LE and recovery may be more likely due to the parallel decrease in cholesterol rather than triglycerides (table 2).

High levels of total cholesterol and LDL-cholesterol are activating platelet function and platelets are aggregating more rapidly in the presence of increasing LDL-cholesterol[1, 5]. Together with the finding that an impaired LE is correlated to total cholesterol and LDL-cholesterol but not to HDL-cholesterol, it remains to be assessed whether the LE was due to an impairment in platelet membrane composition. We thus wondered, whether LDL removal reduces platelet activity and whether hypo-beta-lipoproteinemia (a condition associated with low-total cholesterol and LDL-cholesterol), where platelets aggregate subnormally, may change the behaviour.

Table 2. Hypertriglyceridemia in 15 patients (11 males, 4 females; 36 - 57 a) without ATH (8 - 12 weeks diet)

	before	after
CH	281 ± 36	217 ± 14 *)
TG	1475 ± 361	286 ± 39 **)
LE	84.7 ± 7.3	86.9 ± 5.7
REC	60.7 ± 5.8	61.9 ± 6.1
SUR	167.3 ± 12.4	175.0 ± 10.3 *)

CH... cholesterol; TG... triglycerides; LE... labeling efficiency; REC... recovery; SUR... survival
X ± SD; *) $p < 0.01$; **) $p < 0.00001$

3 Primary hypo-beta-lipoproteinemia

Primary hypo-beta-lipoproteinemia is a condition with a total cholesterol below 100 mg/dl, LDL-cholesterol below 50 mg/dl and triglycerides below 100 mg/dl. We adressed this question in 9 patients (5 males, 4 females; 5 - 61 years) discovered during a cholesterol screening examining the influence of platelets and plasma in a series of cross-incubation experiments using 111Indium-labeling. The lipid parameters (table 3) showed the typical range while the platelet activity was subnormal. Comparing platelets of hypo-beta-lipoproteinemic patients with those of patients with higher total cholesterol,there is clearly an inverse relation between LE and cholesterol (table4). Incubating platelets of HC (table 5) in hypo-beta-lipoproteinemics plasma as compared to their autologous plasma did not show a significant difference further indicating no relevant influence of the plasmatic environment on LE. Cross- incubation experiments clearly indicate that platelets derived from hypo-beta-lipidemic patients show a very high LE, even if incubated in the plasma derived from hypercholesterolemics (total cholesterol above 300 mg/dl) (table 6). In contrast, platelets from HC exhibited an impaired LE which is not improved by incubation in hypolipidemic plasma. Summarizing, these data demonstrate that LE and recovery improved in hypo-β-lipoproteinemia. This effect is due to an altered platelet membrane composition rather than to the plasmatic environment. The labeling results (data not shown) are comparable for indium oxine, oxine sulfate, tropolone and MPO, stabilization with either prostaglandin I_2 or nitric oxide does not further improve the labeling yield (data not shown).

Table 3. Lipids, LPs and platelet function in hypo-β-lipoproteinemia

CH	91.4 ± 3.9	mg/dl
HDL-CH	56.4 ± 6.3	mg/dl
LDL-CH	20.4 ± 10.4	mg/dl
TG	72.0 ± 20.2	mg/dl
plt	249.6 ± 36.3 x	10E3/μl
MDA	2.64 ± 0.72	mM/10E9 pl
TXB2	189.2 ± 18.5	ng/ml
βTG	7.6 ± 2.07	mg/dl

HDL...high-density lipoprotein; LDL...low-density lipoprotein; plt...peripheral platelet count;_MDA...malondialdehyde; TXB2...thromboxane B2; βTG...β-thromboglobulin; mean X ± SD; n=9

Table 4. Labeling efficiency (LE)

CH	LE (%)	n
Hypo-β-LP	95.0 ± 0.7 *)	5
< 250 mg/dl	90.3 ± 1.7 *)	6
< 300 mg/dl	71.2 ± 5.7 **)	6

*) $p < 0.01$; **) $p < 0.001$;
Inc.: 37°C, 5 min; X ± SD

Table 5. Hypo-β-LP plasma does not improve LE

CH	LE (%)	in Hypo-β-LP
< 400 mg/dl	21.6 ± 5.3	23.7 ± 6.2
< 350 mg/dl	39.7 ± 7.4	40.7 ± 8.0
< 300 mg/dl	68.6 ± 6.9	71.3 ± 7.2
< 250 mg/dl	89.3 ± 2.1	88.8 ± 2.4
< 200 mg/dl	90.1 ± 1.4	91.1 ± 1.0

n = 8 (each group); mean ± SD

Table 6. Cross incubation (platelets vs. plasma)

plat	/	plasma	LE (%)
Hypo-β	/	Hypo-β	94.7 ± 1.1
Hypo-β	/	< 300	92.8 ± 6.0
< 300	/	Hypo-β	74.7 ± 1.9 ***)
< 300	/	< 300	72.0 ± 7.5

mean ± SD; ***) $p < 0.0001$

4. Hyperthyroidism

Hyperthyroidism is associated with a decrease in cholesterol and triglycerides. Patients suffering from hyperthyroidism successfully treated by thyreostatics, however, did not show a significant change in labeling parameters and recovery, the extent of change in cholesterol being apparently not sufficient to cause a change in labeling parameters in contrast (table 7).

Table 7. Hyperthyroidism

	before	after
CH	219.6 ± 18.7	248.7 ± 22.3 *)
TG	175.5 ± 25.3	194.3 ± 26.8
T4	17.6 ± 1.2	10.7 ± 1.2 *)
LE	89.7 ± 5.1	88.7 ± 4.3
REC	65.2 ± 5.3	64.9 ± 6.1
SUR	184.6 ± 12.4	182.2 ± 10.7

T4...tetraiodothyronine;
$X \pm SD$; n = 16; *) $p < 0.01$

5. Hypothyroidism

Hypothyroidism is associated with high cholesterol. A triglyceride normalization by hormonal substitution in 11 patients resulted in a significant decrease of total cholesterol and triglycerides (table 8) as well as a significant improvement of LE and REC in parallel. Cross incubation experiments again show (table 9) that the platelets are responsible for the labeling yield achieved rather than the plasmatic environment.

Table 8. Hypothyroidism

	before	after
CH	374.3 ± 32.8	281.4 ± 20.6 *)
TG	283.6 ± 35.2	203.6 ± 21.7 *)
T4	1.7 ± 0.5	10.2 ± 1.0 *)
LE	21.8 ± 5.2	63.5 ± 6.7 *)
REC	8.7 ± 2.6	41.0 ± 7.2 *)
SUR	149.8 ± 18.7	167.8 ± 10.6 *)

$\bar{X} \pm SD$; n = 11; *) $p < 0.01$

6. Omega-3 fatty acid supplement

In 19 patients (15 males, 4 females; 56 - 69 years) suffering from peripheral vascular disease we studied the influence of omega-3 fatty acid supplement (18 mg 20:5 [100 mg fish oil] + 400 mg evening primrose oil). Interestingly enough, although cholesterol is not changed (table 10) and normally a moderate decrease (with a wide variation) in TG is observed, LE and REC show a significant improvement indicating a beneficial change in the platelet membrane allowing a higher uptake. Cross incubation experiments again reveal (table 11) the key importance of platelet membrane composition as compared to the plasma. While these differences can be seen in hyperlipidemics (table 11), they are not apparent in normolipidemics (table 12).

Table 9. Hypo-vs. normothyroidism
(platelets vs. plasma)

plat.	/ plasma	LE (%)
Hypo	/ Hypo	23.7 ± 4.9 *)
Hypo	/ Normo	25.2 ± 5.6 *)
Normo	/ Hypo	88.7 ± 2.2
Normo	/ Normo	89.4 ± 1.9

$\bar{X}$ ± SD; n = 8 each; *) p < 0.01

Table 10. Omega-3 FA-supplement

	before	after
CH	265.5 ± 26.4	261.7 ± 25.0
TG	374.2 ± 84.1	331.5 ± 51.2
LE	67.3 ± 8.1	78.6 ± 4.9 *)
REC	42.6 ± 5.2	54.9 ± 5.0 *)
SUR	142.6 ± 15.8	158.9 ± 10.7 *)

$\bar{X}$ ± SD; *) p < 0.01

Table 11. Omega-3 vs. hyperlipidemics (HL)
(platelets vs. plasma)

plat.	/ plasma	LE (%)
Omega-3	/ Omega-3	78.6 ± 3.3
Omega-3	/ HL	76.9 ± 3.5
HL	/ Omega-3	67.3 ± 4.7 *)
HL	/ HL	65.8 ± 5.1 *)

Cholesterol: 250-300 mg/dl; $\bar{X}$ ± SD; n = 8 each; *) p < 0.01

Table 12. Omega-3 vs. normolipidemics (NL)
(platelets vs. plasma)

plat.	/ plasma	LE (%)
Omega-3 /	Omega-3	90.6 ± 1.3
Omega-3 /	NL	90.2 ± 1.6
NL /	Omega-3	88.7 ± 1.9
NL /	NL	89.8 ± 1.5

$\bar{X}$ ± SD; n = 8 each

Table 13. Role of LDL and oxydated LDL on LE

	mg/dl	LE (%)
LDL	141.8 ± 8.4	91.7 ± 1.3
ox.LDL	141.8 ± 8.4	88.2 ± 2.2
LDL	236.5 ± 15.6	56.3 ± 3.8
ox.LDL	236.5 ± 15.6	45.8 ± 4.1 *)

$\bar{X}$ ± SD; n= 8 each; *) p<0.01

B) In-vitro Experiments

1. The effect of oxydization of LDL is not detectable in a range of normal cholesterol values[11] while it becomes apparent and significantly different in patients with extremely elevated LDL (table13).

DISCUSSION

These findings demonstrate that an increase in blood lipids, and in particular LDL-cholesterol is paralleled by an impairment in platelet labeling which is predominantly associated with the platelets rather than the plasma[9]. An improvement in LP values in one particular patient leads to normalization in the labeling parameters. The fact that the highest correlation can be observed between LE and LDL-cholesterol indicates a binding of the tracer to the LP which has not been qualitatively and quantitatively assessed yet. The finding that the highest correlation between LE and LDL-cholesterol is found in type IIa patients and to a lesser extent in type IIb- and even less in type IV patients further underlines the predominant role of LDL-cholesterol.

TG apparently do not exhibit any influence on the labeling parameters. Interestingly, an alteration in omega-3 fatty acids although not causing significant changes in cholesterol but only in TG-levels is associated with an improved labeling yield. This makes it very likely that both, a change in platelet membrane composition as well as a tracer-LP binding is responsible for the impairment in LE and recovery. The fact that oxydized LDL[11] at a higher range do impair the labeling yield may indicate that oxydized LDL may show a more severe tracer binding than normal LDL.

ACKNOWLEDGEMENTS

The valuable help of Dr. P. Angelberger (Dept. of Chemistry, SGAE Seibersdorf, Austria) in providing the radiotracer and of Eva Unger in preparing and typing this manuscript is gratefully acknowledged.

REFERENCES

1. Boberg, M., M. Vessby and L.B. Croon. Fatty acid composition of platelets and of plasma lipid esters in relation to platelet function in patients with ischemic heart disease. *Atherosclerosis* 58: 49-63 (1985).
2. Jäger, E., H. Kolbe, K. Silberbauer, H. Sinzinger and R. Höfer. Technik der radioaktiven Markierung autologer menschlicher Thrombozyten mit 111-Indium-Oxin und 111-Indium-Oxin-Sulfat und deren klinische Anwendung. *Wr Klin Wschr* 96:106-112. (1984).
3. Kaliman, J., G. Kostner, O. Kraupp, M. Kunze, H. Sinzinger and K. Widhalm. Richtlinien zur Prävention der Atherosklerose. *Wr Klin Wschr* 99: 589.
4. Neumann, I., E. Strobl-Jäger, P. Angelberger, J. O'Grady and H. Sinzinger. A comparison of 111-In-oxine with 111-In-oxine-sulphate for human platelet labeling. *Thromb Haemost Disorders* 5: 5-10 (1992).
5. Shastri, K.M., A.C.A. Carvalho and R.S. Lees. Platelet function and platelet lipid composition in the dyslipoproteinemia. *J Lipid Res* 21: 467-472 (1980).
6. Sinzinger, H., P. Angelberger, and R. Höfer. Platelet labeling with In-111-oxine- benefit of prostacyclin (PGI₂)- addition for preparation and injection. *J Nucl Med* 22: 292 (1981).
7. Sinzinger, H., P. Angelberger and H. Kolbe. Influence of incubation time and temperature on indium-111-oxine uptake by human platelets. *Thromb Haemost* 45: 295 (1981).
8. Sinzinger, H., H. Kolbe, E. Strobl-Jäger and R. Höfer. A simple and safe technique for sterile autologous platelet labelling using "Monovette" vials. *Eur J Nucl Med* 9: 320-322 (1984)
9. Sinzinger, H., J. Flores, K. Widhalm, and S. Granegger. Platelet viability (aggregation, migration, recovery) after radiolabelling from hypercholesterolemics using various tracers (oxine, oxine-sulphate, tropolone, MPO). *Eur J Nucl Med* 14: 358-361 (1988).
10. Sinzinger, H., and I. Virgolini. Nuclear medicine and atherosclerosis. *Eur J Nucl Med* 17: 160-178 (1990).
11. Sinzinger, H., J. O'Grady, Ch. Pirich, and B.A. Peskar. Oxydized low-density lipoproteins and platelet products secreted during activation impair platelet labeling efficiency with 111-Indium-oxine. (in preparation) (1992).

CLINICAL APPLICATIONS OF 111In-TROPOLONATE LABELLED PLATELETS

H. Louwes and J.J.Schuurman

From the Department of Nuclear Medicine
Martini Hospital
Groningen, the Netherlands

INTRODUCTION

This article will discuss the clinical relevance of thrombocyte labelling. It should become clear to clinicans with experience in the field of thrombocytopenia which role this Nuclear Medicine technique can play in diagnosing and managing your patients. The main purpose of the investigation was to use indium labelling to distinguish between thrombocytopenia caused by a failure of platelet production and thrombocytopenia caused by platelet destruction. This obviously is a distinction that cannot always be made on clinical grounds,

The article consists of three parts:

* A review of the clinical diagnosis of thrombocytopenia will be briefly reviewed.

* A few highlights of the separation and labelling techniques will be explained. Some comments on possible quality control procedures will be made. For practical reasons the discussion will be limited to the key points.

* The measurement of Mean Platelet Life (MPL), Platelet Production Rate (PPR), and Initial Recovery (IR) will be described and how these values in patients with trombocytopenia compare with the values in normal individuals.

The clinical relevance of these measurements will be discussed, as well as measurements of platelet uptake by the liver and spleen.

THROMBOCYTOPENIA

In patients who have decreased numbers of platelets or defective platelet function, thrombocytopenia is associated with petechial and purpuric bleeding into the skin. These patients may also have bleeding from the capillaries of the mucosal surfaces in the nose, the mouth, or the digestive tract. In a patient with purpura, skin and mucous membrane bleeding is the most common manifestation. Small petechial spots are usually concentrated on the legs and on areas where the patient's clothing exerts pressure. In general, we see these signs only when the platelet count has dropped below 30 x 10^9 per litre. With a further drop to 20 x 10⁹ spontaneaous hemorrhage becomes increasingly likely.

There are three main causes of thrombocytopenia.

Thrombocytopenia may occur as a result of a decreased platelet production, as a result of increased splenic platelet pooling, or as a result of an increased rate of platelet destruction. A failure to produce platelets may result from generalized bone marrow failure. Bone marrow production may decrease in patients with infiltration by metastatic cancer cells, in patients with Hodgkin's disease, and in patients with vitamin B12 deficiency. Alternatively, selective depression of the stem cells may be induced by radiation, by drugs, by alcohol, or by other chemicals. And in rare cases, we may encounter hereditary thrombocytopenia for example, the Wiskott Aldrich syndrome.

The second cause of thrombocytopenia abnormal platelet distribution may arise, for example, from platelet pooling in an enlarged spleen.

The final cause of thrombocytopenia increased platelet destruction usually results either from an immune disease or from the use of such drugs as heroin, morphine, or anticonvulsants. Less commonly, increased platelet destruction may reflect a disturbance in the coagulation process itself.

PATIENT MANAGEMENT

Patients with thrombocytopenia are generaly managed in the following ways:

A failure of platelet production can be treated with transfusions of platelet suspensions.

For splenomegaly in general, there is no possible treatment.

Increased destruction of platelets by antibodies can be managed in two phases. The first step is treatment with corticosteroids. If the condition recurs, the next option is splenectomy. This is effective in 70 % of patients. And obviously, if platelet destruction is drug-induced, the patient should stop taking the culprit drug. Most cases of drug-induced thrombocytopenia are reversible.

TECHNIQUE FOR LABELING PLATELETS

To separate the cells, the procedure outlined below is followed:

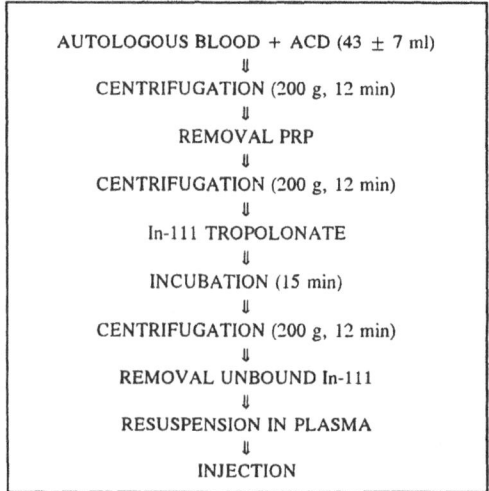

```
AUTOLOGOUS BLOOD + ACD (43 ± 7 ml)
                ⇓
   CENTRIFUGATION (200 g, 12 min)
                ⇓
          REMOVAL PRP
                ⇓
   CENTRIFUGATION (200 g, 12 min)
                ⇓
        In-111 TROPOLONATE
                ⇓
        INCUBATION (15 min)
                ⇓
   CENTRIFUGATION (200 g, 12 min)
                ⇓
      REMOVAL UNBOUND In-111
                ⇓
      RESUSPENSION IN PLASMA
                ⇓
           INJECTION
```

Its important to use autologous blood because injection with labelled donor cells gives an increased MPL. From experience and over the years it has become clear that virtually every hospital developed its own method for separating and labelling cells. Although this is understandable, it represents a serious obstacle not only to standardizing the method, but more importantly to comparing clinical results. The method recommended by the International Committee on Standardization in Hematology (ICSH) in 1988 is the same. In this context, it will be interesting to dwell a little longer

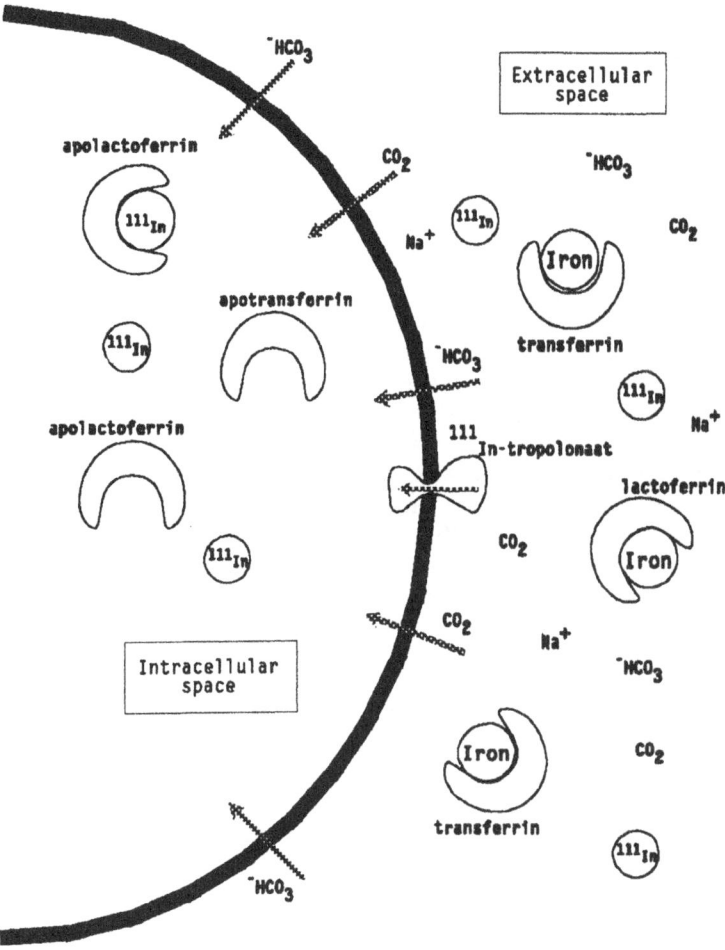

Figure 1.

on the 111Indium tropolonate preparation that is in use and how the labelling to the cells is actually taking place. The preparation is a saturated sodium bicarbonate solution containing carbon dioxide, with a much lower concentration of Indium tropolonate than the one recommended by the ICHS.

Bicarbonate ions are necessary for metals to bind to plasma transferrins. Thus, by supplying bicarbonate ions, the binding of indium to transferrin is favoured, at the expense of indium binding to cells. What accounts for this? After indium passes the double lipoid membrane of the cell, it is captured by protein-like structures called lactoferrins. The lactoferrins, which resemble transferrins, also need bicarbonate ions in order to bind the indium. When carbon dioxide is added to the cell incubation mixture, the intracellular availability of bicarbonate ions is increased, since outside the cell there already exists an excess of bicarbonate and carbon dioxide. In fact, by adding carbon dioxide, the partition equilibrium of indium is shifted away from the plasma and more into the cell. In this way, the binding of indium to the cell is encouraged rather than to plasma. This theory has been confirmed in cell labelling experiments that were carried out in the complete absence of plasma. The result was, that when incubation mixture was flushed with carbon dioxide, the efficiency of cell labelling was greatly enhanced. Without carbon dioxide, only 30 % of the cells could be labelled, but by adding carbon dioxide the labelling efficiency could be boosted to more than 80 %.

QUALITY CONTROL

It is possible to perform a number of quality control tests before giving the radiolabelled cells to the patient. The first and most obvious quality control test is, of course, determination of labelling efficiency. In addition platelet function and viability tests are of vital importance. A large variety of tests is available, and the sheer number of choices only underscores the fact that no one of these tests really stands out above the others as sufficient in itself. However, in practice we observed abnormal results were observed even with intact platelets. When platelets are manipulated during the labelling process-especially during centrifugation, pelleting, and suspension they may lose some ADP and require additional ADP in order to aggregate. This loss of ADP is reversible. A partial degranulation process does not impair platelet survival. If membrane integrity is intact, IR, MPL, and uptake by the liver and spleen are not affected. The major problems with all of these these tests are that they are nonfunctional in-vitro tests and they are rather time consuming as well. The conclusion must be that, at the moment, there is no completely satisfactory method for testing platelet function in vitro.

RESULTS: SUBJECTS

Two hundred and thirty persons were investigated with 111In-tropolonate labelled platelets, 14 normals and 216 patients (table 1).

BLOOD SAMPLING

Mean Platelet Life (MPL), Initial Recovery (IR), and Platelet Production Rate (PPR) are calculated in whole blood samples. These samples are taken at regular intervals of 1,3 and 5 hours after injection of the patients with radiolabelled platelets and twice a day for four days thereafter. It should be mentioned that when a shortening of mean platelet life is expected, additional blood samples are taken on the first day. The MPL is calculated using a gamma function model, according to ISCH recommendations.

MPL AND PPR IN NORMALS AND THROMBOCYTOPENIC PATIENTS (table 1)

In normal individuals, mean platelet life is about 9 days. In contrast, patients with splenomegaly or decreased platelet production have an MPL af 4 to 5 days. In patients with idiopathic platelet destruction, however, platelet life span is dramatically shortened to less than 2 days. Patients with decreased platelet production have a production rate less than half the normal value. In patients with ITP or recurrent disease the range of production rates is very wide, and so the standard deviation is considerable. This probably reflects that fact that the diagnosis of ITP is made by exclusion criteria and the underlying cause is difficult to establish. In contrast to what might be expected, no compensatory mechanism of production is present in these patients.

Table 1. Platelet Kinetics in normals and in patients with thrombocytopenia

Subjects (n = 216)		Normals (n = 14)	Thrombocytopenia			
			Hyper-splenism (n = 39)	Decreased Production (n = 73)	ITP (n = 92)	Recurrent (n = 12)
Platelets	$10^9 l^{-1}$	224 ± 47	79 ± 23	58 ± 38	47 ± 34	58 ± 44
MPL	days	9.2 ± 1.3	4.3 ±1.7	4.9 ± 2.3	1.5 ±1.1	1.9 ±1.8
IPR	%	58 ± 12	37 ± 12	54 ± 14	52 ± 14	67 ± 15
TPPR	$10^9 d^{-1}$	220 ± 60	260 ±140	99 ± 54	344 ±300	234 ±165
k_{12}	10^{-3} min^{-1}	51 ± 8	130 ± 31	67 ± 15	65 ± 15	15 ± 10
STT	min	11.0 ± 1.3	15.5 ±2.5	12 ± 5.8	11.9 ± 6.0	11.5 ±5.2
SBF	ml.min^{-1}	260 ± 80	650 ±150	300 ±295	300 ±235	40 ± 45

MPL = Mean Platelet Life, IPR = Initial Platelet Recovery, TPPR = Total Platelet Production Rate, k_{12} = Transport constant (Blood -> Spleen), STT = Spleen Transit Time, SBF = Splenic Blood Flow

ORGAN UPTAKE MEASUREMENTS (table 2)

Hepatic and splenic uptake is measured with a Large-Filed-Of-View gamma camera (LFOV) interfaced with a computer. Immediately after the labelled platelets are injected, 60 one-minute digital frames are recorded in the posterior position. After the dynamic investigation, static acquisition is begun for 5 minutes in the anterior an posterior positions. Twice a day, these views are repeated and blood samples taken to calculate absolute uptake in the liver and spleen.

As expected, patients with splenomegaly show increased splenic uptake after one hour, expressed as a percentage of the injected dose.

Patients with recurrent disease after splenectomy with an accessory spleen show hardly any uptake, because they have so little splenic tissue.

Liver uptake is much the same in all patients, except those with recurrent disease.

Table 2. Organ Uptake (%) in normals and patients with thrombocytopenic disorders

time after injection (hr)	Normals (n = 14)	Thrombocytopenia			
		Hypersplenism (n = 39)	Decreased Production (n = 73)	ITP (n = 92)	Recurrent (n = 12)
SPLEEN					
1	35 ± 3	59 ± 12	34 ± 14	37 ± 12	6 ± 3
4 - 5	36 ± 3	58 ± 11	34 ± 13	40 ± 14	10 ± 7
21 - 28	35 ± 3	59 ± 13	35 ± 13	45 ± 15	12 ± 7
48 - 54	36 ± 3	59 ± 11	35 ± 13	48 ± 17	15 ± 9
72 - 80	36 ± 3	59 ± 12	36 ± 14	48 ± 17	16 ± 10
LIVER					
1	9 ± 3	8 ± 3	12 ± 4	13 ± 2	31 ± 16
4 - 5	9 ± 2	8 ± 3	11 ± 4	13 ± 3	35 ± 17
21 - 28	9 ± 2	8 ± 3	12 ± 4	14 ± 4	43 ± 14
48 - 54	9 ± 2	8 ± 3	13 ± 5	15 ± 4	48 ± 20
72 - 80	9 ± 3	8 ± 3	14 ± 6	16 ± 4	53 ± 20

The reason for this exception is that, after splenectomy, the liver takes over platelet pooling and destruction. The pattern of the results in normal individuals and in all four patient groups is summmarised in table 3.

In normal individuals, hepatic and splenic uptake remains relatively constant during the five days following administration of indium-111 labelled thrombocytes. Uptake of activity by the spleen during the first hour after injection may reflect pooling. In contrast, increased uptake by the liver during the next few days is a sign of increased platelet destruction. The relative stability of absolute uptake in controls suggests that destruction and pooling are continuous processes that run in parallel. The rate of destruction is sometimes called the destruction/pooling ratio (D/P). But it might make more sense to replace the D/P ratio with a da/dt ratio in which dt is a function of time and da is a function of the absolute increase in activity in both organs. Like destruction and pooling in the spleen, pooling of damaged platelets also takes place in the liver during the first 10 minutes. Normally the heart and liver uptake curves are more or less identical. However, when the cells are damaged, liver uptake increases. These findings are in agreement with the results of the Hammersmith Hospital (London, UK). Both groups believe that dynamic imaging immediately following injection of radiolabelled platelets is a sensitive method for detecting minimal cell damage and/or activation induced during labelling. Maintaining the platelets in plasma helps to minimize this activation.

KINETICS

By means of a two compartmental model the splenic transit time (STT) and splenic blood flow are calculated as proposed by Peters in 1980. The uptake of activity in the normal spleen is fast and has a half time of about 5 minutes. In normals the transportkonstant blood to spleen is approx. 0.051 per minute. This means that 5.1 % of the blood enters the spleen per minute: this represents splenic blood flow. If platelets within the spleen blood flow are in dynamic equilibrium with the circulating platelets, it may be concluded that splenic blood flow dependant upon two factors: size of the spleen and the transit time. In normal individuals (table 1) the STT is about ten minutes, SBF is about 260 ml/min. In patients with hypersplenism the STT and SBF are significantly increased in comparison with the control group. In patients with ITP and decreased production the range of STT and SBF is very wide.

Table 3. Pattern of results

Thrombocytopenia	MPL	TPPR	Spleen after: 1 hour	5-7 days	Liver after: 1 hour	5-7 days
ITP	↓↓↓	↓n↑	var	↑(78%)	n	↑(11%)
Decreased production	↓	↓↓	var	n	n	↑(11%)
Hypersplenism	↓	n	↑↑	id	↓n	id
Recurrent	↓↓	n	-	-	↑	↑↑

MPL = Mean Platelet Production Rate, ↓ = decreased, ↑ = increased, var = variable, n = normal, id = identical

EFFECTS OF THERAPY

Table 4 is representative of what is found in about 70 % of patients with ITP before and after treatment. It should be noticed that, before therapy, the patient has an extremely low platelet count, a markedly shortened MPL, and a normal to high production rate. During prednisolone therapy, both an increase in the number of platelets is observed and in the production rate, as prednisolone activates stem cell production. But there is no change in MPL. After splenectomy, all of these values become nearly normal. You will probably agree that these results confirm what Stratton has said in the New England Journal of Medicine : Noninvasive, physiologic measurements of liver and spleen uptake in the nuclear medicine department can help clinicians know what to expect from drug treatment of surgery. As shown, prednisolone activates platelet production and splenectomy brings the MPL back to normal. How could these results be applied in managing your patients? These patterns may be used to clearly distinguish between patients with ITP and patients with decreased production: In patients with ITP, the MPL is always dramatically shortened to about 2 days and the PPR has a wide range. This means that these patients must be carefully calculated, since the diagnosis is based on exclusion criteria. In addition, these patients show an

Table 4. Effects of Therapy

	Before Therapy	During prednisone	After splenectomy
Platelet count($10^9 1^{-1}$)	15	125	200
MPL (days)	1.0	1.1	7.2
TPPR ($10^9 1^{-1}$)	280	600	220

increased Destruction/Pooling ratio of 70 - 80 % over the spleen. On the other hand, in patients with decreased production, the MPL is only slightly shortened, to about 4-5 days, the PPR range is much better defined, and organ uptake is normal.

CONCLUSION

It's not always possible to distinguish between ITP and decreased platelet production on clinical grounds, since there is no relationship between the number of megakaryocytes and platelet production. Morphologically normal bone marrow does not discriminate between an failure of platelet production and increased platelet destruction. However, the cause of thrombocytopenia can be distinguisted using thrombocyte labelling. This physiologic nuclear medicine technique can also be used to predict the results of therapy. So, it will be clear that thrombocyte labelling can play an important dual role in the diagnosis and treatment of your thrombocytopenic patients.

REFERENCES

1. Danpure HJ, Osman S, Brady F. The labelling of blood cells in plasma with 111In-tropolonate. *BR J Radiol* 55: 247-249 (1982).
2. Peters AM, Klonizakis Y. Dynamic studies with 111Indium labeled platelets. *Br J Radiol* 53; 923 (1980).
3. Peters AM, Savermuttu SH, Malik F, Ind PW, Laverder JP. Intrahepatic Kinetics of Indium-111 Labelled Platelets. *Thrombosis and Haemostasis* 45: 595-602 (1985).
4. ICSH panel on diagnostic application of radioisotopes in Hematology: Recommended method for 111In platelet survival studies. *Journal of Nuclear Medicine,* 29: 564 (1988).
5. Heyns du PA, Badenhorst PN, Pieters H, Lotter MG, Wessels P, Kotze HF. Platelet Turnover and Kinetics in Immune Thrombocytopenic Purpura: Results with Autologous 111In-labeled Platelets and Homologous 51Cr.Labeled Platelets Differ. *Blood* 67: 86-92 (1986).
6. Gernheimer P, Stratton J, Ballem PJ, Slichter SJ. Mechanisms of response to treatment in autoimmune Thrombocytopenic Purpura. *N Engl J Med* 320: 974-980 (1989).

PLATELET-EMBOLI FROM ARTERIAL FILTER AND OXYGENATOR: MAJOR SOURCE OF EMBOLIC COMPLICATIONS DURING CARDIOPULMONARY BYPASS (CPB)

M.K. Dewanjee[1], G.M. Palatianos[2], M. Kapadvanjwala[3], S. Novak[2], D. Sarkar, L. Hsu[4], S. Ezuddin[1], A.N. Serafini[1] and G.N. Sfakianakis[1]

Departments of [1]Radiology, [2]Surgery, [3]Computer Science and Biomedical Engineering
University of Miami, School of Medicine, Miami, Florida
[4]Bentley Laboratories, Irvine, California

ABSTRACT

We developed a direct technique for the estimation of parameters related to half-life ($T_{1/2}$) and rate constants of embolization (RCE) and quantitation of amount of emboli of three size (small, medium and large) shed from the oxygenator and of arterial filter during cardiopulmonary bypass (CPB). CPB was performed in 16 Yorkshire pigs, systemic heparin group (SHG:6); systemic heparin/heparinized circuit group (SH/HCG:5) and Iloprost (2ng/kg/min)/heparinized circuit group (IHCG:5) with 111In labeled autologous platelets. The anesthetized pigs underwent CPB at 2.5-3.0 L/min for 3 hours. Pigs were injected with 111In platelets (300-420 μCi), 24 hours prior to CPB. During CPB, thrombosis and embolization on oxygenator and filter were monitored by a calibrated Geiger probe. The radioactivity in the oxygenator and filter reached a peak value at 25-45 min. post-CPB; the radioactivity then declined for oxygenator, but remained at steady state for filter suggesting continous embolization at the same rate of trapping. The curve-stripping technique of the normalized radioactivity-time curve of the oxygenator was used for the RCE-estimation of different size of emboli shed from the oxygenator; 42% of thrombus embolized from oxygenator in SHG with 3 rate constants with a $T_{1/2}$ of 12 min, 42 min and 13 hr; SH/HCG embolized 35% with $T_{1/2}$ of 78 min and IHCG embolized 30% with a $T_{1/2}$ of 22 min, indicating that there is less embolization in the IHCG. By direct continuous monitoring, we developed a sensitive technique for quantitation of rate of embolus-shedding during CPB.

INTRODUCTION

Thromboembolic complications in patients post-cardiopulmonary bypass were identified[1-5]. Although the foci of thrombus formation and embolization in the oxygenator and arterial filter were recognized, no quantitative information about the rate, size and amount of emboli shed from oxygenator and filter and the inter-relationship of trapping of emboli in arterial filter and thrombi formed and emboli shed from arterial filter was available. Although considerable improvement occurred in oxygenation of blood (bubbling or diffusion of oxygen through membrane or hollow-fiber), no significant improvement was made in arterial filter. Screen-filter rather than depth-matrix filter was used for trapping emboli. The short distance between membranes separating thrombi and filtered blood and high concentration gradient of platelet-releasate and activated clotting factors resulted in thrombus formation and down-stream embolization from arterial filter.

The autologous platelets labeled with 111Indium helped us in identifying the site and amount of adherent thrombi on cardiovascular prostheses and amount of trapped emboli in lung, heart, brain and kidneys by biodistribution[5, 6]. In addition, the non-invasive imaging technique permitted us to follow the dynamic nature of thrombus-buildup and embolization from cardiovascular implants or devices used during extracorporeal circulation for oxygenation or hemodialysis. The radioactivity-time curve was obtained by continuous monitoring of 111In radioactivity on oxygenator and arterial filter during CPB. Assuming the random probability of thrombosis and their embolization from oxygenator and arterial filter, we developed a mathematical model and defined exponential equations to calculate the rate constant of embolization (RCE) during CPB. The normalized radioactivity-time curve was stripped according to the half-life ($T_{1/2}$) of clearance of emboli of different size from oxygenator for quantitation of amount, approximate size and $T_{1/2}$ of emboli from oxygenator.

MATERIALS AND METHODS

The details of blood collection, platelet labeling with 111In tropolone and static and dynamic measurements of adherent thrombi to oxygenator and arterial filter and emboli in lung, brain, heart and kidneys by imaging with gamma camera, ionization chamber, gamma counter and Geiger probe are described in details before[15 - 8].

A. The Labeling of Autologous Platelets with 111Indium Tropolone

The porcine platelets were labeled according to the method of Dewanjee et al.[16]. Sixty milliliters of whole blood were collected from anesthetized Yorkshire pigs in 10 ml of modified ACD anticoagulant solution; the platelets separated by differential centrifugation were incubated with 111In tropolone (600-700 μCi) for 20 minutes and washed by centrifugation. The 111In labeled platelets were measured with an ionization chamber (Capintec CRC-5RH3) and injected via the ear-vein. The platelet harvesting efficiency of typically (40-45)% and labeling efficiency of (80-95)% were obtained routinely.

B. Extracorporeal Circulation with Hollow-fiber Oxygenator and Arterial Filter in the Pig Model

The components of the CPB circuit containing the oxygenator (Bentley CM 50, 5.0 m²) and arterial filter (Bentley AF 1025, 0.5 m²: uncoated control and heparin-coated) were assembled and CPB was carried out for three hours in three groups of sixteen pigs; systemic heparin group (SHG:6); systemic heparin/heparinized circuit group (SH/HCG:5) and Iloprost (2ng/kg/min)/heparinized circuit group (IHCG:5). The details were described before[14]. The anesthesia was induced with ketamine (20 mg/kg

I.M.) and sodium pentobarbital (5-7 mg/kg I.V.)[2-6] and maintained with intravenous infusion of 0.25% sodium pentobarbital. During CPB, the activated clotting times were maintained above 400 seconds. Each animal was sacrificed by exsanguination. The radioactivity in organs (kidneys, lung, heart, brain, liver and spleen) and tissue samples was measured with the ionization chamber and gamma-counter.

C. Dynamic Measurement of Radioactivity of 111In Platelets in the Oxygenator and Arterial Filter during CPB

The radioactivity in the oxygenator and arterial filter during CPB was measured with a lead-collimated Geiger probe detector (Johnson Associates Inc.). The background radioactivity was subtracted from the total radioactivity of adherent thrombus in oxygenator and trapped embolus in the arterial filter and the net radioactivity was plotted with time of CPB.

D. Scintiphoto of Platelet Deposition with the Gamma Camera, Ionization Chamber and Gamma-well Counter

The components of the arterial filter and hollow-fiber oxygenator were removed from the circuit. The intact device and components were imaged with the gamma camera (Siemens, Gammasonics V). The radioactivity in the components was measured in the ionization chamber (Capintec CRC-5R). The samples of fibers and filter-membrane were weighed in a microbalance and the radioactivity was determined with a gamma-well counter in the 111In channel. All the detectors were calibrated with standard sources of 111In to convert the microcurie into counts/min and calculate the percent of injected dose of 111In platelets deposited in components of device, organs and tissues.

E. Algebraic Equations for Normal and Abnormal Platelet Consumption and Platelet-survival Time and Platelet Turn-over Rate

The normal consumption of single platelet will be accelerated by consumptive process of platelet adhesion, aggregation and platelet-fragmentation during CPB. The disappearance of single platelets and platelet-aggregates are described by the following equations:

$$D_{Sp} = N_{Sp}\lambda_{Sp}$$

$$\frac{dN_{Pa}}{dt} = \lambda_{Sp}N_{Sp} - \lambda_{Pa}N_{Pa}$$

$$(D_{Pa})_t = \lambda_{Pa}N_{Pa}$$

$$= \frac{\lambda_{Pa}(D_{Pa})_o(e^{-\lambda_{Sp}t} - e^{-\lambda_{Pa}t})}{(\lambda_{Pa} - \lambda_{Sp})}$$

The disappearance rate constant of single platelet, λ_{Sp}, is described by the following equation:

$dN_{Sp}/dt = D_{Sp} = -\lambda_{Sp}*N_{Sp}$; $T\frac{1}{2}$ (Single platelet for human and pig: 4-5 and 3 days); disappearance rate (D_{Sp}) is proportional to the number of single platelet (N) and λ is the rate constant.

The disappearance rate constant of platelet-aggregates, λ_{Pa}, is described by the following equation:

$$dN_{Pa}/dt = - \lambda_{Pa} * N_{Pa}$$

The net disappearance rate, λ_{Pa}, is the summation of the three embolization rates of three average size of large, medium and small emboli:

$$\lambda_{Pa} = \lambda_{Pa(S)} + \lambda_{Pa(M)} + \lambda_{Pa(L)}$$

G. Arterial Filter in Cascade with Oxygenator in CPB circuit: Steady State for Thrombosis and Embolization

After 25-35 minutes of CPB, a steady state is reached at the arterial filter, where the rate of trapping by filter is equal to that of embolization from oxygenator.

H. Analysis of Radioactivity-time Curve by Curve-stripping Technique for Estimation of Half-life and Determination of Rate Constants of Embolization

The assumptions we have made for modeling the process of platelet-thrombosis and embolization from a device are:
(1) Single platelet disappears from blood at a fixed rate with a fixed half-life and the disappearance rate (D_{Sp}) is proportional to the number of platelets.
(2) The disappearance rate of platelet-aggregate of a group in a specific size range (D_{Pa}) from a device is also proportional to the number of platelet-aggregates in the specific size range and
(3) The net disappearance rate constant for platelet-aggregates of three size range (small, medium and large) from a device is a additive process.

The normalized radioactivity-time curve [counts per min/injected 111In radioactivity (μCi)] of embolization, (the latter part of radioactivity-time curve after the peak value), can be represented by the sum of three exponential terms for 3 size of emboli and a constant A representing the level of single platelets in circulation. The net activity A(t) at time t is described by

$$A(t) = A + A_S * e^{-t*\lambda(S)} + A_M * e^{-t*\lambda(M)} + A_L * e^{-t*\lambda(L)}$$

where A_S, A_M and A_L are intercepts on the Y-axis, indicating the abundance of emboli of three average size (large:L, medium:M and small:S), A is the level of circulating single platelet and lambda-values ($\lambda(S)$, $\lambda(M)$ and $\lambda(L)$) are the corresponding rate constants of embolization. This stripping technique was applied to the embolization curve generated from oxygenator-radioactivity during CPB (Figure 1).

The simplest method of curve-fitting is by curve-peeling or stripping[12]. The tail-end portion of the semi-log plotted A(t) curve is extrapolated to t=0 to give A_L. The half-life of this straight line gives the rate constant $\lambda(L) = 0.693/T_{1/2}(L)$. The calculated values of this exponential function are subtracted from the net curve A(t) to obtain the second half-life and rate constant for medium emboli: $\lambda(M) = 0.693/T_{1/2}(M)$. The process is repeated for $\lambda(S) = 0.693/T_{1/2}(S)$, until there are no more points left. The semi-log straight line at each stage is drawn to best represent the experimental values that seem to belong to tail-end portion of that stage. Lipid-soluble 111In tropolone label randomly platelets of all ages.

RESULTS AND DISCUSSION

This dynamic embolization from oxygenator and steady state level of adherent thrombus in the arterial filter observed by continuous monitoring are shown in the schematics (Figure 1). Significant decrease of thrombus formation and embolization with Iloprost infusion was noted. These significant findings suggest that at 30-40 minutes post-CPB, the arterial filter sheds emboli at the same rate of trapping, supporting preliminary data of increased screen-filter pressure[3] at similar time frame. The half-life of thrombus relates to the time of build-up and adhesivity via the platelet-receptors and fibrinogen and the adsorbed adhesive proteins on the surface of polypropylene and polyester net-work; the final retention-time may be dependent on the extra-platelet organization, fibrinolytic activity and platelet-cytoskeleton[13].

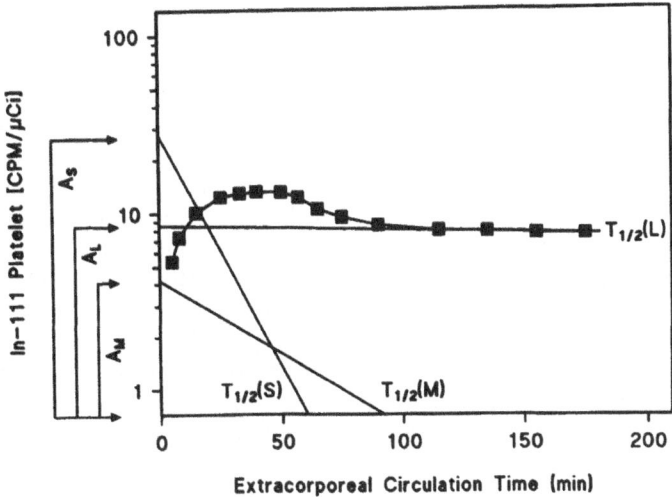

Figure 1. The curve-stripping technique for the estimation of half-life and magnitude of emboli (A) of three different size (small:S, medium:M and large:L) from oxygenator during CPB in a pig model.

The principles of computational fluid mechanics helped us in identifying the transport of cellular elements of blood, differential distribution i.e. near-wall excess of platelets and areas of disturbed flow in cardiovascular systems (bifurcation, stenosis or aneurysm) or prostheses[3, 4]. But it failed to account for the interaction of activated clotting factors adsorbed on damaged vessel wall or cardiovascular prostheses and cellular elements of blood resulting in thrombus formation and embolization[1 - 5]. The interpretation of the kinetics of platelet aggregation and embolization remains tentative in the absence of rational formulations of these two aspects of dynamic pathology. We describe a kinetic scheme to derive the rate equations for platelet aggregation and embolization; the former process was originally described by Jamaluddin and Krishnan[9]. The dynamic nature of thrombosis and embolization on cardiovascular prostheses was investigated with 111In labeled platelets by several investigators[3 - 8]. The normal values of platelet survival time and platelet turn-over rate were studied by several investigators[8].

Assuming the random probability of thrombosis and their embolization from oxygenator and arterial filter, we developed a mathematical model and defined equations to calculate the half-life and rate constant of embolization (RCE) from oxygenator and arterial filter with 111In labeled platelets, during CPB in pig model. The higher sensitivity at higher depth of field of Geiger probe over that of NaI(Tl) detector and sufficient number of adherent thrombi in 55,000 hollow-fiber and large surface area in arterial filter, provided statistical accuracy of measurements of radioactivity during CPB procedure. The exponential equations were originally developed by Rutherford and Sodee[10] and Bateman[11], for describing the probability of decay of single radionuclide and radionuclides in cascade. These type of equations are also used for describing the surviving cell-fractions post-irradiation. We pinpointed the major site of embolic complications as the arterial filter. The thrombi/meter^2 in the filter is ten-fold higher than that of oxygenator. Peak thrombus-time (25-45 min) was almost identical for both oxygenator and arterial filter, suggesting that during CPB, same thrombus-level was maintained on the arterial filter by continuous embolization at the same rate. The normalized radioactivity-time curve was stripped according to the half-life $T_{1/2}$ of clearance of emboli of different size from oxygenator and arterial filter. The sequential stripping technique resulted in 3 values of half-lives. The oxygenator embolized 42% of total thrombus with $T_{1/2}$ values of 12 min, 42 min, and 13 hr, for 3 size of emboli; $T_{1/2}$ is directly related to emboli-size and rate constant of embolization is inversely proportional to $T_{1/2}$. By direct continuous monitoring and data analysis on the basis of this model, we developed a new technique for quantitation of amount and $T_{1/2}$ of emboli from oxygenator. Maximum embolization occurred with systemic heparin, during 30-90 min period post-initiation of CPB; this is also the period of highest risk for embolization. We estimated that 2-4% of total platelets embolized at a rate of $1.2\text{-}2.4\text{X}10^6$/min with an average size of 180-210 μm, having 1 x 10^6 platelets in each aggregate, to occupy and occlude the 200 μm diameter of fiber-lumen[6].

Although the oxygenator has been perfected to a large extent, and the thrombus level dropped significantly from 20% (bubble oxygenator) to 2-3% (hollow-fiber oxygenator), no major simultaneous improvement occurred in the arterial filter (gasoline filter). The current filter uses pleated dacron (polyester hydrophobic surface) fiber network (porosity 25 μm). The accordion configuration with lateral (side-to-side) as opposed to end-to-end blood flow results in a less favorable hemorheology and thrombus-formation both inside and outside of the filter and the trapping of emboli in distal organs[5, 6]. The capacity for thrombus formation by this filter is high and the capacity for thrombus retention is low. Similar steady state also was obtained in lung tissue due to emboli-trapping and platelet-disaggregation; this process may be ongoing in the arteriole, capillary networks and venule during CPB procedure. After 30 minutes of oxygenation, the thrombus level reached a steady state. Considering the average size of platelets of 2.5 μm, about 80 platelets will almost occlude the 200 μm lumen of hollow-fiber and forbid formation of larger aggregates. Thus in the fiber-lumen, only medium size emboli (200 μm) could be generated. However, larger emboli are found to form on the exit port of oxygenator. During CPB, circulating platelets are a burden.

These emboli generated localize in the hippocampus (short-term memory loss) and other sensitive parts of brain, lung, heart and kidneys causing thromboembolic complications induced by ischemia and cell-death. The growth of platelet-aggregate depends specifically on shear rate and platelet-releasate (ADP, serotonin, thromboxane A_2 etc). By decreasing the number of platelets before CPB and redesigning the arterial filter for facilitating the dilution of these aggregating agents, the thrombosis and subsequent embolization could be significantly reduced. The radiolabeled platelets and hollow-fiber oxygenator provided simple tools for monitoring the large number of thromboembolic events to elucidate the theory of embolization.

ACKNOWLEDGEMENTS

The supports of NHLBI (Shannon Award: HL47201), Baxter Healthcare Corporation, Department of Energy grant DE-FG05-88ER60728 and Florida High Technology and Industry Council are gratefully acknowledged. The expertise of James S. Robertson, M.D.,Ph.D. in the modeling calculations was highly appreciated. The authors appreciate the assistance of Messers. Bob Burke and Kennneth R. Kitchens in making the photographs.

REFERENCES

1. Kirklin JK, Kirklin JW. Cardiopulmonary bypass for cardiac surgery. Chapter 32, Vol II; In "Surgery of the Chest". Eds. Sabiston DC and Spencer FC. Saunders Co. Philadelphia, 1990; pp 1107-1125.
2. Guidoin RG, Kenedi RM, Galleti P, et al. Thrombus formation and microaggregate removal during extracorporeal membrane oxygenation. *J Biomed Mat Res* 13: 317-335 (1979).
3. Folie BJ, McIntire LV. Mathematical analysis of mural thrombogenesis: concentration profiles of platelet-activating agents and effects of viscous shear flow. *Biophysical J.* 56: 1121-1141 (1989).
4. Goldsmith HL, Turitto VT. Rheological aspects of thrombosis and haemostasis. Basic principles and applications. *Thromb Haemostsis.* 55: 415-535 (1986).
5. Dewanjee MK, Vogel SR, Peterson KA, et al. Quantitation of platelet consumption on oxygenator and stabilization of platelet membrane with prostacyclin and ibuprofen during cardiopulmonary bypass surgery in dogs. *Trans ASAIO* XXVII: 197-202 (1981).
6. Dewanjee MK, Palatianos GM, Kapadvanjwala M, et al. Rate constant of embolization and quantitation of emboli from hollow-fiber oxygenator and arterial filter during cardiopulmonary bypass. *ASAIO Journal* 39: M317-M321 (1992).
7. Dewanjee MK, Rao SA, Didisheim P: Indium-111 tropolone, a new high affinity platelet label:Preparation and evaluation of labeling parameters. *J Nucl Med* 22:981-987 (1981).
8. Robertson JS, Ezekowitz MD, Dewanjee MK, Lotter MG, Watson EE. Radiation absorbed dose estimates for radioindium labeled autologous platelets (MIRD Dose Estimate No. 15). *J Nucl Med* 33: 777-780 (1991).
9. Jamaluddin MP, Krishnan LK. A rate equation for blood platelet aggregation. *J theor Biol* 129: 257-261 (1987).
10. Rutherford E and Soddy F. The cause and nature of radioactivity. Part I. *Phil Mag* 4: 370-396 (1902).
11. Bateman H. Solution of a system of differential equations occurring in the theory of radio-active transformations. *Proc Cambridge Phil Soc* 15: 423-427 (1910).
12. Lassen NA and Perl W. Compartmental analysis, Chap. 10, in Tracer kinetic methods in medical physiology. Eds. Lassen NA and Perl W. Raven Press, N.Y., pp 137-155, 1979.
13. Dewanjee MK. Platelet consumption in health and disease. (ISORBE Proc., Barcelona, 1992).

THE FATE OF EMBOLI POST-RECANALIZATION OF THROMBUS-OCCLUDED ARTERY AND VEIN IN YORKSHIRE PIGS

M.K. Dewanjee, G. Panoutsopolous, M. Kapadvanjwala, W. Ganz, A.N. Serafini, G. N. Sfakianakis and R. Diaz[1]

Departments of Radiology, Surgery and Biomedical Engineering University of Miami, School of Medicine, Miami, FL USA
[1]Dow Corning Wright Theratek Inc., Miami Lakes, Miami, FL USA

SUMMARY

Aged thrombi (4-day old) could neither be disaggregated by thrombolytic enzymes nor removed by balloon thrombectomy. Metabolic fate of thrombi post-recanalization was determined with 111In labeled platelets. Aged (4-day) labeled platelet-emboli were induced in the femoral, carotid artery and jugular vein in twelve Yorkshire pigs. The thrombi were pulverized with a high speed impeller (80,000 RPM) and the debri generated were flushed with the effluent with heparinized saline and allowed to localize in the down-stream perfusion beds of lungs, liver, legs or brain. The debri generated during recanalization of occluded vessels were also analysed for size distribution by differential filtration (5, 12, 75, 500 and 1000 μm) and radioactivity was determined with a Geiger probe. Autologous platelets were labeled with 111In tropolone (400-500 μCi); 111In labeled platelet-thrombi were induced by thrombin addition in segments (4-5 cm of ligated vessels in femoral/carotid artery and jugular vein. The residual thrombi were monitored with a Geiger probe and gamma counter. The emboli in the leg-muscle, lungs and brain were imaged with a gamma camera and quantified with an ionization chamber. Filtration indicated the average size of emboli (75 μm). Most of debri from the jugular vein were found in the lungs and liver. Small amount of debri from carotid and femoral artery was found in brain and leg muscle respectively. Labeled platelets provided a simple technique for determination of the fate of emboli generated by recanalization in the pig model.

INTRODUCTION

Despite impressive achievements in the reduction of cardiovascular mortality and the decrease in the incidence of atherosclerosis due to improved nutrition and preventive care, thrombosis and atherosclerosis remain the number one cause of death in western countries. Although thrombectomy, balloon angioplasty and atherectomy devices are extensively used in 600,000 patients every year, the reocclusion rate of (30-35)% is high[1, 2]. For the recanalization of vessel or synthetic vascular graft occluded by thrombi, concerns remain about the complications of ischemic damage induced by the size and amount of debri generated by the thrombectomy device[1, 2, 10 - 13].

The objective of this study is to determine the distribution and fate of emboli generated by mechanical thrombolysis with 111In labeled platelets. This tracer was successfully used in a variety of cardiovascular prostheses for quantificaion of thrombi and drug interventional studies. Although the acutely formed thrombi (within 6-8 hours), could be dissolved by thrombolytic therapy with streptokinase and tissue plasminogen activator or removed by balloon thrombectomy, the aged thrombi (5-7 days old) could not be degraded or removed by either of the techniques and the occluded vessel could be recanalyzed only by mechanical thrombolysis with a rotating thrombolytic catheter which generates small emboli (70-100 μm). The high-speed rotating (60,000-100,000 RPM) catheter (Dow Corning Wright Theratek) with an elliptical stainless cam/impeller is fitted with a helical drive shaft powered by a motor. The cam/impeller pulverizes and emulsifies the thrombi into microparticles that are washed out by the sterile buffer; these microparticles localize at the distal vascular bed till they get wedged; ultimately they are broken down into smaller aggregates and metabolized by the phagocytic cells. Another high speed catheter (Rotablator™, Heart Technology) with diamond-tipped brass burr is being evaluated for atherectomy by several medical centers. Considering the size of the catheter tip (4 Fr-8 Fr), they sould be able to make lumen of 0.5-1.5 mm in thrombosed vessels (small artery, vein and A-V shunt).

The metabolic fate and quantitation of their distribution in the distal perfusion bed (distal limb or brain, in the case of artery or pulmonary bed in the case of venous occlusion) is not known. Twelve pigs in two groups (4-day aging in the femoral and carotid artery and vein group) will be used in this protocol.

MATERIALS AND METHODS

The healthy Yorkshire pigs weighing 25-30 kg (age 4-5 months old, male or female) were used for the thrombolysis study. Swine coagulation, fibrinolytic systems and complement system are similar to those of the human. Also, swine blood reacts to systemic heparinization in a similar manner as the human blood[3]. The animals were sacrificed with an overdose of barbiturate and biodistribution was quantified with a gamma counter. This study was conducted in accordance with the requirements of the Good Laboratory Practice (GLP) regulations, 21 GFR 58. The pigs were immobilized with ketamine (25 mg/kg, IM) and anesthetized with Na-pentobarbital (30 mg/kg).

GENERAL METHODS OF RADIOLABELING AND MAPPING OF THROMBI AND EMBOLI

A(i). Autologous Platelet Labeling with 111Indium-Tropolone

Three hours prior to the vessel ligation, the platelets of each pig were labeled with 111Indium tropolone according to the method of Dewanjee et al.[4]; 43 mls of whole blood from each pig were collected in 7 ml of modified ACD anticoagulant solution (NIH-A, Fenwal Lab); 111Indium-chloride was were mixed with 25 micrograms of tropolone (Aldrich Chemical Co.) in 25 microliters of sterile isotonic saline. The platelets were incubated with 800-1000 μCi of 111In tropolone (Amersham

Inc., Arlington Heights, IL) for 20 minutes. The free 111In was removed by centrifugation at 1500 G for 10 minutes. The platelet harvesting efficiency of 40-45% and labeling efficiency of 80-95% were routinely obtained by the above mentioned procedures in our laboratory[5-7].

A(ii). Ligation of Vessels and Formation of Aged Thrombi in the Ligated Vessels with Thrombin

The pig was anesthetized, the femoral and neck areas were sterilized with betadine; incisions were made in the groins and neck and femoral artery, femoral vein, common carotid artery and jugular vein (6 cm long, 3-4 mm ID) in Yorkshire pigs were isolated. The adventitia of vessels was cleaned and the small branches are ligated by silk sutures. The distal and proximal ends of vessel was ligated with two silk sutures. The blood was aspirated and mixed with autologous 111In platelets (250-350 μCi) were injected in the middle of lumen of each ligated vessel with a 22 G needle; 100 units of thrombin (0.2 ml, Sigma Chemical Co., St. Louis), were added. The suture around the needle (22 G) was pulled to prevent leakage and left in place for a period of aging (4-day). The skin incisions were closed with silk sutures and animal was allowed to recuperate for 4 days. The legs, heart, brain, liver, spleen and kidneys and lungs were imaged at 3, 6, 24, 48, 72 and 96 hours with a gamma camera (Siemens Inc., Gammasonics V, IL). The camera spectrometer was adjusted to include the 151- and 245-keV photo-peaks of 111In radionuclide.

A(iii). Recanalization of Occluded Vessels with Theratek Catheter in the Yorkshire Pig Model

After 4 days of thrombus-aging, the thrombotic occlusion was opened up by mechanical thrombolysis. The pig was anesthetized, and ligated vessels were isolated. Sutures were placed around the vessels to lift and align them properly for recanalization. Small incision was made in the neck of the ligated vessel and the catheter was introduced via a catheter sheath introducer. During the operation, the heparinized saline (10 IU/ml) was infused through the catheter at a rate of 10 ml/min; after thrombolysis, the debri were flushed at a rate of 0-60 ml/min with a flush volume of 0-60 ml. Actual run times in these groups of pigs ranged from 50-586 seconds. The tip of the thrombolysis catheter was placed in front of the occluded vessel and the system was programmed to rotate at 80,000 RPM and reversed; in some studies of smaller vessels, we started with smaller catheter (Fr 5) and changed to a larger size catheter (Fr 8). The forward and reverse movement was continued for 2-3 minutes, till 50-80% of the thrombi was removed from ligated vessel. The loss of radioactivity was monitored with the Geiger probe and gamma camera. During thrombolysis, the rate of thrombus removal and build-up of emboli at the distal muscle bed, lung or brain were monitored with a Geiger probe. The animal was sacrificed with an overdose of barbiturate and organs were harvested, weighed with a balance (Mettler). The samples of tissues were taken and the radioativity was measured with a gamma counter. The calculation of biodistribution was carried out with a spread-sheet (LOTUS 123) and IBM PS/2.

A(iv). Size Distribution of Emboli Generated by Trac Wright Catheter Using Differential Filtration Technique

The ligated vessels, suspended in phosphate-buffered saline were placed on a horizontal mount and recanalized. The effluent suspension was collected in a teflon flask and sequentially filterred with filters of different porosity (Spectrum and Poretics Inc., 5, 12, 70, 500 and 1000 μm). The radioactivity on the filters was measured with the calibrated Geiger probe and the percent of distribution was calculated with a IBM PS/2 computer.

RESULTS AND DISCUSSION

The size distribution of radiolabeled platelet-emboli on filters of different porosity post-recanailzation of 4-day thrombi is shown in Figure 1. The amount of 111In labeled platelets retained post-mechanical recanalization of ligated vessels varied between 30-65%. No regional hot spot of significance in the cerebral perfusion bed for major arteries was identified by embolization of 111In labeled platelet-emboli from the ligated carotid artery.

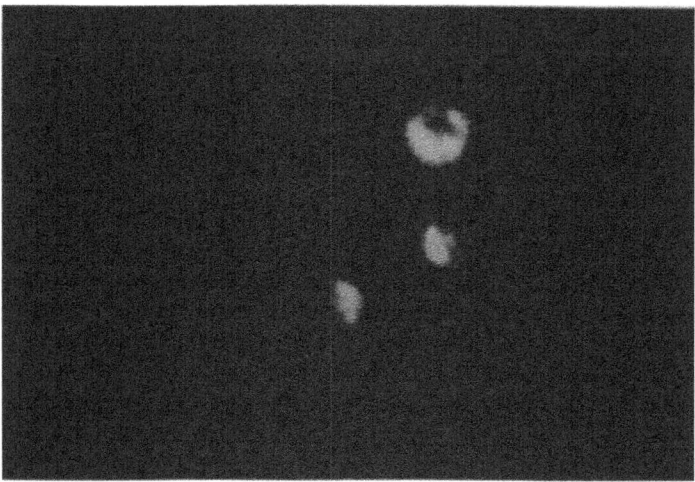

Figure 1. Distribution of radiolabeled platelet-emboli on filters of different porosity, post-recanalization of 4-day thrombi. Note higher amount of thrombi retained on the 75 μm filter.

The distribution in the legs, brain and lung was uniform suggesting the trapping of small emboli. No hot spot was observed in the scintiphotos of lung, pelvis and brain (0.08%). Liver uptake was higher than lung uptake (2.2%), suggesting that smaller emboli (< 10-12 μm) escaped trapping by the capillary networks of lungs. Similar results were obtained from the histogram of radioactivity distribution on the filters of different porosity (Figure 1). The majority of the particles were of the average size of 75 μm[10-13]. The catheter should always be in the center of the lumen to avoid wall-perforation. Although no thrombolytic enzymes were used, small emboli were generated which spontaneously resolved without ischemic damage. This catheter may provide a new tool for the removal of emboli from A-V shunt or occluded vessels.

REFERENCES

1. Simpson JB, Selmon MR, Robertson GC et al. Transluminal atherectomy for occlusive peripheral vascular disease. *Am J Cardiol* 61: 96G-101G (1988).
2. Tobis JM, Smolin M, Mallery J, MacLeay L. Laser-assisted thermal angioplasty in human peripheral artery occlusions: mechanisms of recanalization. *J Amer Coll Cardiol* 13:1547-1554 (1989).
3. Addonizio VP Jr, Edmunds LH Jr, Colman RW. The function of monkey (M. mulatta) platelets compared to platelets of pig, sheep and man. *J Lab Clin Med* 91:989-997 (1978).
4. Dewanjee MK, Rao SA, Didisheim P: Indium-111 tropolone, a new high affinity platelet label: Preparation and evaluation of labeling parameters. *J Nucl Med* 22:981-987 (1981).
5. Dewanjee MK: Methods of assessments of thrombosis in vivo. Blood in Contact with Natural and Artificial Surfaces. Vol. 516, Theme 4, Part one. Eds. Leonard EF, Vroman L, Turitto VT. New York Academy of Science, New York, N.Y. 1987, pp. 541-571.
6. Dewanjee MK, Fuster V, Rao SA, Forshaw PL, Kaye MP: Noninvasive radioisotopic technique for detection of platelet deposition on mitral valve prostheses and quantitation of visceral microembolism in dogs. *Mayo Clin Proc* 58:307-314 (1983).
7. Dewanjee MK, Tago M, Josa M, Fuster V, Kaye MP: Quantification of platelet retention in aortocoronary femoral vein bypass graft in dogs treated with dipyridamole and aspirin. *Circulation* 69:350-356 (1984).
8. Kessler C, Kelly AB, Suggs WD, Weissman JD, Epstein CM, Hanson SR, Harker LA. Induction of transient neurologic dysfunction in baboons by platelet microemboli. *Stroke* 23:697-702 (1992).
9. Dewanjee S, Dewanjee, Dietrich WD, Prado R, Watson BD, Dewanjee MK. Direct method of quantitation of platelet-embolus and residence time in brain with radiolabeled platelets formed by photodenudation of endothelial cells of carotid artery in a rat model. Proc. ISORBE, Barcelona, 1992.
10. Salinas-Zeballos ME, Zeballos GA, Gootman P. A stereotactic atlas of pig brain. Swine in Biomedical Research, Vol 2, Plenum Press, New York, 1985; pp 887-906.
11. Snyder SO, Wheeler JR, Gregory TR, Gayle RG and Parent FN. Peripheral vascular experience with the Trac-Wright atherectomy device.
12. Desbrosses D, Petit H, Torres E, Barrionuevo D, Figueroa A, Wenger JJ, Ramenah B and Kieny R. Percutaneous atherectomy with the Kensey catheter: Early and midterm results in femoropopliteal occlusions unsuitable for conventional angioplasty. Proc. of Annual Meeting of Societe de Chirurgie Vasculaire de Langue Francaise, June 23-24, 1989. *Annals of Vasc Surg* 4: 550-552 (1990).
13. Schmitz-Rode T and Gunther RW. Percutaneous mechanical thrombolysis. A comparative study of various rotational catheter systems. *Invest Radiol* 26(6): 557-563 (1991).
14. Kensey KR, Nash JE, Abrahams C and Zarins CK. Recanalization of obstructed arteries with a flexible, rotating tip catheter. *Radiology* 165(2): 387-389 (1987).

DIRECT METHOD OF QUANTITATION OF PLATELET-EMBOLUS AND RESIDENCE TIME IN BRAIN WITH RADIOLABELED PLATELETS FORMED BY PHOTODENUDATION OF ENDOTHELIAL CELLS OF CAROTID ARTERY IN A RAT MODEL

S. Dewanjee, W.D. Dietrich, R. Prado, B.D. Watson and M.K. Dewanjee

Departments of Neurology and Radiology
University of Miami School of Medicine
Miami, Florida, USA

ABSTRACT

Platelet-thrombus was induced in Wistar rat (300-350 gm) model by photoactivation of common carotid artery. Heterologous blood were collected in ACD-anticoagulant and platelets were separated and labeled with 111In tropolone; 50-100 μCi of 111In platelets were infused in anesthetized rats and carotid injury was induced for 6 minutes of laser-irradiation at 20-30 minutes of equilibration time. The rats were heparinized and sacrificed by decapitation at 30 and 180 minutes after injury and brain was removed and sectioned for measurement of regional radioactivity. The sections were weighed in a microbalance and radioactivity was measured in a gamma-counter in the 111In channel. The ratios of normalized radioactivity of 16 sections of brain to blood are higher in the thrombus-trapping areas of middle cerebral arteries. The ratio of radioactivity of right to left brain (control) and platelet-density per gram of tissue was calculated. The ratios at 15 minutes was higher in the posterior brain and similar values at 180 minutes, suggesting that these emboli may not resolve without pharmacological intervention with fibrinolytic agents. This tracer technique provided a simple technique for monitoring the size of thrombus, their cerebral distribution, right/left assymetry and residence time providing a baseline for interventional therapy.

INTRODUCTION

Although 111In labeled platelets were used in a variety of studies in animal models and patients[1-4], to localize the site of thrombus formation, no quantitative study was carried to trace the emboli. Previous studies of experimentally induced brain ischemia in the rat model have provided morphological evidence of blood brain barrier alteration[5-9]. Quantification of embolization in the rat brain has been accomplished by photochemical damage of vascular endothelium and subsequent intravenous administration of 111Indium-tropolone labeled platelets in the rat. Because of the existence of thrombolytic substances produced by the endothelial cells released into the blood, it was hypothesized that embolization will decrease with time spontaneously[9].

The regional emboli-distribution in rat brain formed from thrombus formed on carotid artery was never quantified. The 111indium labeled platelets provide a simple and sensitive technique for measurement of platelet-distribution and estimation of cerebral emboli as a focal point of higher radioactivity. The suitable gamma ray energies of 111In also permits non-invasive imaging of cerebral distribution of emboli and residence time in rat and human brain and evaluation of pharmacological intervention on the extent of embolization and reduction of ischemic brain injury. The abundance of low energy conversion and Auger electrons generated in the vicinity of the 111In labeled emboli provide high resolution autoradiography[10-13].

MATERIALS AND METHODS

A. Platelet Labeling with 111In-Tropolone

Heterologous platelets of rats were labeled according the method of Dewanjee et al.[1]. Sterility was maintained throughout the following procedure. A total of 36 mL of blood were withdrawn from two male Wistar rats (250-400g) into two 30 mL syringes containing a total of 6 mL of acid citrate dextrose (ACD) solution (maintaining a 6:1 ratio of whole blood to ACD). The whole blood was centrifuged for 10 minutes at 200 g, and the supernate, platelet enriched plasma (PEP), was transferred to a conical centrifuge tube with a pipet. The PEP was centrifuged for 10 minutes at 1600 g, and the supernate was discarded. The platelet pellet was resuspended in 1 mL of ACD/saline; 25 μg of tropolone were added to 200 μCi of 111In chloride in a conical centrifuge tube and vortexed. The resuspended platelets were added to 111In-tropolone and allowed to incubate for 30 minutes at room temperature after resuspending in an additional 1 mL of ACD/saline solution. The suspension of labeled platelets was centrifuged at 1600 g for 10 minutes, the supernate was removed and saved for calculating labeling efficiency, and the platelet pellet was resuspended in 3 mL of ACD/saline solution. After centrifugation at 1600 g for 10 minutes, the supernate was removed and saved for calculating labeling efficiency; the labeled platelets were resuspended in 2 mL of ACD/saline solution. A 1 mL fraction of the 111In labeled platelets per rat was withdrawn into a 10 mL syringe. The remaining fraction of labeled platelets was saved to determine harvesting efficiency by platelet count with a Coulter counter. The radioactivity of labeled platelets was measured with an ionization chamber.

B. Photochemical Activation with Rose Bengal and Denudation

Twelve heparinized male Wistar rats weighing between 250 and 300 g in four groups were used in this protocol. Rats were initially anesthetized with 3% halothane for 3-5 minutes, and maintained on 1.5% halothane and a mixture of 70% nitrous oxide-30% oxygen delivered by a closely fitting face mask. Femoral artery and venous catheters were inserted for the measurement of arterial blood pressure and blood gases and for fluid administration. The right common carotid artery (CCA) of rats were exposed using an operating microscope. Rats were intubated and mechanically ventilated. The rats were placed on their back, and the exposed CCA was aligned with the beam of a tunable argon laser (514.5 nm, peak power = 1.5 W). The 111In-tropolone labeled platelets were injected and allowed to incubate for 25 minutes. The photosensitizing dye, rose bengal (40 mg/kg in 0.9% saline), was injected. The CCA was irradiated with the laser for 6 minutes. Ten minutes (or 2 hours and 55 minutes) after irradiation, 5 mL of blood was withdrawn from the rat and saved to determine platelet counts and free Indium levels. Rats were then heparinized to prevent post-mortem clot formation and sacrificed with an overdose of halothane (3%).

C. Measurement of Regional Radioactivity in Rat Brain

After sacrificing the rats, the segments of carotid arteries and brain were sponged to remove adherent blood. Five millimeter segments were surgically removed from the left (control) and right (irradiated) CCA of the rats, and placed in gamma counter tubes. The brain was carefully removed and dissected into 16 sections (Table 1, 8 in the left hemishpere and 8 in the right hemisphere). These tissues along with samples of heart, lungs, liver, spleen, kidneys, and leg muscle were harvested, weighed in a microbalance, and measured for radioactivity in the gamma counter (Cobra II, model 5003, Packard Inc.,). The percent of injected dose and ratios of radioactivity in left and right hemispheres were calculated.

D. Autoradiography of Platelet Emboli in Rat Brain

After sacrificing the rats, the brains were carefully removed from the skull and frozen over liquid nitrogen. Frozen sections (10 μm) were made in a cryostat and exposed to Kodak SB-5 x-ray film for 5-7 days. The film was developed and fixed[13]. The regional density of the foci of platelet-emboli on the ipsilateral and contralateral sections at 5 levels of 12.2-, 9.7-, 6.2- and 2.7 mm anterior and posterior to the interaural line of brain was determined by counting the silver grains with a dissecting microscope[7, 8].

RESULTS AND DISCUSSION

The distribution of emboli in 4 groups of rat brain (15 min control, 180 min control, 15 min irradiated and 180 min irradiated) is determined by measurement of radioactivity and autoradiography. The regional radioactivity in sections of rat brain (Frontal cortex:FC, Frontal-parietal coretc:FPC, Striatum:Str, Posterior occipital cortex: POC, hippocampus:Hip, Thalamus:Thal, Cerebellum:cereb, Brain stem:BSt) at 15 and 180 min post-irradiation is shown below (Table 1):

Table 1

RB/LB	FC	FPC	Str	POC	Hip	Thal	Cereb	BSt
15 min	1.6	1.73	1.40	1.46	2.35	1.17	1.24	1.14
180 min	1.05	1.22	1.43	1.40	1.00	1.15	0.83	1.00

The regional radioactivity, specifically in the regions of middle cerebral artery, increases from baseline values due to trapping of emboli; in a similar fashion, the right/left assymetry also represents higher level of trapping of emboli in the right hemispheres than left hemispheres due to injury induced in the right carotid artery.

Regional platelet distribution in cerebral hemispheres is almost uniform in control rats giving rise to a ratio of the radioactivity/gram of right to left brain of unity. In the photodenuded group (right carotid artery) of rats at 15 minutes, this ratio is higher than 1.5-2.5, indicating higher embolus trapping in the zones of frontal cortex and hippocampus

Table 2. The energy and abundant of photons and electrons in the decay of 111In radionuclide; the abundance low energy electrons are suitable for high resolution autoradiography[12]

	Average energy (MeV)	Yield/decay	Range (microns)
γ_1	1.71E-01	9.06E-01	
γ_2	2.45E-01	9.37E-01	
IC 1 K	1.45E-01	8.24E-02	2.05E+02
IC 1 L	1.67E-01	1.00E-02	2.72E+02
IC 2 M,N...	1.71E-01	1.40E-03	2.83E+02
IC 2 K	2.19E-01	5.21E-02	5.20E+02
IC 2 L	2.41E-01	9.10E-03	6.09E+02
IC 2 M,N...	2.45E-01	1.90E-03	6.22E+02
Auger KLL	1.91E-02	1.03E-01	8.21E+00
Auger KLX	2.23E-02	3.94E-02	1.08E+01
Auger KXY	2.55E-02	3.60E-03	1.36E+01
CK LLX	1.83E-04	1.51E-01	8.69E-03
Auger LMM	2.59E-03	8.35E-01	2.87E-01
Auger LMX	3.06E-03	1.90E-01	3.75E-01
Auger LXY	3.53E-03	1.09E-02	4.73E-01
CK MMX	1.25E-04	9.15E-01	6.35E-03
Auger MXY	3.50E-04	2.09E+00	1.64E-02
CK NNX	3.88E-05	2.54E+00	2.50E-03
Auger NXY	8.47E-06	7.82E+00	2.51E-04
X-ray K_{A1}	2.32E-02	4.63E-01	
X-ray K_{A2}	2.30E-02	2.40E-01	
X-ray K_{B1}	2.61E-02	7.88E-02	
X-ray K_{B2}	2.66E-02	1.86E-02	
X-ray K_{B3}	2.61E-02	3.82E-02	
X-ray K_{B5}	2.63E-02	1.10E-03	
X-ray L	3.23E-03	4.99E-02	
X-ray M	3.56E-04	3.00E-03	

Total yield of Auger and CK electrons per decay = 14.7
Total yield of IC electrons per decay = 0.16
Total yield x-rays per decay = 0.89
Total yield of γ-rays per decay = 1.84 Total energy released per decay = 419205 eV
Auger and CK energy released per decay = 6750 eV
IC energy released per decay = 25957 eV
X-ray energy released per decay = 19966 eV
γ-ray energy released per decay = 366532 eV

(sensitive to ischemia). The radioactivity ratio is lower in most of the hemispheres at 3 hours post photodenudation, suggesting the spontaneous resolution of emboli by endogenous platelet-disaggregating agents and vasodilators.

In addition to the low and medium energy gamma rays of 171 and 245 keV, the decay of 111In radionuclide results in an abundant number of medium and low energy conversion and Auger electrons[10-12]. The radionuclide has high photon abundance (percent, % of photons and electrons are indicated in parentheses) with gamma rays of 171.3(90.5%) and 245(94.0%) keV. Although the conversion [144.6(8.4%), 168(1.3%), 218.6(5.0%), 242.1(1%)] and Auger electrons [18.57-25.44(14%), 3.0-3.7(31%), 2.5-3.5(73%), 0.51(191%)] and x-rays 23.1(68%), 26.2(14.6%) increase radiation dose in clinical studies, the low energy electrons are superb for high resolution autoradiography (Table 2). These low energy electrons have ranges in tissue of 0.0025-622 μm[12] and the number of electrons are 14.7 per decay; majority are Auger and Coster-Kronig electrons; only 0.16% are conversion electrons. The brain of thrombosed rats at 15 min of photo-irradiation, demonstarted dense radioactivity overlying the pial surface and brain parenchyma; platelet-emboli appeared bilaterally in the frontal cortex. In the posterior sections, the emboli were seen primarily in the areas of brain perfused by the irradiated right common carotid artery. The level of platelet-emboli reduced significantly in the 180 min group, probably due to resolution of loosely adherent emboli.

The knowledge of the regional emboli distribution and residence time of emboli in the rat brain, will permit pharmacological interventional studies for enhancing the early embolus-dissolution sparing the ischemic brain tissue[16].

Since the spatial therapeutical window is short (5 minutes) in ischemic brain, this tracer technique and the data-base of emboli distribution and residence time in the rat model will play a critical role in future mechanistic and interventional studies promoting drug development for patients undergoing stroke.

This direct technique of emboli-localization in rat brain with 111In labeled platelets suggest that thrombi in common carotoid artery predispose them to the zones of middle cerebral artery and frontal cortex. The thrombus formed by laser-induced photodenudation are relatively small in size and emboli trapped reslove in a period of less than 3 hours suggesting that platelet-disaggregating agents in vivo (endothelial derived relaxation factor: EDRF, prostacyclin, plasmin, etc.) may play a protective role in reduction of ischemic brain damage by emboli.

REFERENCES

1. Dewanjee MK, Rao SA, Didisheim P. Indium-111 tropolone,a new   high affinity platelet label: Preparation and evaluation of labeling parameters. *J Nucl Med* 22:981-987 (1981).
2. Pumphrey CW, Fuster V, Dewanjee MK, Chesebro JH, Vlietstra RE, Kaye MP: Comparison of the antithrombotic action of calcium antagonist drugs with dipyridamole in dogs. *Amer. J. Cardiol* 51: 591-595 (1983).
3. Dewanjee MK, Fuster V, Rao SA, Forshaw PL, Kaye MP: Noninvasive radioisotopic technique for detection of platelet deposition on mitral valve prostheses and quantitation of visceral microembolism in dogs. *Mayo Clin Proc* 58:307-314 (1983).
4. Dewanjee MK: Methods of assessments of thrombosis in vivo. Blood in contact with natural and artificial surfaces. Vol. 516, Theme 4, Part one. Eds. Leonard EF, Vroman L, Turitto VT. New York Academy of Science, New York, N.Y. 1987, pp. 541-571.
5. Nagashima G, Nowak TS, Joo F, Ikeda J, Ruetzler C, Lohr J, Klatzo I. The role of the blood-brain barrier in ischemic brain lesions. Chapter 29, In Pathophysiology of the Blood-Brain Barrier. Fernstrom Foundation Series. Eds, Johansson BB, Owman C and Widner H. Elsevier Amsterdam 1990, pp 311-321.
6. Watson BD, Dietrich WD, Prado R, Ginsberg MD. Argon laser-induced arterial photothrombosis. *J Neurosurg* 66: 748-754 (1987).
7. Dietrich WD, Prado R, Watson BD, Nakayama H: Middle cerebral artery thrombosis: Acute blood-brain barrier alterations. *J Neuropath Exp Neurol* 47:, 443-451 (1988).
8. Dietrich WD, Prado R, Watson BD, Busto R, Ginsberg MD. Hemodynamic consequences of common carotid artery thrombosis and thrombogenically activated blood in rats. *J Cereb Blood Flow Metabol* 11: 957-965 (1991).
9. Kessler C, Kelly AB, Suggs WD, Weissman JD, Epstein CM, Hanson SR, Harker LA. Induction of transient neurologic dysfunction in baboons by platelet microemboli. *Stroke* 23:697-702 (1992).
10. Jonsson B-A, Strand S-E, Larsson BS. A quantitative autoradiographic study of the heterogenous activity distribution of different ^{111}In-labeled radiopharmaceuticals in rat tissues. *J Nucl Med* 33: 1825-1835 (1992).
11. Sparrman P, Marelius A, Sundstrom T, Petterson H. Conversion coefficients of transitions in ^{111}Cd by a new precision method. *Zeit Physik* 192: 439-448 (1966).
12. Howell RW. Radiation spectra for Auger-electron emitting radionuclides: Report No. 2 of AAPM Nuclear Medicine Task Group 6`. *Medical Physics* 19: 1371-1383 (1992).

13. Dewanjee MK. Autoradiography of live and dead cells in tissue culture with Tc-99m tetracycline. *J Nucl Med* 16: 315-317 (1975).

14. Paxinos G, Watson C. The rat brain in stereotaxic coordinates. Academic Press, New York, 1982.

15. Andrews RK, Fox JEB. Platelet receptors in hemostasis. *Current Opinion in Cell Biology.* 2: 894-901 (1990).

16. Lie JT. Pathology of occlusive disease of the extracranial arteries. In "Occlusive cerebrovascular disease. Diagnosis and surgical management." Ed. TM Sundt. WB Saunders Co. 1987, pp 19-37.

MULTICOMPARTMENTAL COMPUTER ANALYSIS OF 111In-TROPOLONE LABELLED BLOOD PLATELET KINETIC DATA IN NORMAL HUMANS

M.A. Sweetlove[1], H.F. Kotzé, M.G. Lötter[1], P.N. Badenhorst, J.P. Roodt and H. Pieters

Department of Haematology
[1]Department of Biophysics
University of the Orange Free State
Bloemfontein, South Africa

INTRODUCTION

Scintillation camera imaging of the in vivo distribution of platelets labelled with 111In has become a routine investigative procedure. Computer assisted image analysis further enables one to determine the radioactivity in an organ and to quantify the percentage of whole body radioactivity in that organ[1]. The limitation of imaging is that, within an organ, there is no distinction between platelets that are functional from those that have been injured during collection, or have been sequestrated[1,2]. Since imaging cannot distinguish between these components of organ radioactivity, we used compartmental

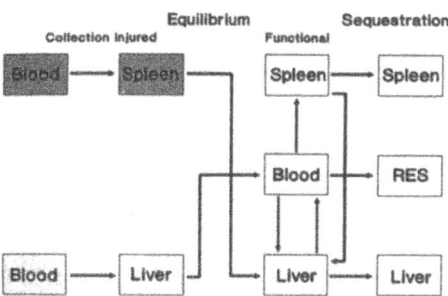

Figure 1. Compartmental model to simulate platelet movement in the body during both the equilibrium and sequestration phases. In Model 1, no compartment were included that simulated collection injured platelets. It was assumed that labelled platelets will equilibrate between the blood and the spleen and liver, and that labelled platelets from the spleen will enter the blood via the liver. Model 2 included a compartment to simulate collection injured platelets in the liver where they will accumulate transiently. Model 3 included compartments to simulate collection injured platelets in both the spleen and liver, and injured platelets in the spleen will enter the blood via the liver.

analysis (Figure 1) in order to attempt to quantify the contribution of each of the components to organ radioactivity. The SAAM program (simulation analysis and modelling) was used for this purpose.

METHODS AND RESULTS

Platelet kinetic data from 5 normal human subjects were used. Autologous platelets were labelled with 111In-tropolone and reinjected[2]. Standard methods were used to determine the mean platelet lifespan and in vivo distribution of the labelled platelets[1, 2].

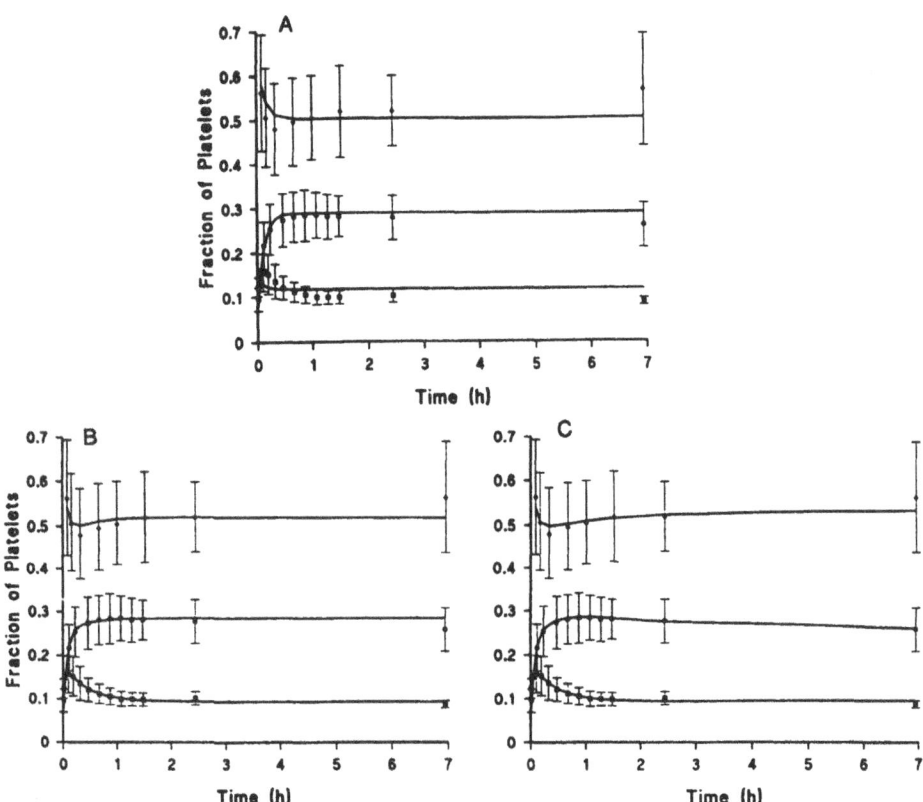

Figure 2. Simulation of the equilibrium phase with Models 1(A), 2(B), and 3 (C). The data points represent the mean experimental data (± 1 SEM) and the curves the simulated data.

When reinjected, labelled platelets redistribute between blood and organs until equilibrium between circulating and injected labelled platelets are reached. Some platelets accumulate transiently in the liver as a result of the collection injury (Figure 2). As labelled platelets age in the circulation, the senescent platelets are selectively sequestered by the macrophages of the monocyte-macrophage system, and thus disappear from the circulation (Figures 3). To simulate this, the platelet kinetic data were analysed in two phases. The first phase, the equilibrium phase, included the data that were measured

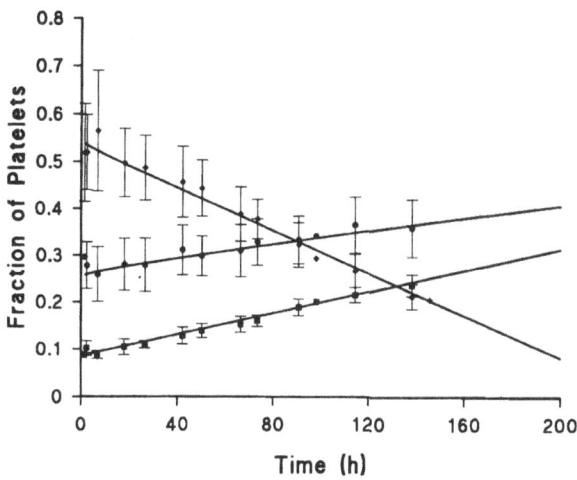

Figure 3. Simulation of the sequestration phase. The mean experimental data (± 1 SEM) is represented by the data points and the simulated data by the curves.

during the first 7 hours following reinjection of the labelled platelets (Figure 2). The second, the sequestration phase, included the data that were measured from 7 hours until the end of the platelet lifespan (Figure 3).

The first model (Model 1) that was used to simulate the equilibrium phase was rather simple. We assumed that platelets distribute from the blood to the spleen and liver, and that platelets re-enter the blood from the spleen via the liver (Figure 1). No compartment to simulate the movement of collection injured platelets was included. The fit of this model is given in Figure 2A. This model did not simulate the data well. In the second model (Model 2) a compartment to simulate the movement of collection injured platelets in the liver was added (Figure 1). Thus, collection injured platelet will accumulate transiently in the liver. The fit of this model is given in Figure 2B. Spleen and liver radioactivity, but not heart radioactivity, was simulated well. The third model (Model 3) included a compartment to simulate the movement of collection injured in both the spleen and the liver (Figure 1). Inclusion of this compartment improved simulation of heart radioactivity (Figure 2C). The constants obtained from the SSAM program with Model 3 gave the kinetics of labelled platelets through the spleen and liver. Accordingly, approximately 20% of the labelled platelets were collection injured. Of these, 10 % (range 5- 16%) accumulated transiently in the liver, and their transit time was 29 min (range 20-38 min). The normal transit time of platelets through the liver was 0.3 min. Nine per cent (range 5-12%) of the labelled platelets accumulated transiently in the spleen. Their transit time was 208 min (range 60-47 min), significantly longer than the 5 min of uninjured platelets.

Modelling of the sequestration phase was approximated by the Dornhorst function. We assumed that platelets were sequestrated by a random and age dependent process. The fit of the sequestration model is given in Figure 3. The simulated data fitted the experimental data well. When the mean platelet lifespan was calculated from the compartmental model, the estimate compared favorably with that calculated using standard mathematical curve fitting techniques, i.e. 205 hours (range 188-255 hours) versus 227 hours (range 203-250 hours) respectively. The estimates of the in vivo distribution at equilibrium and the sites of sequestration of senescent platelets also compared favorable (Figure 3).

DISCUSSION

We have developed a compartmental model that can be used to quantify the movement of platelets in the body. The third model as shown in its entirety in Figure 1 allows one to determine the contribution of the different sources of radioactivity to total organ radioactivity, i.e. radioactivity from functional circulating platelets, senescent sequestrated platelets and collection injured platelets. We were also able to show that collection injured platelets accumulate transiently in the spleen. An advantage of modelling of the platelet kinetic data may be that platelet survival can be more reliably determined by using the results of the disappearance of labelled platelets from the circulation and their simultaneous appearance in the spleen and liver.

REFERENCES

1. Heyns A du P, Lötter MG, Badenhorst PN. Platelet imaging. In: Methods in Haematology, LA Harker, TS Zimmerman (Eds) Churchill livingstone (Edinburgh): 216-234 (1983).
2. Kotzé HF, Heyns A du P, Lötter MG, Pieters H, Roodt JP, Sweetlove MA, Badenhorst PN. Comparison of oxine and tropolone methods for labelling platelets with indium-111. *Journal of Nuclear Medicine* 32: 62-66 (1991).

INFLUENCE OF PLATELET MEMBRANE SIALIC ACID AND PLATELET ASSOCIATED IgG ON AGEING AND SEQUESTRATION OF BLOOD PLATELETS IN BABOONS

H.F. Kotzé, V. van Wyk, A. du P Heyns[1], J.P. Roodt, M.G. Lötter and P.N. Badenhorst

Department of Haematology
University of the Orange Free State, Bloemfontein
[1]South African Blood Transfusion Services, Johannesburg
South Africa

INTRODUCTION

Blood platelets circulate for approximately 10 days in normal humans. The macrophages of the monocyte-macrophage system then recognise them as old and phagocytose and destroy them. The mechanism through which the macrophages recognise the "old" platelets is not known. A hypothesis to explain red cell ageing and sequestration implicates that membrane sialic acid may play a role. According to this view, red cells loose sialic acid while they are circulating. This exposes a senescent cell antigen on the red cell membrane. IgG recognises and binds to the antigen. Once sufficient antibody-antigen complex is formed, the macrophages recognise the red cells as "foreign" and phagocytose and destroy them[1].

We investigated if a similar mechanism of recognition exists for senescent platelets. Enzymatic removal of platelet membrane sialic acid shortens their mean platelet lifespan markedly[2], and a senescent cell antigen, similar to that identified for red cells, was identified in old platelets[1].

METHODS

Normal, healthy baboons were used in this study. Blood was collected, and the platelets harvested by differential centrifugation. An aliquot of the platelet rich plasma was removed to determine platelet sialic acid and platelet associated IgG. The platelets were then treated with neuraminidase to remove sialic acid (0.002 U/ml for 30 min at 37°C). An aliquot was again removed to determine platelet sialic acid and platelet associated IgG. The treated platelets were then labelled with 111In-oxine, reinjected and their recovery from the circulation and mean lifespan determined[3,4]. In all baboons, the lifespan of normal untreated platelets was determined within a month after the studies with treated platelets.

RESULTS

The treated, labelled platelets were viable. Their recovery in the circulation, 81 ± 24%, was not significantly different from that of the untreated platelets, 85 ± 12%. Also, in vitro aggregation in response to ADP and collagen was not different form that of untreated platelets.

The disappearance of treated and untreated labelled platelets from the circulation is given in Figure 1. This was determined in 19 baboons. A mean of 20 ± 15% of the sialic acid was removed. There were two subpopulations of treated labelled platelets. The first, approximately 22%, was removed from the circulation within the first 3 hours after their injection. It is likely that enough sialic acid was removed to signal that this subpopulation was old, and must be destroyed by the macrophages. The remaining subpopulation had a linear, but shorter than normal survival curve. This indicates that these platelets were removed as a result of senescence. The linearity further implicates that equal amounts of sialic acid was removed from platelets of all ages.

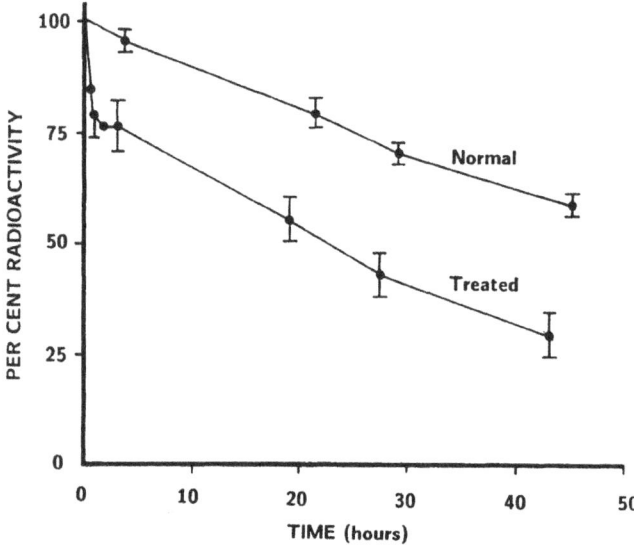

Figure 1. Platelet survival curves of normal (untreated) and neuraminidase-treated 111In-labelled platelets. The untreated platelets disappeared from the circulation in an age-dependent manner; this is reflected by the linear survival curve. The disappearance curve of the treated platelets shows two components; an exponential rapid clearance, and a second phase parallel to that of normal platelets.

Figure 2 illustrates the relationship between the shortening in platelet lifespan as a result of the removal of sialic acid and the amount of sialic acid removed. The exponential relationship is consistent with the view that only a given amount of sialic acid have to be removed to signal platelet senescence and thus permanent removal of the platelets from the circulation.

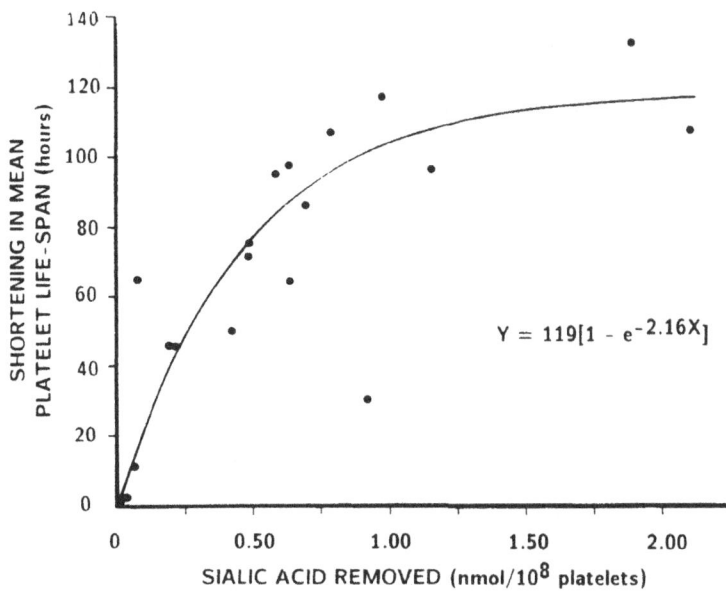

$$Y = 119[1 - e^{-2.16X}]$$

Figure 2. The relationship between decrease in the sialic acid content of the platelet membrane after treatment and the shortening in platelet survival as a result of the removal of sialic acid indicates that the removal of sialic acid shortens platelet survival.

Removal of sialic acid resulted in an increase in platelet associated IgG. In 26 studies, the linear relationship between the amount of sialic acid removed and the increase in platelet-associated IgG was

sialic acid removed = 0.14 + 0.068 x increase in IgG (r = 0.621)

The relationship between the shortening in mean platelet lifespan after sialic acid was removed and the increase in platelet-associated IgG is illustrated in Figure 3. The exponential relationship is consistent with the view that only a given amount of IgG have to attach to platelets to signal senescence, and thus sequestration and permanent removal of the platelets from the circulation.

CONCLUSIONS

The results of this study strongly suggest that platelet sialic acid and platelet-associated IgG plays a role in platelet ageing and subsequent sequestration by the macrophages. We hypothesize that platelets loose sialic acid from their membranes while they are circulating. The loss of sialic acid exposes a neo-antigen, presumably similar to the senescent cell antigen described in red cells. An antibody recognises the exposed antigen and binds to it to from an antigen-antibody complex. Once sufficient IgG is bound to the platelet membrane, this signals that the platelet is aged. This signal to phagocytose and destroy the "old" platelets is recognised by the macrophages of the monocyte-macrophage system, especially those located in the spleen, liver and bone marrow.

This hypothesis is logical. It suggests that the monocyte-macrophage system will recognise an aged cell in the circulation as "foreign". It is therefore not necessary to postulate a new mechanism specifically aimed at the recognition of senescent platelets. Macrophages will only be performing their normal task of surveillance against foreign cells when they remove senescent platelets from the circulation.

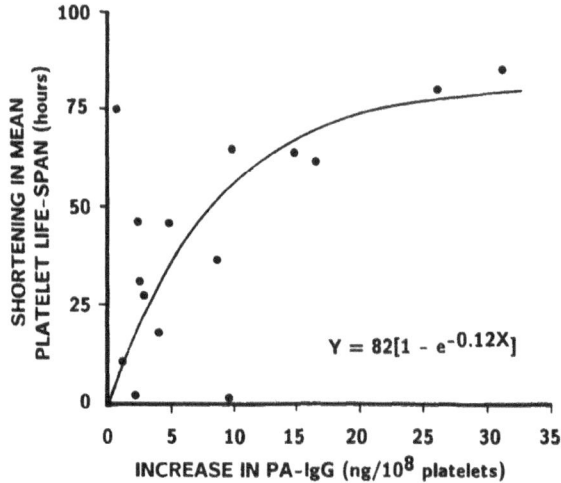

Figure 3. There is a correlation between the increase in platelet-associated IgG after removal of sialic acid and the shortening in mean platelet lifespan. This supports the view that removal of sialic acid and the resultant increase in platelet-associated antibody induces sequestration of platelets.

REFERENCES

1. Kay MMB. Isolation of a phagocytosis-inducing IgG-binding site in senescent somatic cells. *Nature* 289: 491-494 (1981).
2. Greenberg JP, Packham MA, Cazenaeve JP, Reimers HJ, Mustard JF. Effect on platelet function of removal of sialic acid by neuraminidase. *Laboratory Investigation* 32: 476-484 (1975).
3. Kotzé HF, Lötter MG, Badenhorst PN, Heyns A du P. Kinetics of In-111-platelets in the baboon. I. Isolation and labelling of a viable and representative platelet population. *Thrombosis and Haemostasis* 53: 404-407 (1985).
4. Kotzé HF, Lötter MG, Badenhorst PN, Heyns A du P. Kinetics of In-111-platelets in the baboon. II. In vivo distribution and sites of sequestration. *Thrombosis and Haemostasis* 53: 408-410 (1985).

UPTAKE OF RADIOLABELED META-IODOBENZYLGUANIDINE BY HUMAN PLATELETS

S. Granegger, M. Banyai and H. Sinzinger

Department of Nuclear Medicine, University of Vienna
Ludwig Boltzmann Institute for Nuclear Medicine, and
Wilhelm Auerswald Atherosclerosis Research Group, Vienna, Austria

INTRODUCTION

(123I, 131I)-meta-iodobenzylguanidine (mIBG) is routinely used for diagnosis and treatment of enolase positive tumors (phaeochromocytoma [Sisson et al. 1981], neuroblastoma [Kimming et al. 1984], a. o.) of neural crest origin.

Scintigraphy with 131I-mIBG, a norepinephrine analogon acting at the postganglionar synapse, is frequently performed for diagnostic reasons. MIBG cannot be quantitatively determined, however, as its metabolism is different (not via monoamino-oxidase, catechol-o-methyltransferase [Manger et al.1986]). Platelets may accumulate mIBG via the adrenergic mechanism.

Drugs interfering with the adrenergic system are known to interfere with tumor uptake of mIBG (Solanki et al. 1992).

Limited information, however, is available so far on the interaction of platelets with mIBG; Sisson et al. (1988) reported that 131I-mIBG used for treatment of neuroblastoma caused a dose dependent thrombopenia. Munkner et al. (1985) found, that the platelet uptake of 131I-mIBG, used for scintigraphy of neuroblastomas, was thrice as high as in plasma, while Feldman et al. (1984) observed that the 131I-mIBG uptake in platelets could only be inhibited by extremely high doses of serotonin.

Therefore, we assessed the question,whether platelets do (selectively) accumulate mIBG in vitro, and whether there is a relevant in vivo uptake; finally we examined, whether an influence of drugs can be observed, and if, to a clinically relevant extent.

MATERIAL AND METHODS

In-vitro Study

The uptake of radioiodinated mIBG by freshly isolated platelets from healthy volunteers (incubation for 6 hours at 37°C) was evaluated. In parallel experiments, the influence of calcium channel blockers, beta-blockers and of the unlabeled compound on the platelet uptake of radioiodinated mIBG was investigated.

In-vitro Part of the In-vivo Study: Platelet rich plasma (PRP) was prepared after anticoagulation (acid citrate dextrose; 9:1) by centrifugation at 150 x g for 10 minutes at 22°C. Platelet poor plasma (PPP) and a platelet pellet were obtained by differential centrifugation (500 x g; 10 min). The platelet bound and free radioactivity was subsequently determined in a gamma-counter.

Quality Assurance

Quantification of free iodine was done by paper electrophoresis (Whatman 3MM; 0.05 M HOAc/NaOAc pH 4.5, 300 V, 6 min). Free iodine amounted usually less than 1 %, allowing direct formulation with sodium-citrate and sterile filtration. In case free iodine was above 3%, purification on a RP-C18 column was performed. Assessment of radiochemical purity was done by RTLC (Merck S n-propanol: 10 % NH4OH = 3:1; Rf mIBG = 0.45).

In-vivo Study (Diagnostic Scintigraphy)

Patients received intravenously 0.5 mCi (18.5 MBq) 131I-mIBG/1.73 m^2 body surface. They were positioned under a LFOV-gamma camera equipped with a high energy parallel hole collimator. Static images were recorded 3, 5, and 7 days after tracer administration. Blood samples were drawn throughout the whole period of investigation in order to determine the pharmacokinetics of mIBG and to monitor the peripheral platelet count.

RESULTS

Platelets show a relevant time-dependent (figure 1) uptake of mIBG both in-vitro (20-30 %) and in-vivo (20-40 fold higher than plasmatic activity), which can be inhibited in-vitro by the addition of unlabeled mIBG (figure 2). Due to the time course of mIBG platelet uptake, there is evidence for 2 uptake mechanisms, a specific intravesicular, sodium- and energy- dependent (persistent 24 - 36 h), without metabolism and an unspecific, extraneuronal, low affinity-, high capacity- one, with a washout of 3 to 4 hours. In patients without any drug known to interfere with the mIBG-uptake (Solanki et al. 1992) a selective in-vivo uptake by platelets (77 % at mean at day 3, 60 % at day 7) is associated with a significant ($p < 0.01$) drop (figure 3) in platelet count (207 ± 59 x 10^3 / μl vs. 286 ± 104 x 10^3 /μl [prevalue]). In contrast, in presence of β-blockers the platelet uptake was much less extensive (figure 4), while the peripheral platelet count was unaffected in these patients. While two β-blocking agents examined (propanolol, atenolol) resulted in a significant inhibition of mIBG-uptake (figures 5, 6), nifedipine, a calcium antagonist (at least in 3 patients examined), showed no interference at all.

DISCUSSION

As there is a selective and rather high uptake of mIBG by platelets, the knowledge of the peripheral platelet count is advisable prior to administration of any diagnostic and - even more - therapeutic mIBG-dose. It is not known at present, whether mIBG is taken up by platelets, or probably also by megacaryocytes. As

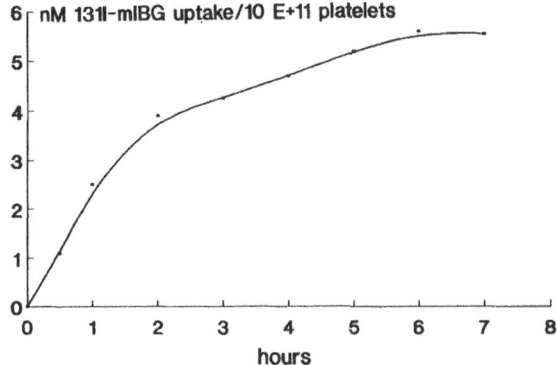

Figure 1. mIBG uptake by platelets.

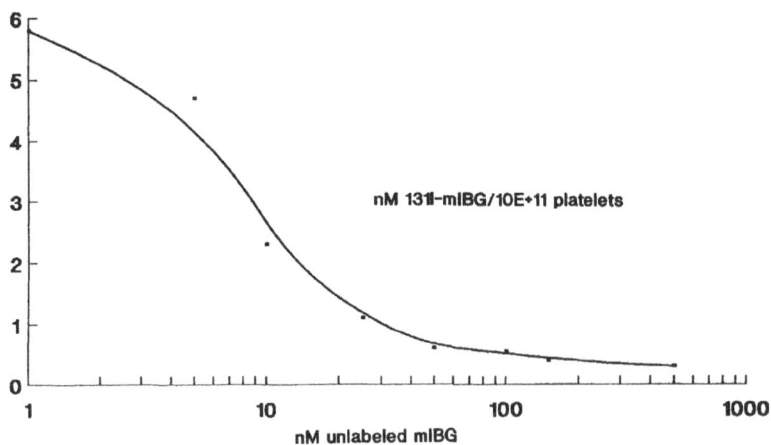

Figure 2. Inhibition of mIBG uptake by the unlabeled compound.

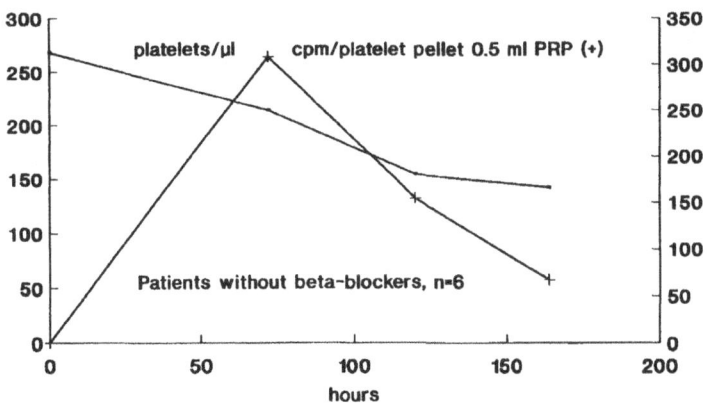

Figure 3. Platelet-associated activity after intravenous administration.

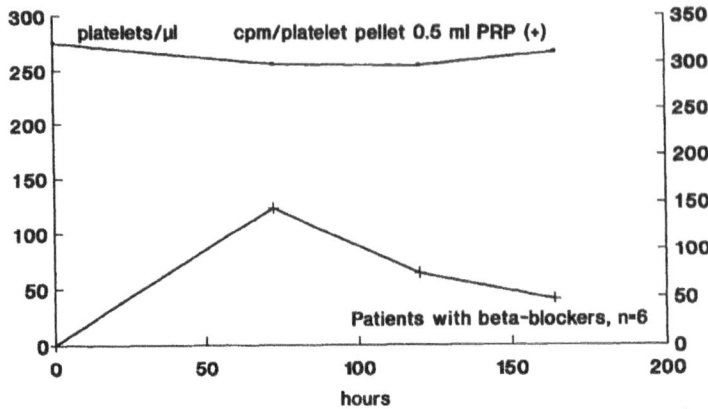

Figure 4. Platelet-associated activity after intravenous administration.

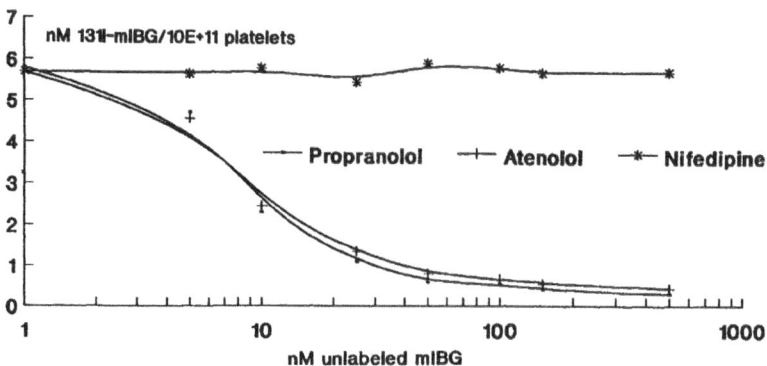

Figure 5. Inhibition of mIBG uptake by other compounds.

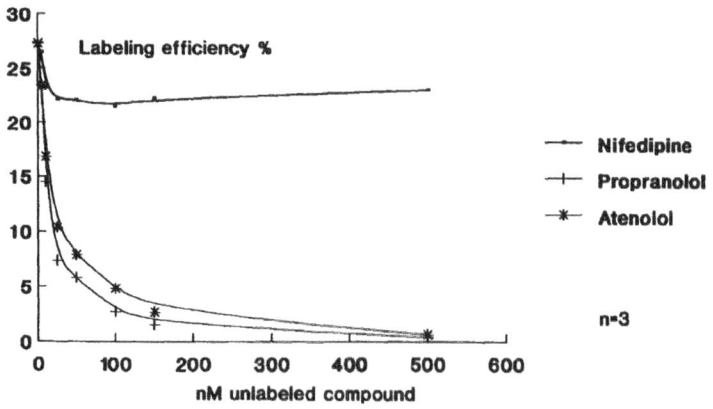

Figure 6. Reduction of labeling efficiency by other compounds.

thrombocytopenia may occur (Sisson et al.1988) or show further deterioration, other bone marrow damaging (chemo-) therapy should be administered with a certain time interval. The in-vitro and in-vivo mIBG-uptake by platelets can be drastically diminished by beta-blockers. In 3 patients on a calcium channel blocker, however, this effect could not be achieved. Preliminary data show that the platelet mIBG-uptake may follow the same criteria (Solanki et al.1992) as in other tissues, the question, which of the many substances interfering with tissue mIBG-uptake interferes with platelet accumulation and to which extent, still remains to be assessed. We thus conclude, that due to the highly selective uptake mechanism of mIBG by the platelets, therapeutic doses might potentially be harmful to patients, a fact which should be carefully considered.

REFERENCES

Banyai M., Sinzinger H, 1992. Selective uptake of the guanethidine analogue 131I-meta-Iodobenzylguanidine by platelets is inhibited by beta-blockers. 4th Erfurt Conference on Platelets, Abstract p. 30.

Banyai M., Sinzinger H., 1992. Selective accumulation of the guanethidine analogue 131I-meta-Iodobenzylguanidine in platelets in diagnostic scintigraphy. *Coagulation* 2: 47.

Feldman J.M., Frankel N., Coleman R.E., 1984. Platelet uptake of the pheochromocytoma - scanning agent 131I-meta-iodobenzylguanidine. *Metabolism* 33: 397.

Kimming B., Brandeis W.E., Eisenhut M., et al, 1984. Scintigraphy of neuroblastomas with 131I-mIBG. *J Nucl Med*25: 773-775.

Mangner T.J., Tobes M.C., Wieland D.W., et al., 1986. Metabolism of I-131 metaiodobenzylguanidine in patients with metastatic pheochromocytoma. *J Nucl Med* 27: 37-44.

Munkner T., 1985. 131I-meta-iodobenzylguanidine scintigraphy of neuroblastomas. *Sem Nucl Med* 15: 154.

Sisson J.C., Frager M.S., Valk T.W., et al., 1981. Scintigraphic localization of pheochromocytoma. *N Eng J Med* 305: 12-17.

Sisson J.C., Hutchinson R.J., Carey J.E., Shapiro B., Johnson J.W., Malleth S.A., Wieland D.M., 1988. Toxicity from treatment of neuroblastoma with 131I-meta-iodobenzylguanidine. *Eur J Nucl Med* 14: 337-340.

Solanki K.K., Bomanji J., Moyes J., Mather S.J., Trainer P.J., Britton, K.E., 1992. A pharmacological guide to medicines which interfere with the biodistribution of radiolabelled meta-iodobenzylguanidine (MIBG). *Nucl Med Commun* 13 : 513-521.

GRANULOCYTE KINETICS

A.M. Peters

Department of Diagnostic Radiology
Hammersmith Hospital
London, United Kingdom

INTRODUCTION

The kinetics of granulocytes have been extensively studied using non-imaging radionuclides such as di-isopropylfluorophosphonate labelled with 32P, tritiated thymidine and 51Cr. With the development of 111In labelling of granulocytes and the recognition of the need to avoid granulocyte activation during labelling, came the opportunity to identify the principal sites of physiological granulocyte margination. The phenomenon of granulocyte margination has been known for several decades and was inferred from observations by Wintrobe's group[1] that following infusion of radiolabelled granulocytes to normal volunteers only about 50 % of the dose could be accounted for in the circulating blood. The other 50 % were thought to have entered a marginating granulocyte pool (MGP). The physiological validity of this conclusion was demonstrated by the simultaneous administration of adrenalin, which increased recovery from 50 % to about 80 %.

With the availability of 111In, we were able to "map" the distribution of the MGP in man, showing that about 40 % of it was in the spleen, with most of the remainder being accounted for by the liver (30%) and lung (10%)[2]. The bone marrow probably contributes a substantial fraction to the remainder. The techniques we used included compartmental analysis, deconvolution analysis and comparison of gamma camera signals over organs of interest following sequential intravenous injections of 111In labelled red cells and 111In labelled granulocytes with those in the peripheral blood, thereby expressing granulocyte mean transit time through an organ as a quotient of mean red cell transit time. Deconvolution analysis, based on peripheral blood time-activity curves as the input function, gave mean granulocyte transit times through the liver and spleen which were in agreement with those based on the transit time of labelled red cells.

PULMONARY GRANULOCYTE KINETICS

The mean transit time through the lung of radiolabelled granulocytes is about 2.5

that of red cells, indicating that the ratio of the marginating to circulating pools in the lung is about 1.5, similar to the value for the whole body[1]. The mean transit time immediately after cell injection is about 5, and it takes 30-40 minutes for this to decrease to the resting value of 2.5, suggesting a minor element of activation even after isolation and labelling in plasma based media[3].

Although there is evidence to the contrary, exercise in our studies failed to demarginate the few marginating granulocytes in the lungs[3]. There was, in fact, an increase in the lung granulocyte signal in normal volunteers undergoing four minutes of vigorous exercise one hour after injection of the cells, but this was the passive result of a substantial release of radiolabelled granulocytes from the splenic pool. The findings of Hogg's group[4] were contradictory to these, in that exercise in their subjects caused a decrease in the lung signal and a simultaneous increase in the liver and splenic signals. Their subjects performed exercise before equilibration of the granulocytes throughout the marginated pools, and possibly before the recovery of the granulocytes from the apparent early element of activation (see above). The decrease in the lung activity may, therefore, have been due to release of relatively "stiff" cells trapped in the lung.

If the lung is a relatively minor site of granulocyte margination, it should be possible to identify circumstances in which the lung MGP could be increased. McNee et al[5] demonstrated an increase in lung 111In labelled granulocyte content as a result of acute cigarette smoking, although, as in Hogg's studies, the stimulus was applied during the period of granulocyte equilibration, in fact during the infusion of the labelled cells. Asking volunteers to smoke one hour after injection of the labelled granulocytes, i.e. following their equilibration, we observed no change in the count rate from the lung (unpublished observations). Cigarette smoking may cause a reduction in splenic blood flow, which as a result of diversion of cells from the splenic pool, could result in an increased count rate originating from the lung circulating granulocyte pool if the stimulus was applied during equilibration. The analogous phenomenon with 111In labelled platelets and intravenous adrenalin infusion has been clearly demonstrated by Wadenvik and Kutti[6].

In contrast to cigarette smoking, inhalation of the cytokine, platelet activating factor (PAF) does cause an almost immediate and substantial increase in the lung MGP[7]. Thus, the lung signal approximately doubled while the circulating activity decreased to about one half of baseline levels. The native peripheral granulocyte count was faithfully followed by the blood 111In labelled granulocyte concentration, indicating normal function of the labelled cells. There was rebound neutrophilia which was not, however, accompanied by an increase in the labelled granulocytes, suggesting that it was due to the release of new cells from the bone marrow pool.

An expanded pulmonary MGP can be demonstrated in some diseases, including systemic vasculitis[8], inflammatory bowel disease (IBD)[9], graft versus host disease involving the gut (unpublished observations) and, of more common knowledge, the adult respiratory distress syndrome. Whereas in the latter, the pulmonary granulocytes are thought to contribute significantly to the lung disorder, no over lung damage is apparent in the other three conditions, although Lecouffe et al[10] claim to have demonstrated an increase in alveolar permeability to inhaled 99mTc aerosol in otherwise asymptomatic patients with IBD. It may be that extracellular migration is required before lung damage occurs. Certainly, Henson's group has shown that intravenous C5a injection in the experimental animal led to increased granulocyte margination in pulmonary capillaries, but there was no extravascular migration, no increase in the number of lavaged neutrophils and no change in pulmonary endothelial permeability to radioionated protein[11]. In contrast, C5a given by inhalation produced marked extravascular migration, an increase in lavaged neutrophils, an increase in protein permeability and histological evidence of gross lung damage. Granulocyte margination by itself, however, does not appear to cause lung injury.

Recently, we have been able to confirm in IBD that, in addition to an increased marginated pool, there is evidence of increased migration[12], and this is almost certainly also true for systemic vasculitis. Sensitive tests for lung damage will be required to study the effects of marginating granulocytes, and low levels of migration, on lung integrity. It is of some interest that, whereas an increase in the lung MGP can readily be induced by intravenous injection of cytokines and extravascular migration induced by deposition of chemoattractants in the alveolar air spaces, it has been more difficult to induce migration by the intravenous administration of agents, or by pretreatment of granulocytes, or by a combination of the two. Nevertheless, Worthen et al[13] demonstrated that whereas FMLP and LPS given alone caused no increased accumulation of granulocytes in the interalveolar septal tissue, the two given together did. Clearly, much more work needs to be done on the mechanisms and the consequences of increased granulocyte intravascular margination and of significant migration into the interstitial tissues of the lung.

One such approach may be to use monoclonal antibodies which recognise activated endothelial cell adhesion molecules. One such antibody, an anti-E-selectin, is under development in our own unit in collaboration with Dr D O Haskard[14], and will be used as a marker of vascular activation, including the pulmonary vasculature, in man. In pigs, marked accumulation of the 111In labelled monoclonal antibody can be seen in the lungs and the liver following vascular stimulation by intravenous injection of the cytokine, interleukin-1. Increased upregulation of E-selectin has also been demonstrated in the skin in response to intradermal injection of IL-1 and other cytokines, including PMA, phorbol ester and TNF. These radiolabelled monoclonal antibodies may be very useful for the detection of inflammations of various levels of chronicity in man.

THE SPLEEN

The spleen is interesting in the different way it handles the formed elements of blood. The mean transit times through the spleen of plasma, red cells, leucocytes and platelets are all different. The spleen is, in effect, a cell sorter. A cell pool can be said to exist if the transit time of the cell through the pool, relative to plasma transit time, is greater than a reference ratio of transit times elsewhere, e.g. whole body circulation times. The mean transit time of red cells through the spleen is 40-60 seconds, and intrasplenic haematocrit is higher than the whole body haematocrit. Reducing red cell deformability, by heating, lengthens this transit time to 10-15 minutes. granulocytes and platelets have similar mean intrasplenic transit times of 8-10 minutes. Lymphocytes and monocytes almost certainly have transit times of this order or higher.

The concept of the spleen as a cell sorter is reinforced when the effects of interventions, such as vigorous exercise are studied[15]. A four minute period of intense exercise results in plasma volume contraction. There is also a thrombocythaemia and leucocytosis, even after correction for the haemoconcentration. Radiolabelled cell studies have demonstrated that the major source for these circulating cell increments is the spleen[15]. Red cells are also expelled from the spleen during exercise with a time course that is different from those seen with platelets and granulocytes. Thus, more red cells are initially expelled, but, after completion of the exercise, they return to the organ sooner. In contrast platelets and granulocytes continue to leave the spleen for 5-10 minutes after the termination of exercise, before returning. These different time courses can be explained on the basis of the different mean transit times of the cells through the spleen. Thus, if exercise was to produce an abrupt fall in splenic blood flow, this would represent a disturbance to the dynamic equilibrium existing between cells in the blood and splenic pool. Rates of re-equilibration will be determined by mean cell intrasplenic transit times. So cell expulsion from the spleen is probably the passive result of a decrease in splenic blood flow, and this would be consistent with the paucity of smooth muscle in the splenic capsule of humans. The spleens of "athletic" animals like cats, dogs and race horses are quite different in that they do contain capsular smooth muscle and actively contract to expel blood cells.

Because of the significant granulocyte pool in the spleen, splenomegaly may cause granulocytopenia. The splenic pooling of granulocytes can also be appreciated in patients with severe sepsis or inflammatory bowel disease, in whom splenic counts drop significantly between early (1-3 hours) and late (24 hours) 111In labelled granulocyte scans, more than in controls. This is because pooled cells are continuously diverted towards migration into the inflammatory foci. Indeed, Moisan et al[16] used this fall in splenic counts as a measure of disease activity in IBD.

THE LIVER

The liver is difficult to study with respect to granulocyte kinetics because of its sensitivity to granulocyte damage or activation. In this respect, it is rather similar to the lung. This can be appreciated from the early sharp fall usually seen in liver activity between 40 minutes and 3 hours, which is out of phase with splenic and circulating activities, and which presumably represents the release of reversibly activated cells. This phenomenon can be turned to clinical advantage in patients having white cell scans for sepsis in or around the liver. Thus whereas liver activity falls sharply, activity in pus rises, or at least remains unchanged between 40 minutes and 3 hours. The liver continues to accumulate activity between 24 and 48 hours in all subjects, unlike the bone marrow and spleen (wherein it becomes constant after 24 hours), almost certainly as a result of continued uptake of non-cell-bound, eluted, 111In.

THE BONE MARROW

The bone marrow usually gives quite an impressive signal from an early stage after injection of radiolabelled granulocytes, particularly 99mTc HMPAO cells, suggesting that it marginates granulocytes. This has been more difficult to recognise in comparison with the spleen because, as a result of on-going cell destruction in the bone marrow reticuloendothelial system, the bone marrow signal continues to rise between 3 and 24 hours. However, it does not rise as much as would be anticipated if all the contained activity was due to cells destroyed there. This can be confirmed by comparing the 3/24 hour activity ratio in bone marrow with that in an enclosed abscess in which the same ratio is significantly less (unpublished observations). Although not well recognised, this phenomenon could be used to distinguish bone marrow activity from migrated activity in an infection site in patients with suspected osteomyelitis, especially infected hip prosthesis. Thus the 3/24 hour activity ratios would be different. We are currently investigating this approach as an alternative to the separate injection of 99mTc colloid for defining bone marrow[17, 18]. Since 99mTc gives such a clear image of bone marrow, a modification of this approach would be to give cells doubly labelled with 99mTc HMPAO and 111In tropolone, using the 99mTc signal for early imaging and the 111In signal for late imaging. This is technically quite feasible, as both radionuclides are taken up by granulocytes in suspension, without cross-chelation, in the presence of HMPAO and tropolone.

CONCLUSION

Cell kinetics, and especially granulocyte kinetics, are not only of physiological interest, but important to understand for the clear interpretation of white cell scans. As in the examples shown above, a good understanding of granulocyte kinetics can be used to extract additional clinical information from routine white cell scans.

REFERENCES

1. Athens JW, Mauer AM, Ashenbrucker H, Cartwright GE, Wintrobe MM. Leukokinetic studies III. The distribution of granulocytes in the blood of normal subjects. *J Clin Invest* 40: 159-164 (1961).
2. Peters AM, Saverymuttu SH, Bell RN, Lavender JP. Quantification of the distribution of the marginating granulocyte pool in man. *Scand J Haematol* 34: 111-120 (1985).
3. Peters AM, Allsop P, Stuttle AWJ, Arnot RN, Gwilliam M, Hall GM. Granulocyte margination in the human lung and its response to strenuous exercise. *Clin Sci* 82: 237-244 (1992).
4. Muir AL, Cruz M, Martin BA, Thommasen HV, Belzberg A, Hogg JC. Leukokinetics in the human lung: role of exercise and catecholamines. *J Appl Physiol* 57: 711-719 (1984)
5. Mc Nee W, Wiggs B, Belzberg A, Hogg JC. The effects of cigarette smoking on neutrophil kinetics in human lungs. *N Engl J Med* 321: 924-928 (1989).
6. Wadenvik H, Kutti J. The effect of adrenaline infusion on splenic blood flow and intrasplenic platelet kinetics. *Br J Haematol* 67: 187-192 (1987).
7. Tam FWK, Clague J, Dixon CMS, Stuttle AWJ, Henderson BL, Peters AM, Lavender JP, Ind PW. Inhaled platelet activating factor (PAF) causes pulmonary neutrophil sequestration in normal man. *Am Rev Respir Dis* (in press).
8. Jonker N, Peters AM, Gaskin G, Pusey CD, Lavender JP. A retrospective study of granulocyte kinetics in patients with systemic vasculitis. *J Nucl Med* 33: 491-497 (1992).
9. Jonker ND, Peters AM, Carpani de Kaski M, Hodgson HJ, Lavender JP. Pulmonary granulocyte margination is increased in patients with inflammatory bowel disease. *Nucl Med Commun* 13: 806-810 (1992).
10. Lecouffe P, Vendel H, Huglo D, Colombel J-F, Wallaert B, Marchandise X. Pulmonary and intestinal permeabilities in Crohn's disease. *Eur J Nucl Med* 16: S180 (abstr) (1990).
11. Henson PM, Larsen GL, Webster RO, Mitchell BC, Goins AJ, Henson JE. Pulmonary microvascular alterations and injury induced by complement fragments: synergistic effect of complement activation, neutrophil sequestration and prostaglandins. *Ann N Y Acad Sci* 384: 287-300 (1982).
12. Ussov W Yu, Peters AM, Hughes JMB, Hodgson HJ. Quantitative study of pulmonary neutrophil trapping. *Nucl Med Commun* (in press) (abstr).
13. Worthen GS, Haslett C, Rees AJ, Gumbay RS, Henson JE, Henson PM. Neutrophil-mediated pulmonary vascular injury. Synergistic effect of trace amounts of lipopolysaccharide and neutrophil stimuli on vascular permeability and neutrophil sequestration in the lung. *Am Rev Resp Dis* 136: 19-28 (1987).
14. Peters AM, Keelan E, Licence S, Binns R, Haskard DO. Imaging inflammation and vascular activation with a labeled monoclonal antibody against E-selectin. *J Nucl Med* (in press) (abstr).
15. Allsop P, Peters AM, Arnot RN, Stuttle AWJ, Deenmamode M, Gwilliam ME, Myers MJ, Hall GM. Intrasplenic blood cell kinetics in man before and after brief maximal exercise. *Clin Sci* 83: 47-54 (1992).
16. Moisan A, Bretagne JF, LeCloriec I, Darnault P, Bourguet P, Gastard I, Herry JY. A new isotopic index of disease activity in inflammatory bowel disease: a splenic activity fall of In-111 labelled granulocytes. *J Nucl Med* 28 (suppl): 688 (abstr) (1987).
17. King AD, Peters AM, Stuttle AWJ, Lavender JP. Imaging of bone infection with labelled white blood cells: role of contemporaneous bone marrow imaging. *Eur J Nucl Med* 17: 148-151 (1990).
18. Palestro CJ, Roumanas P, Swyer AJ, Chun KK, Goldsmith SJ. Diagnosis of musculoskeletal infection using combined In-111 leukocyte and Tc-99m SC marrow imaging. *Clin Nucl Med* 17: 269-273 (1992).

EXPERIENCES IN IMMUNOSCINTIGRAPHY OF LEUKOCYTES

W. Becker[1], R. Kinne[2], F. Emmrich[2], G.R. Burmester[3], A. Schwarz[4] and F. Wolf[1]

[1]Department of Nuclear Medicine
[2]Max Planck Research Group Rheumatology/Immunology
[3]Department of Medicine III
University of Erlangen-Nuremberg
[4]Radiochemisches Labor, Behring Werke-Höchst AG
Frankfurt/Main, Germany

IN-VITRO DATA

EPITOPES

During the selection of monoclonal antibodies (Mab) raised against purified carcinoembryonic antigen (CEA) two Mabs were identified which immunoprecipitated a glycoprotein of 95kD present in perchloric acid extracts of normal lung and on the surface of normal granulocytes. One of these antigens had a molecular weight of 55kD, the other one of 95kD. When tested on frozen sections of colon carcinomas, normal spleen, lung and pancreas each type of Mab gave a clearly different pattern of reactivity. The Mab binding NCA-55 stained granulocytes as well as bronchiolar and alveolar epithelial cells in lung and inter- and intralobular duct apithelial cells in pancreas, whereas the Mab binding on NCA-95 stained only the granulocytes[1]. NCA-95 is expressed in dependence from the maturation stage of the studied cells[2] and is codey by CGM6 gene codes[3,4]. Although much is known concerning the structure and tissue distribution of these antigens, only recently have researchers reported possible biological roles for NCA and CEA. OIKAWA et al.[5] proposed that NCA functions as a homotypic adhesion molecule, a function similar to that suggested for CEA[6]. His conclusions were based on the observation of an increase in cell-cell aggregation of Chinese hamster ovary cells following transfection of NCA cDNA. LEUSCH et al[7] recently described the bacterial binding properities of CEA and provided evidence that NCA has similar properities. The relevance of these findings as it relates to NCA on granulocytes, however, remains to be determined.

GRANULOCYTE FUNCTION TEST

The antigranulocyte antibodies BW250/183 binds approximately 10^5 epitopes per granulocyte which express NCA-95[9]. The binding does not lead to a significant internalization of the Mab into the cytoplasma (during 2h at 37°C incubation). Despite its strong binding capacities, BW250/183 does not significantly influence granulocyte-mediated functions (enzyme release, pinocytosis, chemiluminescence)[10]. Furtheron the antibody does not induce any lytic effects to epitope positive cells via human complement or peripheral blood monocytes. So the antibody does not influence the normal physiologic capacities of human granulocytes to perform exudative burst[10].

SPECIFICITY, IMMUNOREACTIVITY, ASSOCIATION CONSTANT AND BINDING KINETICS

MASCHEK et al[12] demonstrated in blood specimens of patients after antibody injection an antibody binding in circulating blood and in granulocytes of infected hip joints. About 20.000, resp. 70.000 antibodies can be bound per granulocyte. The affinity constant of BW250/183 was given with 2×10 l/mol[14].

LABELLING TECHNIQUE

For BW250/183 labelling in a first step the antibody is reduced by a thiol reagent (2-mercaptoethanol or 2-aminoethanethiol-hydrochlorid). The reduced antibody is lyophilized in the presence of phosphate buffer (pH 7.2). The 99mTc-labelling is accomplished by adding small amounts of a labelling unit such as pyrophosphate, di-tri- or tetraphosphonates and IDA-compounds. The lyophilized tin-II containing compound is dissolved in physiologic saline. An aliquot(1ml) of this solution corresponding to about 10ug tin, is transferred into the vial, containing the lyophilized mab and finally 99mTc- eluate is added. The labelling yield was higher than 95% [15].

IN-VIVO USE

KINETICS OF ANTIGRANULOCYTE ANTIBODIES (BW250/183)

Using the 99mTc-labelled antibodies BECKER et al.[17] have calculated the amount of labelled antibody binding to circulating granulocytes. These data correlate well with in-vitro experiences of the 123I labelled AK-47[11] which demonstrate that after the first 1-2h no more than 10-20% of injected or added antibodies bind to circulating granulocytes. Comparable results were reported by JOSEPH et al.[10], who found 24.2% of the administered antibodies bound to granulocytes.

In 1984 DILLMAN et al.[18] recommended, that it seems imperative to rigorously exclude binding to circulating cells of all types of Mabs with potential human application, because all circulating blood cells opsonized with Mab are rapidly removed from the circulation by the reticulo-endothelial system. He found after injection of 5mg of anti-CEA antibody a rapid drop of peripheral leukocytes accompanied with chill and fever. Using the BW250/125 in a dose between 250ug to 1000ug we never could measure a significant alteration of the number of circulating leukocytes[17].

In a comparative human study of the recovery rate if 111In-oxine labeled

148

granulocytes, of in-vitro antibody (BW250/183) labelled granulocytes and of intravenously injected 99mTc-antibodies the recovery rate of the 111In-oxine-granulocytes and of the in-vitro antibody labelled cells was comparable during 180min after injection of the radioactivity[17]. This demonstrates the unaltered functional behaviour of granulocytes in vivo after binding these specific antibodies. It has been demonstrated as well that antibody labelled cell can be activated in vivo. For this reason a sham dialysis model in patients undergoing regular dialysis treatment was used[17]. During hemodialysis a granulocytopenia has been observed in patients. The basic mechanism for the granulocytopenia is a granulocyte sequestration into the lung due to an increased expression of an adhesion promoting surface glycoprotein after the start of dialysis with a cuprophane membrane. This increased migration of leukocytes into the lung could be demonstrated with 111In-oxine leukocytes in febrile patients[17]. 99mTc-anti-NCA-95 antibody labelled granulocytes demonstrated the same in-vivo behaviour with activation of peripheral, antibody labelled cells, and migration into the lungs. These in-vivo kinetic data with 99mTc-anti-NCA-95 antibodies demonstrate that antibody labelled granulocytes in vivo have a comparable kinetic behaviour in normal (recovery rate) and activated (sham dialysis model) conditions.

WHOLE BODY DISTRIBUTION

Tab.1 gives the data of the whole body distribution of 99mTc-labelled anti-NCA-95 4h and 24h after injection in whole body scans of 10 patients without detectable infectious diseases and without hematological diseases. This degree of bone marrow activity can well be explained as a migration of the labelled precursurs (4h) of the granulocytes out of the marrow (20h) after differentiation to normal granulocytes.

Table 1. Whole body distribution of 99mTc granulocyte antibody at 4 h and 24 h p.i.

body compartment	4 h	24 h
bone marrow	55% +/- 7%	40% +/- 5%
liver	10% +/- 2%	11% +/- 3%
spleen	6% +/- 2%	6% +/- 3%
circulating granulocytes	10% +/- 3%	
free circulating antibody	19% +/- 4%	

FOCUS UPTAKE OF ANTIGRANULOCYTE ANTIBODIES

10% of the injected antibody binds to circulating granulocytes, which are functionally not disturbed and may focus an infection as antibody labelled granulocytes. 19% of the injection antibody is free immunoglobulin in circulation, which has the same potential than 111In labelled nonspecific human IgG in rats with deep thigh infections[21]. So the uptake of the circulating immunoglobulin is not antigen related. Looking at the potential of monoclonal antibodies in detection of infectious diseases and the given data about their in-vivo behaviour the actual hypothesis about the uptake mechanism of this antibody as follows:

1. migration of antibody labelled circulating granulocytes to the focus due to their undisturbed chemotactic behaviour.
2. unspecific antigen unrelated uptake of free antibody due to the increased capillary permeability in the focus. The resulting image quality with high target-to-background ratios is due to the specific binding of high amounts of the injected antibodies to epitopes in bone marrow and spleen and the resulting low back ground activity. This rapid endogenous background subtraction allows the detection of small lesions with an excellent image quality.

CLINICAL APPLICATIONS

After the first reports of the human application of 99mTc-labelled anti-NCA-95 antibodies no adverse reactions could be demonstrated. Both reporting groups found a high diagnostic accuracy in unselected patient groups with this technically easy to perform method.

IMAGE PROTOCOLL

In a study of 56 patients BECKER et al.[22] examined the diagnostic accuracy of this method at different times after antibody injection.

For most clinical questions planar scintigraphy is sufficient, due to the high target-to-background ratio, specially in abdominal infections. SPECT seems to be obligatory in patients with suspected endocardits[23], skull infections and for an exact anatomical localization of other lesions[24]. But it has to be stressed that some lesions only can be detected 20h p.i., when reliable SPECT studies are difficult to perform with the usual injected activities of 555 MBq 99mTc.

BONE INFECTIONS

In patients with hip-prosthesis infection is one of the most serious complications with a frequency of 1%-4%[25]. The confirmation of infection demands explantation of the prosthesis; therefore an accurate method for determination of infection is necessary. Modern imaging modalities like MRI and CT are not helpful in regions with metallic implants. Conventional x-ray studies may detect loosening, but the periprosthetic bone resorption and other loosening signs are not specific for the differentiation for sepsis and loosening[25].

In a series of 43 patients SCIUK et al[25] studied the diagnostic value of 123I and Tc-99m-antigranulocyte antibodies in these patients in comparison to the three phase bone scan. The perfusion and blood pool scan in these series had a sensivity, specificity and diagnostic accuracy of 67%, 71% and 70%, the late bone scan of 92%, 24% and 48%. Anyway normal bone scans are always recommended before immunoscintigraphy, because a normal bone turnover in the region of prosthesis rules out septic loosening with a very high probability. The immunoscintigraphy in their series had a sensitivity of 89%, a specificity of 84% and an accuracy of 86% and are comparable with previous studies using 111In-oxine-labelled granulocytes[26,27]. The diagnostic problems of immunoscintigraphy are also comparable to conventional leukocyte scintigraphy. False positive scans are found in periprosthetic granulomas, damage of the polyethylene surface of the prosthesis and metallosis. Other problems are bone marrow islands. The distribution of red bone marrow varies widely and may occur at any location around the prosthesis, very often at the tip of the prosthesis. Two possible ways exist to solve this problem. PALESTRO et al.[29] proposed to use 99mTc-sulfur colloid scanning, which is taken up in normal bone marrow but not in infectious lesions, which is due to colloid size. The more simple way is the information of the dynamic behaviour of the monoclonal antibodies, whose accumulation in the focus of infection tends to increase from 4h to 24 h p.i., while the binding to marrow epitopes is constant. In most of our examined patients the 24h uptake was higher than the uptake in the adjacent bone marrow. This underlines the importance of the 24h scan.

Another clinical problem are postsurgical infectious complications, because at the one hand hematomas and necrotic tissue in the surgical area are favourable conditions for bacterial growth and on the other hand normal wound healing covers early symptoms of infection. REULAND et al[30] examined prospectively 106 patients after orthopedic surgery. They reported an accuracy of 81% in the hips, 81% in the thigh, 84% in the knees and 100% in the tibia. The problem in these situations is the nonspecific deposition of leukocytes in hematomas, contusions and in aseptic inflammation. The authors reported that the uptake of labelled granulocytes tends to be more intense and localized in septic complications.

Another result in their study was, that immunoscintigraphy does not work well in the spine[30]. An observation which was shared by others as well[31,32]. This problem is known from 111In-oxine leukocyte scintigraphy[33], where the sensitivity decreases the more an infection is located near the spine. The reason for this behaviour may be a decreased blood flow due to an extended fibrosis of the medullary, chronic spondylitis and the development of peripheral connective tissue membranes which can not be passed by leukocytes[34].

SOFT TISSUE AND ABDOMINAL INFECTIONS

In patients with soft tissue and abdominal diseases we found[22] a diagnostic accuracy wich 99mTc-anti-NCA-95 scanning of up to 100%, which was clearly higher than in patients with bone infections (84%). The reason for the higher accuracy could be a better vascularization of soft tissue infections, a higher prevalence of accute infections in these patients and, especially in abdominal diseases, an excellent target-to-background ratio in the abdominal cavity with no excretion of activity in the bowel[35]. For this reason we have prospectively examined the relevance of intestinal activity in patients undergoing immunoscintigraphy with this specific antibody[35]. We found that intestinal activity was always diagnostic for an infectious or inflammatory bowel disease. Regarding the kinetic behaviour of 99mTc-NCA-95 antibodies in chronic inflammatory bowel disease[33]. We found that in none of these patients the diseased segments could be detected, 2h p.i. already 49% of the segments, 5h p.i. 55% and 20h p.i. 91% of the diseased segments could be detected. In another prospective study in chronic inflammatory bowel disease (CIBD) SEGARRA et al[36] found sensitivities, specificities and accuracies of 61%, 100% and 78% at 4hours p.i. and 79%, 92% and 85% at 24 hours. They reported a high concordance in a segmental analysis between 111In-oxine leukocytes (93%) and immunoscintigraphy (89%). Both of the reviewed studies did not find any transmural antibody kinetic in the intestine, which was primarily expected because this is a well known fact in 111In-oxine leukocytes studies[37]. This could also be measured objectively in three patients with ulcerative colitis, in whom MAHIDA et al. measured a maximum of 0.9% of fecal excretion, which probably is due to an unspecific 99mTc-excretion and not due to CIBD, because in 111In-oxine studies pathologic fecal excretions start at levels higher than 2% of the injected activity[39]. In conclusion to these findings early scans in CIBD seemed not necessary in 99mTc-anti-NCA-95 immunoscintigraphy, 24h are diagnostic.

Using 111In-oxine granulocytes the kinetic behaviour of these cells allow a differentiation between diseased bowel segments and abdominal abscesses[37]. This differentiation is not possible with immunoscintigraphy because of the missing intestinal transmural kinetic.

There are only a small number of studies reporting clearly defined soft tissue diseases, which have been examined by immunoscintigraphy. In an already mentioned study we found a very high sensitivity up to 100%[22] in soft tissue infections including patients with CIBD (Fig. 1). LIND et al.[41] found 8 true positive, 2 true negative and one false negative scan in a small number of patients with soft tissue infections.

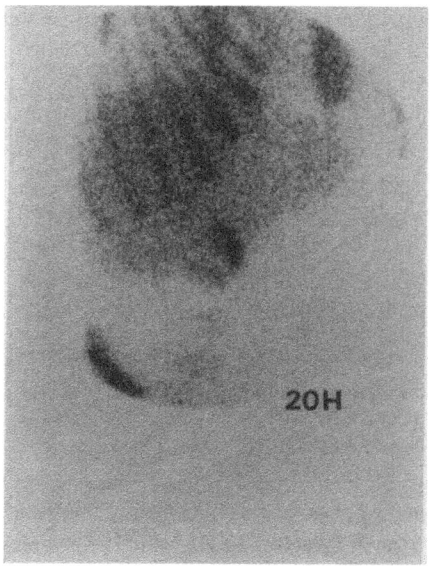

Fig. 1. Patient with fever of unknown origin and pathologic 99mTc-NCA-95-antibody uptake (20 h p.i.) in the gallbladder with surgical proven acute cholecystitis.

VASCULAR GRAFT INFECTIONS

Prosthetic vascular graft infection is an infrequent, but severe complication of vascular reconstructive surgery with mortality rates ranging from 25% to 75%[42]. The low incidence of graft infections might be the reason for the sparse data on the effectiveness of leukocyte scintigraphy in these cases[43]. The diagnosis of a graft infection is always a clinical diagnosis. The complete extend of the infection has to be given by imaging procedures. Immunoscintigraphy with specific antigranulocyte antibodies offers best assumption to localize vascular graft infections due to the rapid endogenous background subtraction and low vascular activity. CORDES et al[44] reproted a total of 40 examinations in 27 patients with a sensitivity of 94% and a specificity of 85%. Problems were described in the early course after surgery, especially as false negative images. False positive results were observed in perivascular hematoma, especially in the late 24h images, which have to be excluded by sonography and computed tomography.

PROSTHETIC VALVULAR HEART DISEASE

In a previous study with 111In-oxine leukocytes in 29 patients with inflammatory heart diseases[45] it could be demonstrated that scintigraphy might be important in patients with infected prosthetic valvular heart disease only, but not in subacute infective endocarditis. BAIR et al[46] could demonstrate, that also 99mTc-labelled antigranulocyte imaging localizes infective prosthetic valvular disease.

The disadvantage of 111In-oxine granulocytes in the reported studies were the inappropriate physical characteristics for SPECT imaging and so small vegetations could not be visualized. In contrary, 99mTc-/123I immunoscintigraphy offers best characteristics for SPECT.

So MUNZ et al[23] reported, that the combination of immunoscintigraphy with SPECT and echocardiography localizes subacute infective endocarditis in 11 of 15 patients. But the authors stressed, that only the 24h-SPECT scans led to a correct localization of the focus due to the residual blood pool activity at 4-6h. In all these patients echocardiography, especially the transesophageal approach, detects vegetations with confirmed infective endocarditis with a resolution down to 2-3 mm is size. Thus the resolution is far better than that of immunoscintigraphy. On the other hand scintigraphy localizes not only vegetations,but also valvular leaflets, connective tissue infection, endocardium infection and other than cardiac infections as a possible focus of endocarditis.

LUNG DISEASES

The scintigraphic detection of inflammatory lung diseases with 111In-oxine granulocytes offers problems. COOK et all[47] only found infective lung diseases in 52% of patients with a focal lung uptake. A lot of positive uptakes occurs in septic disordes, when activated granulocytes pool in the lung.

Immunoscintigraphy of granulocytes has not yet been systematically examined in patients with pneumonia or other infective lung diseases. To our own experience lung abscesses can well be detected, but we have never localized pneumonias. This runs parallel with single reports about false negative scans in lung abscesses[41]. It is still unproven whether 99mTc-anti-NCA-95 scanning offers an advantage over the potential of 111In-oxine and especially of Ga-67 scanning in lung infections.

HUMAN ANTIMOUSE ANTIBODIES

The large IgG1-molecules are strong inducers of human antimouse antibodies (HAMAS). The HAMAS could make a second administration of the antibody potentially dangerous or could possibly lead to image degradation due to rapid hepatic clearence of the immunoconjugates. Recently evidence, however, indicates that imaging can be performed in the face of HAMAS with worthwhile results[48]. These data demonstrate, that HAMAS are induced but often are of minor importance. Probably the low doses of injected antibodies minimize the HAMA response in these patients.

But also these low HAMA response rates may lead to clinical problems. So the question arises what precisely can be done to make antibody injection more safe. The first and most obvious option for change is the use of small fragments. The production of engineered antibodies, the so called chimeric antibodies, could reduce the HAMA problem. Human monoclonal antibodies would also reduce the production of HAMA. For the use of antigranulocyte antibodies only the first step has been studies in a small number of patients.

99mTc-Antigranulocyte Fab'-Fragments (INCA-90)

Recently BECKER et all[47] reported their experiences with 99mTcFab'-fragments. They used a one vial system with 1.25 mg of lyophilized murine NCA-95-Fab'-fragments(IMMU-MN3;IMMUNOMEDICS,INC). After labelling with 740-900 MBq of 99mTc-pertechnetate they injected 0.5 to 1.25 mg of the labelled fragment after a short incubation period of 5 min. The labelling efficiency was higher than 95%. In 10 patients they compared the immunoscintigraphic images with the results of 111In-oxine or 99mTc-HMPAO labelled leucocyte images. The examined patients suffered from osteomyelitis, abdominal sepsis or sinusitis. The correlation between autologous leucocyte scintigraphy and immunoscintigraphy was good. But in two patients the detection of the focus was possible already one hour after fragment injection, whereas the leucocyte images got positive at 24 h and demonstrated a negative 4 hours scan. Calculating the target to background ratio over the focus the ratio was 1.7 in with both imaging modalities. The ratio decreased in the antibody scans but increased in the leucocyte scans to the 24 h image. All the detected lesions with the fragment could already be detected at 1 h p.i.. The HAMA results in 8 specimens one month after injection were all negative. These preliminary data demonstrate the rapid available diagnosis with a safe procedure, but further results have to prove these promising data.

99mTc-Anti-Lymphocyte Antibodies (IgG1;CD4)

Rheumatoid arthritis is accepted to be an autoimmune disease with a predominant role of CD4 T-cells[62], which appears to initiate and perpetuate inflammation possibly after they have been elicited by contact with environmental antigens and stimulated during encounter of cross-reactive structures unique for the joint cartilage. Persistently stimulated in the inflammatory focus these T-cells might then initiate and perpetuate inflammation. Murine monoclonal anti-CD4 antobodies have been therapeutically used in rheumatoid arthritis and clinical improvement was observed[39]. Based on this considerations we decided to use a 99mTc labelled anti CD4 antibody (MAX.16H5) with high affinity to the human CD4-molecule for scintigraphic imaging[56]. It is not known whether elimination of CD4-cells or merely inhibition of T cell activation are the predominant effects. The latter might be possible because CD4-molecules interact with MHC class II molecule during antigen recognition by T cells[55, 56].

No information is yet available concerning traffic and distribution of CD4 T cells during anti - CD4 therapy which may help clarifying this issue. Moreover present imaging modalities in rheumatoid arthritis, especially in the early disease is disappointing and of minor value in differentiating joint diseases. Radiographs of the joints only show soft tisue swelling[57], joint scintigraphy[58] with 99mTc-pertechnetate is not diagnostic and records only synovia hyperemia with moderate sensitivity and low specificity[53, 66]. The scintigraphy with 99mTc-phosphate-complexes demonstrated the pattern of joint involvement, if subcortical bone metabolism is already involved, and may well establish the diagnosis[64].

154

PATIENTS

4 patients with active, severe rheumatoid arthritis were examined. Long lasting previous conventional therapy was performed with gold salts, penicillamine, and methotrexate in all patients and with endoxane, azulfidine, chloroquine, interferon and lymphapereses in some patients. 4 weeks before scintigraphy the conventional antiinflammatory therapy was stopped, ongoing steroid treatment was retained with less than 10 mg/d. All the patients had a positive rheumatoid factor, positive β-2-microglobulin and hyperimmunoglobulinemia. These patients were part of a study population who underwent experimental anti-CD4 treatment: a therapeutic trial for refrectory rheumatoid arthritis[61].

The Ritchie-index[64] and the number of painful joints were used to monitor the severity and the actual extent of the disease[52]. For this reason we used the joint tenderness score of shoulder, elbow, wrist, metacarpophalangeal, proximal, hip, knee, ankle midtarsal and metatarsal joints. A scoring of other joints and a separate scoring of immediately neighboured joints was not performed, because in the scan grading these joints are only difficult to score separately. The following clinical grading was used:
- grade 0: the patient had no tenderness
- grade 1: the patient complained of pain
- grade 2: the patient complained of pain and winced
- grade 3: the patient complained of pain, winced and withdrew

The joints were furthermore examined for being swollen or not. Swollen joints were judged as 1, not swollen joints as 0. Using this scoring, we had to judge 44 joints (both sides and 5 proximal inter phalangeal joints and so on) of every patient.

Three of these patients were examined with intravenously injected 99mTc-labelled antibodies. One female patient was examined with in-vitro antibody labelled lymphocytes.

Monoclonal Antibodies

Anti-CD$_4$ monoclonal antibodies were produced by immunizing BALB/c mice with the human CD$_4$ + T cell clone 2C11[56]. Spleen cells of immunized mice were fused with the Ag8.653 fusion partner. Hybridoma supernatants were tested in cell-ELISA and cytofluorometric analyses for exclusive binding to CD$_4$ + T cells prepared from peripheral blood. Titration of the anti-CD$_4$ antibody MAX.16H5 subsequent Scatchard-plot analysis om Molt 4 cells revealed a considerably high association constant to the CD4 molecule. MAX.16H5 monoclonal antibody was produced, purified and tested according to the requirement for monoclonal antibodies in therapy[54]. The antibody has been tested at the workshop (T101)[63].

99mTechnetium-Labelling

The monoclonal antibodies were labelled according to the Schwarz method[52]. The antibodies were provided as a kit with 2 mg of the lyophilized, partially reduced antibody together with a Sn(II)-complex. For this reason the antibodies were mildly reduced with 2-mercaptoethanol, purified and stabilized with phosphate buffer and sorbitol. The tin-complex was 1,1,3,3-propantetraphosphonat (PTP).Immediately before application of the antibodies, 2-3.7 GBq of freshly eluted 99mTc-pertechnetate were added to the solution of the lyophilized antibody and the dissolved tin-complex. After an incubation of 15 min at room temperature, 370-550 MBq of the labelled antibodies (200 μg - 300 μg) were slowly intravenously injected. Measured by HPLC there was less than 1% free pertechnetate and less than 1% 99mTc-PTP and incubated at room temperature for 20 min. After washing the cells once more with NaCl 0.15 M the labelling efficiency was determined. In this lymphocyte preparation the labelling efficiency of CD4 expressing cells was no more than 2%. At least 10 MBq of 99mTc antibody labelled cells were reinjected.

RESULTS

There was no adverse reaction observed after the intravenous application of the 99mTc-labelled monoclonal antibody[65].

Organ Activity Distribution

The distribution of the radioactivity [66] of the whole body could be compared 4h and 24 h p.i. After 24 h the total amount of whole body activity after a decay correction was 4% +/- 1.1% lower than 4 hours p.i. The only significant activity excretion was by the kidneys, so about 4% of the applicated activity was presumably renally excreted. The splenic uptake decreased from 4 h (7.5% +/- 0.7% of the total body activity) to 24 h p.i. (4% +/- 0.6%) (p<0.01). This is a decrease of 39%. The liver activity slightly increased from 25% +/- 0.9% at 4 h to 30% +/-0.8 (p<0.01) of the total body activity at 24 h p.i. This is an increase of the liver activity of 30%. The estimation and calculation of the bone marrow uptake is difficult, because the outlining of the bone marrow by different regions is difficult. This is the reason why the rib uptake was not calculated. Regarding the difficulty of delining exactly all bone marrow structures about 50% +/-2.5% of the radioactivity were localised in the bone marrow 4 h and 24 h p.i.. Joints without pathologic activity had uptake values of 0.5% +/-0.09, diseased joints had an uptake of 2% (4 h), which increased up to 2.5% (24 h). This is an increase of 25% (p>0.05). The mean value of the joint uptake of both shoulders, elbows, hips, knees and ankles was 9.5% +/- 0.9% and increased to 12.5% (+/-1.2%). This is an increase of 31.5% (p>0.05). The uptake ratio in the small joints was not calculated from the whole body scan.

Clinical Index, Bone Scan and Immunoscintigraphy

The individual joint infiltrations could be localised not earlier as 90 min p.i.. In all patients both with in-vivo labelled lymphocytes and in-vitro labelled lymphocytes the joints could be clearly delineated 4 to 6 hours p.i. 20 hours p.i. they still could be seen, but there was no additional information in these late scans. The infiltration of the joints with CD_4- labelled lymphocytes was best correlated with the joint swelling and the positive early bone scan (bloodpool scan) (Fig2). The CD_4-scan was only weakly correlated with the Ritchie-index and not significantly with the late bone scan. There were different patterns of joint uptake. We found nearly negative late bone scans with intensive uptake in the CD-scan. On the other hand there was an intense uptake in the bone scan without any positive immunoscintigraphical findings.

CONCLUSIONS

These data demonstrate, that immunoscintigraphy of leukocytes has comparable results as conventional in-vitro labelling techniques of leukocytes. These techniques are

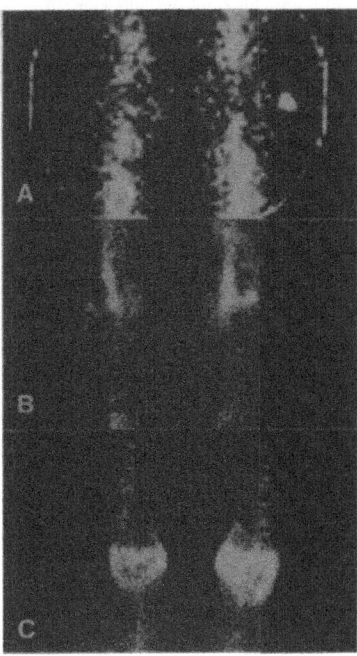

Fig. 2. Three 99mTc-CD4-antibody scans with significant joint uptake differences in a patient in remission of disease (A), a patient with moderate activity (B) and a patient with severe activity of chronic polyarthritis (C).

rapidly available, easy to prepare and offer low radiation exposure to the patients. The HAMA problem is lower as primarily expected and can still be lowered for example by using Fab' fragments.

REFERENCES

1. Buchegger F., Schreyer M., Carrel s., Mach J.P. Monoclonal antobodies identify a CEA crossreacting antigen of 95kD(NCA-95) distinct in antigenicity and tissue distribution from the previously described NCA of 55kD.*Int J Cancer* 3: 643-649 (1984).
2. Noworolska A., Harlozinska A., Buchegger F., Lawinska B., Richter R. Expression of non specific cross-reacting antigen species in myeloid leukemia patients and healthy subjects. *Blut* 58: 69-73 (1989).
3. Berling B., Koblinger F., Grunert F., Thompson J.A., Bromacher F., Buchegger F., von kleist S., Zimmermann W. Cloning of a carcinoembryonic antigen gene family member expressed in leukocytes of chronic myeloid leukemia patients and bone marrow. *Cancer Res*50: 6234-6239 (1990).
4. Watt S.M., Sala Newby G., Hoang T., Gilmore D.J., Grunert F., Nagel G., Murdoch S.J., Tchilian E., Lennox E.S., Waldmann H. CD66 identifies a neutrophil-specific epitope within the hematopoetic system that is expressed by members of the carcinoembryonic antigen family of adhesion molecules. *Blood* 78: 63-74 (1991).
5. Oikava S., Inuzuka C., Kuroki M., Matsuoka Y., Kosaki G., Nakazato K. Cell adhesion activity of non-specific cross-reacting antigen (NCA) and carcinoembryonic antigen (CEA) expressed on

CHO cell surface: homophilic and heterophilic adhesion. *Biochem. Biophys. Res Commun* 164: 39-45 (1989).

6. Benchimol S., Fuks A., Jothy S., Beauchemin N., Shirota K., Stanners C.P. Carcinoembryonic antigen, a human tumor marker, functions as an intercellular adhesion molecule. *Cell* 57: 327-334 (1989).

7. Leusch H.G., Hefta S.A., Drzeniek Z., Hummel K., Markos-Pusztai Z.,Wagner C. Escherichia coli of human origin binds to carcinoembryonic antigen (CEA) and non- specific cross-reacting (NCA). *Febs Lett*261: 405-409 (1990).

8. Solter D., Knowles B.V. Monoclonal antibodies defined a stage specific mouse in ionic antigen (SSEA-1) *Proc. Natl. Acad. Sci USA* 75: 5565-5569 (1976).

9. Bosslet K., Steinsträser A., Schwarz A., Schorlemmer H.U., Krumwieh D., Sedlacek H.H. Generation and functional characteristics of the granulocyte selective monoclonal antobody BW250/183 in:Becker W., Wolf F. Immunoscintigraphy of blood cell elements. *Nukl. Med* 28: 148-159 (1989).

10. Joseph K., Höffken H., Bosslet K., Schorlemmer H.U. In vivo labelling of granulocytes with Tc-99m-anti-NCA monoclonal antibodies for imaging inflammation. *Eur. J. Nucl. Med* 14: 367-373 (1988).

11. Andres R.Y., Schubiger A., Tiefenauer L., Seybold K., Locher J.T., Mach J.P., Buchegger F. Immunoscintigraphic localization of inflammatory lesions: concept radiolabelling and inh-vitro-testing of a granulocyte specific antibody. *Eur. J. Nucl. Med* 13: 582-586 (1988).

12. Maschek W., Neumüller H., Pastl K., Dienstl E., Böhler N., Syre G. Kinetic und immunozytochemische Färbung monoklonaler Tc-99m-markierter Anti-CEA-Antikörper gegen Granulozyten nach intravenöser Applikation. *Nucl Med* 29: 19-23 (1990).

13. Schubiger P.A., Hasler P.H., Novak-Hofer I., Bläuenstein P. Assessment of the binding properities og Granuloszint. *Eur J Nucl ed* 15: 605-608 (1989).

14. Steinsträsser A., Ber berich R., Kuhlman L., Zabori S., Schwarz A. Bindung des monoklonalen Antikörpers BW250/183 an menschliche Granulozyten. *Nukl. Med.* 31: 57-63 (1992).

15. Schwarz A., Steinsträsser A. A novel approach to Tc-99m-labelled monoclonal antibodies *J. Nucl. Med* 28: 721 (1987).

16. Hasler P.H., Seybold K., Andres R.Y., Locher J.T. Schubiger P.A. Immunoscintigraphic localization of inflammatory lesions: pharmacokinetics and estimated absorbed radiation dose in man. *Eur. J. Nucl. Med* 13: 594-597 (1988).

17. Becker W., Borst U., Fischbach W., Pasurka B., Schäfer R., Börner W. Kinetic data of in-vivo labeled granulocytes in humans with a murine Tc-99m-labelled monoclonal antibody. *Eur. J. Nucl. Med* 15: 361-366 (1989).

18. Dillman R.O., Beauregard J.C., Sobol R.E., Royston I., Bartholomew R.M., Hagan P.S. Halpern S.E. Lack of radioimunodetection and complications associated with monoclonal anticarcinoembryonic antigen antibody cross reactivity with an antigen on circulating cells *Cancer Res* 44: 2213-2218 (1984).

19. Becker W., Marienhagen J., Ordnung D., Wolf F. Kinetic of In-111-oxine labelled, Tc-99m-anti-NCA-95-MOAB in-vivo and in-vitro labelled granulocytes. in: Schmidt H.A.E., Chambron J. (eds.) Nuclearmedicine, Schattauer (1990) 311-313.

20. Becker W., Schaefer R., Börner W. In vivo viability of In-111-labelled granulocytes demonstrated in a sham-dialysis model. *Brit J. Radiol* 62: 463-467 (1989).

21.Juweid M., Fischman A.J., Rubin R.H., Baum R. Strauss H.W. Comparision of Tc-99m-labelled monoclonal antigranulocyte antibody and In-111-labelled IgG for the detection of local sites of infections in rats. *Nucl. Med. Comm.*12: 637-644 (1991).

22. Becker W., Saptogino A., Wolf F. The single late Tc-99m granulocyte antibody scan in inflammatory diseases. *Nucl. Med. Comm* 13: 186-192 (1992).

23. Munz D.L., Morguet A.J., Sandrock D., Heim A., Sold G., Figulla H.R., Kreuzer H., Emrich D. Radioimmunoimaging of subacute infective endocarditis using a technetium-99m monoclonal granulocyte specific antibody. *Eur. J. Nucl. Med* 18: 977-980 (1991).

24. Seybold K., Locher J.T., Coosemans C., Andres R.Y., Schubiger P.A., Bläuenstein P. Immunoscintigraphic localization of inflammatory lesions: clinical experience. *Eur. J. Nucl. Med* 13: 587-593 (1988).

25. Sciuk J., Puskas C., Greitemann B., Schober O. White blood cell scintigraphy with monoclonal antibodies in the study of the infected endoprosthesis. *Eur. . Nucl. Med* 19: 497-502 (1992).

26. Becker W., Pasurka B., Börner W. Bedeutung der Leukozytenszintigraphie bei der infizierten Totalendoprothese. *Fortschr. Röntgenstr* 150: 284-289 (1989).

27. Pring D.J., Henderson R.G., Rivett A.G., Krausz T., Coombs R.R.H., Lavender J.P. Autologous

granulocyte scanning of painful prosthetic joints. *J.Bone Joint Surg* 68: 647-652 (1986).

28. Palestro C.J., Swyer A.J. Kim C.K., Goldsmith S.J., Infected Knee prosthesis: diagnosis with In-111 leukocyte, Tc-99m-sulfur-colloid and Tc-99m-MDP imaging. *Radiology* 179: 645-648 (1991).

29. Pring D.J., Henderson R.G., Keshavarzian A., Rivett A.G., Krausz T., Coombs R.R.H., Lavender J.P. Indium-granulocyte scanning in painful prosthetic joint *Radiology* 179: 645-648 (1991).

30. Reuland P., Winker K.-H., Heuchert Th., Ruck P., Müller-Schauenburg W. Weller S., Feine U. Detection of infection in postoperative orthopedic patients with Technetium-99m labeled monoclonal antibodies against granulocytes. *J. Nucl. Med.* 32: 2209-2214 (1991).

31. Hotze A., Briele B., Overbeck B., Kropp J., Gruenwald F., Mekkawy M.A., von Smekal A., Moeller F., Biersack H.J. Technetium-99m-labelled anti-granulocyte antibodies in suspected bone infections.*J. Nucl. Med* 33: 526-531 (1992).

32. Sciuk J., Brandau W., Vollet B., Stücker R., Erlemann R., Bartenstein P., Peters P.E., Schober O. Comparision of technetium-99m polyclonal human immunoglobulin and technetium-99m monoclonal antibodies for imaging chronic osteomyelitis. *Eur. J. Nucl. Med* 18: 401-407 (1991).

33. Schauwecker D.S. Diagnosis with In-111 labelled leukocytes. *Radiology* 171: 141-146 (1989)

34. Kaps H.P., Georgi P. Die Leukozytenszintigraphie mit Indium-111 bei akuter und chronischer Osteomyelitis im Tiermodell-Eine experimentelle Studie. *Nucl. Med.* 25: 61-70 (1986).

35. Becker W., Fleig W., Marienhagen J., Hahne E., Wolf F. Diagnostische Bedeutung der intestinalen Aktivität bei der Immunoszintigraphie mit Tc-99m-NCA-95-Antikörpern. *Nucl. Med.* 229: 47-48 (1990).

36. Segarra I., Roca M., Baliellas C., Vilar L., Ricart Y., Mora J., Puchal R., Martin-Comin J. Granulocyte-specific monoclonal antibody technetium-99m BW 250/183 and Indium-111 oxine labelled leucocyte scintigraphy in inflammatory bowel disease. *Eur. J. Nucl. Med* 18: 715-719 (1991).

37. Becker W., Fischbach W., Reiners C., Börner W. Three phase white blood cell scan: its diagnostic accuracy in abdominal inflammatory diseases. *J. Nucl. Med.* 27: 1109-1115 (1986).

38. Mahida Y.R., Perkins A.C., FrierM., Wastie M.L., Hawkey C.J. Monoclonal antigranulocyte antibody imaging in inflammatory bowel disease: a preliminary report. *Nucl. Med. Comm* 13: 330-335 (1992).

39. Becker W., Fischbach W., Jenett M., Reiners C., Börner W. In-111-oxine labelled white blood cells in the diagnosis and follow-up of Crohn's disease. *Klin. Wschr.* 64: 141-148 (1986).

40. Fischbach W., Mössner J., Seyschab H., Höhn H. Tissue carcinoembryonic antigen and DNA aneuploidy in precancerous and cancerous colorectal lesions. *Cancer* 65: 1820-1824 (1990).

41. Lind P., Langsteger W., Költringer P., Dimai H.P., Passl R., Eber O. Immunoscintigraphy of inflammatory processes with a technetium-99m labeled monoclonal antigranulocyte antibody (MAb BW 250/183). *J. Nucl. Med.* 31: 417-423 (1990).

42. Lawrence P.F., Dries D.J., Alazraki N., Albo D. Indium-111 labelled leucocyte scanning for detection of prosthetic vascular graft infection. *J. Vasc. Surg.* 2: 165-173 (1985).

43. Becker W., Düsel W., Berger P., Spiegel W. The In-111 granulocyte scan in prosthetic vascular graft infections: imaging technique and results. *Eur. J. NUcl. Med* 13: 225-229 (1987).

44. Cordes M., Hepp W., Langer R., Pannhorst J., Hierholzer J., Felix R. Vascular graft infection by I-123 labelled antigranulocyte antibody (anti-NCA-95) scintigraphy. *Nucl. Med.* 30: 173-177 (1991).

45. Becker W., Borst U., Maisch B., Epping J., Börner W., Kochsiek K. In-111-labelled granulocytes in inflammatory heart disease. *Eur. Heart J. (Suppl.)* 1: 307-310 (1987).

46. Bair J., Becker W., Volkholz H.-J., Wolf F. Tc-99m-labelled anti-NCA-95 antibodies in prosthetic heart valve endocarditis. *Nucl. Med.* 30: 149-150 (1991).

47. Cook P.S., Datz F.L., Disbro M.A., Alazraki N.P., Taylor A.T. Pulmonary uptake in indium-111 leucocyte imaging : clinical significance in patients with suspected occult infections. *Radiology* 150: 557-561 (1984).

48. Abdel-Nabi H., Doerr R., Roth S.C. Recurrent colorectal carcinoma detection with repeated infusions of In-111 ZCE - 025 Moab. *J. Nucl. Med* 30: 748 (1989).

49. Bosslet K., Auerbach B., Höffken H., Loseph K. Frequence and relevance of the human antimouse immunoglobulin (HAMA) response in immunoscintigraphy. in: Becker W., Wolf F. Immunoscintigraphy of blood cell elements. *Nucl. Med.* 28: 148-159 (1989).

50. Berberich R., Hennes P., Alexander C. Enzündungsnachweis und HAMA-Bildung nach Applikation des monoklonalen Antikörpers BW 250/183.

51. Becker W., lauer U., Marienhagen J., Goldenberg D.M., Wolf F. Comparison of Tc-99m-antigranulocyte (NCA-95) Fab'-fragments and scintigraphy with In-111-oxine/Tc-99m-HMPAO-labelled leucocytes in infectious diseases. *J. Nucl. Med* 33:903 (1992).

52. Bull, B.S., Westengard J.C., Farr M., Bacon P.A., Meyer P.J., Stuart J. Efficacy of tests used to monitor rheumatoid arthritis. *Lancet* II:965-967 (1989).

53. Coleman R.E., Samuelson C.O., Jr., Baim S., Christian P.E., Ward J.R. Imaging with Tc-99m-MDP and Ga-67 Citrate in patients with rheumatoid arthritis and suspected septic arthritis: concise communication. *J. Nucl. Med* 23: 479-482 (1982).

54. Emmrich F. Empfehlungen für die Herstellung und Prüfung in vivo applizierbarer monoklonaler Antikörper. *Dtsch. Med. Wschr.* 112:194-198 (1987).

55. Emmrich F. Activation of T cells by crosslinking the T cell receptor complex with the differentiation antigens CD4 and CD8. Implications for the generation of MHC-restriction and for repertoire selection in the thymus. *Immunology Today* 9: 296-300 (1988).

56. Emmrich F., Eichmann K., Weltzein H.U. The generation of the repertoire of T cell specificities and functions: towards a concictent model. *Progr. In. Immunol. VI, Toronto* 406-417 (1986).

57. Gilliland B.C., Mannik M. Disorders of the joints and connective tissue in: Harrison's (ed) Principles of Internal Medicine McGraw Hill, Tokio 1872-1880 (1980).

58. Green F.A., Hays M.T. The pertechnetate joint scan. *Ann. Rheum. dis* 31: 278-286 (1976).

59. Herzog Ch., Walker Ch., Pichler W., Aeschlimann A., Wassmer P., Stockinger H., Knapp W., Rieber P., Müller W. Monoclonal anti-CD4 in arthritis. *Lancet* II: 1461-1462 (1987).

60. Hoffer P.B., Genant H.K. Radionuclide joint imaging. *Sem. Nucl. Med.* 6: 121-129 (1976).

61. Horneff G. Burmester G.R., Strobel G., Gramatzki M., Kalden J.R., Emmrich F. Therapie der chronischen Polyarthritis mit einem monoklonalen Antikörper gegen das CD4-Antigen auf T-Helferzellen. *Akt. Rheumatol* 14: 232 (1989).

62. Janossy G., Panay G., Duke O., Bofill M., Poulter L.W., Goldstein G. Rheumatoid arthritis: a disease of T-Lymphocyte/ macrophage immunoregulation. *Lancet* II: 839-842 (1981).

63. Kissmeyer-Nielsen F. (ed). Tissue: histocompatibility and immunogenetics. *Munsgaard*, Kopenhagen, 63 (1989).

64. Ritchie D.M., Boyle J.A., McInnes J.M., Jasani M.K., Dalakos T.G., Grieveson P., Buchanan W.W. Clinical studies with an articular index for the assessment of joint tenderness in patients with rheumatoid arthritis. *Quart. J. Med* 37: 393-406 (1968).

65. Becker W., Horneff G., Emmerich F., Burmester G., Kalden J., Wolf F. Kinetics of Tc-99m-labelled antibodies against CD4 (T-Helper) lymphocytes in man. *Nucl. Med* 31: 84-90 (1992).

66. Becker W., Emmerich F., Horneff G., Burmester G., Kalden J.R., Schwarz A., Wolf F. Imaging autoimmune rheumatoid arthritis specifically with Tc-99m-labelled anti-CD4 (T-Helper lymphocyte) antibodies. *Eur. J. Nucl. Med* 17: 156-159 (1990).

IN VITRO AND IN VIVO COMPARISON OF SOME PROPERTIES OF ANTIGRANULOCYTE ANTIBODIES

J.Th. Locher[1], K. Seybold[1], P.H. Hasler[2], P. Bläuenstein[2] and P.A. Schubiger[2]

[1]Department of Nuclear Medicine, Kantonsspital, Aarau
[2]Radiopharmaca Division, PSI, Villigen-PSI
Switzerland

INTRODUCTION

Our experience with the immunoscintigraphy of infection exceed 600 cases. In 1985 we started with an 123I labeled compound, the anti- CEA antibody Mab-47, which binds to granulocytes in a very specific manner (Locher 1985). It was, thereafter, an useful tool to detect hidden infections either by conventional scintigraphy or by SPET. But, the unsatisfactory supply with 123I should be eliminated by developing the 99mTc labeled Mab 47. We tried several prototypes of 99mTc- kits, from which one was clinically tested. This compound consists of a derivative of Mab- 47, namely a tetraaza ligand coupled with a carboxylate bound to the free amines of Mab 47 and tin tartrate. This kit seemed to be very handy for clinical use (because the labeling was performed in a one-step process only). After the addition of pertechnetate and a single filtration process to eliminate colloidal 99mTc byproducts this agent was ready for injection. The product had identical biokinetical properties as the iodinated form, but, unfortunately, was not stable enough for routine preparations. We found, that the coupling of the ligand to the antibody needed an optimal amount of ligands, which was difficult to get in a water medium without damaging the antibody. It is well known, that in the meantime the BW 250/183, another 99mTc-labelled Mab from Behring, became commercially available and very successful (Joseph 1987). Here the labeling is performed by the Schwarz method, a two step procedure, which works very good for complete (and therefore relatively large) antibody molecules.

METHODS

The *technical datas* of the different reagents used for comparison are summarized thereafter (Table 1). The short physical halflife of 99mTc allowed the application of higher activity doses (15 mCi for our preps, up to 30 mCi for the Bering compound) compared with the 123I-mab. Also the protein content was double or triple when using 99mTc labeled agents, what implies some higher risks of antigenicity (to be discussed in another paper). Our clinical protocol is published elsewhere (Seybold 1988). In case of the dual isotope scintigraphies the gammacamera window setting for the respective energy peaks was very narrow (+/- 5%) in order to keep the effect of contaminatory 123I- radiation into the 99mTc-range neglectable (below 7%).

Table 1. Comparison of technical datas

	123I Mab-47	99mTc Mab-47	99mTc BW 250/183
Injected dose (mCi)	3 - 5	15	15 - 30
Physical halflife (hrs.)	11	6	6
Protein content (mcg)	120	200 - 500	200 - 500
Available form	labeled	kit	kit
Preparation on site	none	1 step	2 steps
Radiochemistry	iodogen	terminal aminogroup	double S- brigde

IN VITRO RESULTS

Plasma binding curves were almost equal in all studies as demonstrated over 48 hours in 5 patients. We measured individual values of 7-17%, what was in a good agreement with the theoretical calculations of Hasler presented at the ISORBE meeting in Vienna (Hasler 1990) and the experiences of others (Becker 1989).

The *blood activity* declined biexponentially using both labels. For all reagents two markedly different halflife have been measured. After the correction for decay the values were almost identical ($t_{1/2}$: 0,73 and 9,28 hrs. ($t_{1/2 \, eff.}$ for the 99mTc-agent: 4,7 hrs.)), what signifies an equal biokinetic behaviour of all preparations during the first hours after injection.

The data of *paper-chromatography* (TLC) of blood and urine samples supported this fact. Up to 24 hours there was a single narrow peak in plasma probes. In contrast urine samples show an identical peak after 6 hours only, whereas after 24 hours a doubling of peaks indicates the appearence of some degradation products. (The excreated activity was at the same R_f value as the 99mTc- tetraaza complex, the rest being mainly pertechnetate and small amounts of unidentified byproducts. On the HPLC (separation by molecular weight) the same results were obtained as with TLC: In the case of 123I the excreated activity was found at the R_f value of iodide.)

For both isotopes the *urine excreation* reached 15-20% of the injected dose after 36 hours, but the cumulative percentage was lesser for 99mTc- preps. Together with some scintigraphic observations we interpret this fact with a substantial liver uptake (because of an in vivo formation of microcolloids, perhaps depending on the quality of the labeling process).

The *biodistributions* in man of both reagents were comparable too. Higher accumulations in the measured organs were seen using the iodinated agent, probably due to the better detectability because of its longer halflife. This result also correspond with some clinical observations.

The whole body and organ specific *clearences* are crucial factors for the diagnostic possibilities of scintigraphy and SPET. The effective halflife is most important. As to be shown, some chronic infections could be better diagnosed with the 123I-Mab-47, because the directing, so called "filling-in" phenomenon takes some time to be seen. On the other hand a shorter effective halflife of the 99mTc-compounds corresponds with lower *radiation doses*.

RESULTS OF COMPERATIVE CLINICAL STUDIES

Dual Isotope Studies

Studies of the whole body distribution of both 99mTc mabs, independently of the labeling method used, showed a typical renal uptake and, in comparison with the 123I-mab, a more prominent concentration of the activity in the liver. It is our experience, yet, that the degree of the liver activity of 99mTc is rather dependent on the quality of the labeling procedure than caused by biokinetical differences. We explain this with an accidental and, therefore, variable formation of microcolloids, which are trapped by the RES. A similar mechanism must be supposed in the case of an adverse immunoreaction because of an exceeded HAMA production (see next paper Seybold).

Comparison of 123I-Mab-47 and BW 250/183

Similar results, as already noted under above, were found in all cases of an acute infection on planar scans. However, in contrast with the iodinated mab, SPECT images were not possible to perform after 24 hours p.i., when for the labeling 99mTc was used (because of the shorter halflife). This is a disadvantage in cases of *chronic osteomyelitis*, in which the tracer accumulation is hampered by the local pathology. Then, the gradual filling-in of the activity into an initial cold lesion could be followed on planar scans only with a much lower chance of detectability. This phenomenon is typical for any form of infection and, therefore, diagnostically important. It is not seen in cases of destruction of bone marrow or scars. (Figure 1).

Comparisons of Both 99mTc Labeled Compounds

In a series of patients we compared the 99mTc labeled Behring compound with our 99mTc labeled mab-47; in other words the classical two step method of labeling with our one step version. Repeated injections within 4 days were necessary for this study. Planar scans as well as SPECT images (figure 2) revealed equal results in all cases at 6 and 24 hours p.i. As already supposed from the blood measurements mentioned above, the clinical results showed a biokinetically identical behaviour of both compared compounds.

The clinical experiences showed comparable methodical accuracies for the 99mTc labeled and the iodinated reagents. Depending on the clinical situation the sensitivities were 91% for the 99mTc-mab and 99% for the 123I-mab, the specificities 96% and 90% respectively.

CONCLUSIONS

The permanent availability of 99mTc and the easy labeling of the testkits together with the better quality of the scans are the main advantages of these compounds. Our comparative in vitro and in vivo studies showed only minor kinetic differences, which were mostly without any diagnostical relevance. Instead, there are some technical difficulties, which influence the use of the different immunotracers. As already said, our 99mTc-labeled mab-47 is not stable enough for the clinical use on a regular basis. We

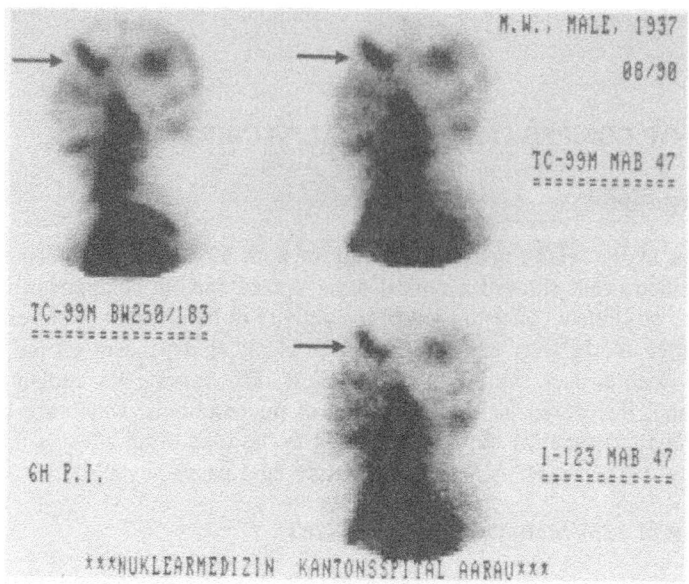

Figure 1. Cranial osteomyelitis. Identical accumulations of labeled mabs. 99mTc BW 250/183 (left); 99mTc-mab-47 and 123I-mab-47 (right)

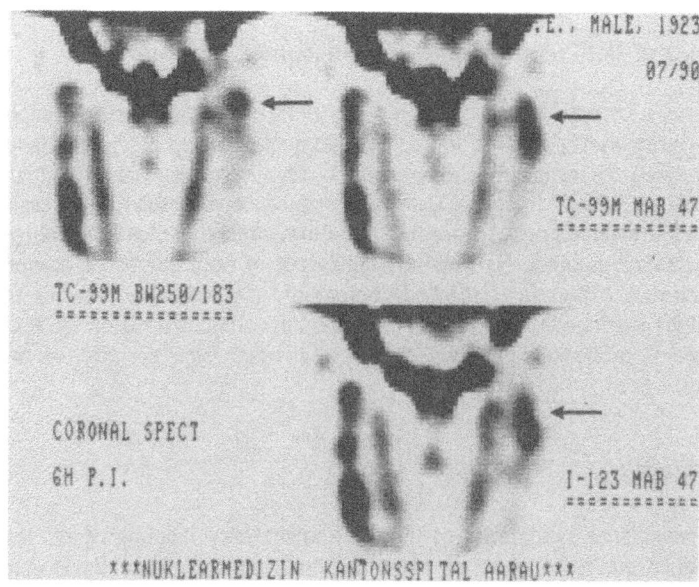

Figure 2. Infected hip prostesis (arrow). Coronal SPECT images at 6 hours p.i. 99mTc BW 250/183 (left); 99mTc-mab-47 and 123I-mab-47 (right)

hope to overcome the problems, which would be crucial for future labelings of other biomolecules or smaller antibody-fragments. Today we use the Bering compound BW 250/183 regularly in all acute cases beside its higher antigenicity and the 123I-mab-47 in more chronic cases, when SPECT and late images are needed.

REFERENCES

Locher JT, Seybold K, Andres RY, Schubiger PA, Mach JP, Buchegger F (1986) Imaging of inflammatory lesions after injection of radioiodinated monoclonal antigranulocytes antibodies. *Nucl Med Comm* 7: 659-670.

Joseph K, Höffken H, Damann V (1987) In-vivo Markierung von Granulozyten mit Tc-99m markierten monoklonalen Antikörpern: erste klinische Ergebnisse. *Nuccompact* 18: 223 - 226.

Seybold K, Locher JT, Coosemans C, Andres RY, Schubiger PA, Bläuenstein P.(1988) Immunoscintigrapic localization of inflammatory lesions: Clinical experience. *Eur J Nucl Med* 13: 587 -593.

Hasler PH, Novak-Hofer I, Bläuenstein P, Schubiger PA (1990) The in-vivo binding behaviour of an I-123 labeled anti-granulocytes antibody. In Sinzinger H, Thakur ML (Eds.) Radiolabelled cellular blood elements. Progr. in clin. biol. Research (Wiley-Liss, New York) Vol 355: 327 -336.

Becker W, Borst U, Fischbach W, Pasurka B, Schäfer R, Börner W (1989). Kinetic data of in-vivo labeled granulocytes in humans with a murine Tc-99m labeled monoclonal antibody. *Eur J Nucl Med* 15: 361- 366.

ANTIGENICITY OF DIFFERENT ANTIGRANULOCYTES ANTIBODIES ASSESSED BY HAMA FOLLOW-UP IN PATIENTS UNDERGOING IMMUNOSCINTIGRAPHIC DETECTION OF INFECTIONS

K. Seybold, M. Trinkler, L.D. Frey and J.Th. Locher

Department of Nuclear Medicine
Kantonsspital Aarau
Aarau, Switzerland

INTRODUCTION

In the last years increasing numbers of patients have being given murine monoclonal antibodies (Mabs) for radioimmunodetection (RID) and for immunotherapy. Especially, since the introduction of the immunoscintigraphy of infections (Locher 1986) antigranulocytes antibodies (AGAb) are administered in a rapidly growing scale for RID of infections and bone metastasis. Due to this, the problem of the potential human immunoreaction against murine Mabs, i.e. production of HAMA (human antimouse antibodies) has become more relevant (Courtenay-Luck 1986, Schroff 1985), because HAMA may influence the diagnostic outcome of immunoscintigraphy (Hertel 1990, Pimm 1985, van Kroonenburgh 1988). Despite that, in the recent literature there are only poor reports on HAMA follow-up in patients undergoing immunoscintigraphy of infections (Lind 1990). So we evaluated the clinical relevance of HAMA, and its determination in a larger number of patients by using various and differently labeled antigranulocytes antibodies.

PATIENTS AND MATERIALS

In 140 patients immunoscintigraphy of infections was performed partially after repeated and/or simultaneous application of various AGAb:
123I-MAb47 [Granuloszint®, PSI, Switzerland] (150 MBq/0.15 mg MAb) (Locher 1986, Seybold 1988), 99mTc-MAb47 (400 MBq/0.4 mg MAb), and 99mTc-BW250/183 [Anti-Granulozyt®, Behring, Germany] (800 MBq/0.4 mg MAb) (Joseph 1987).
From these 140 patients 158 HAMA serum courses were intensively documented after single and repeated injections of 123I MAb47 (n= 49), and of 99mTc BW250/183 (n = 84).10 patients received a simultaneous injection of the dual isotopes-labeled MAb47, while 15 patients got a repeated injection of 123I MAb 47 and 99mTc BW 250/183 within a few days for comparison reasons.

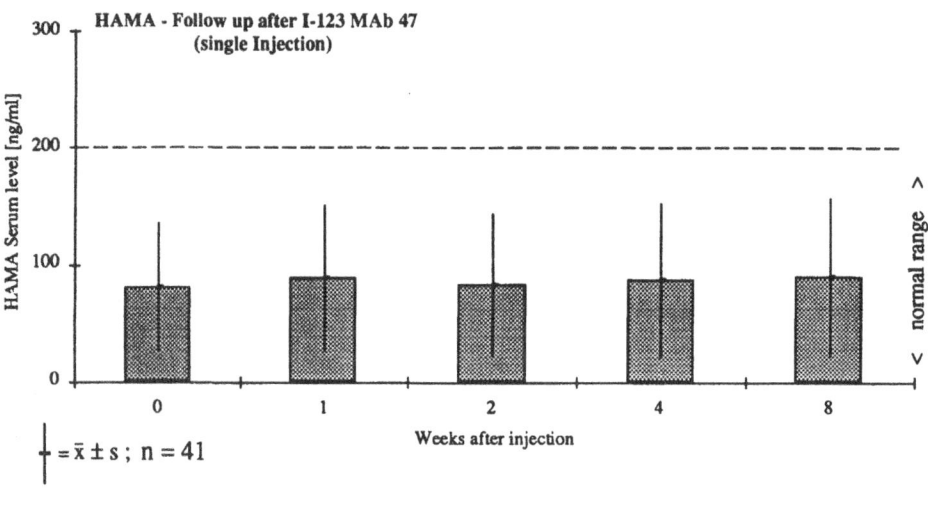

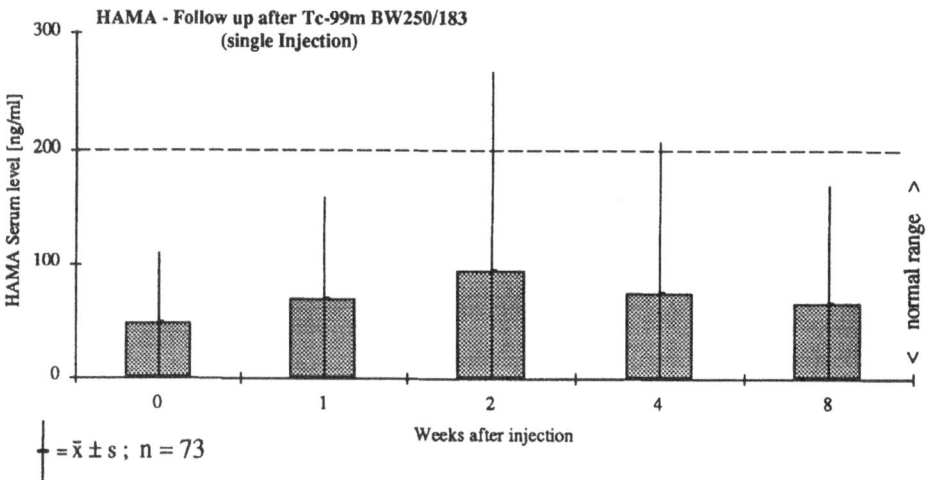

Figure 1. HAMA follow-up (mean values and standard deviations) in patients undergoing immunoscintigraphy of infection after single injection of 123I MAb47 (above) and 99mTc BW250/183.

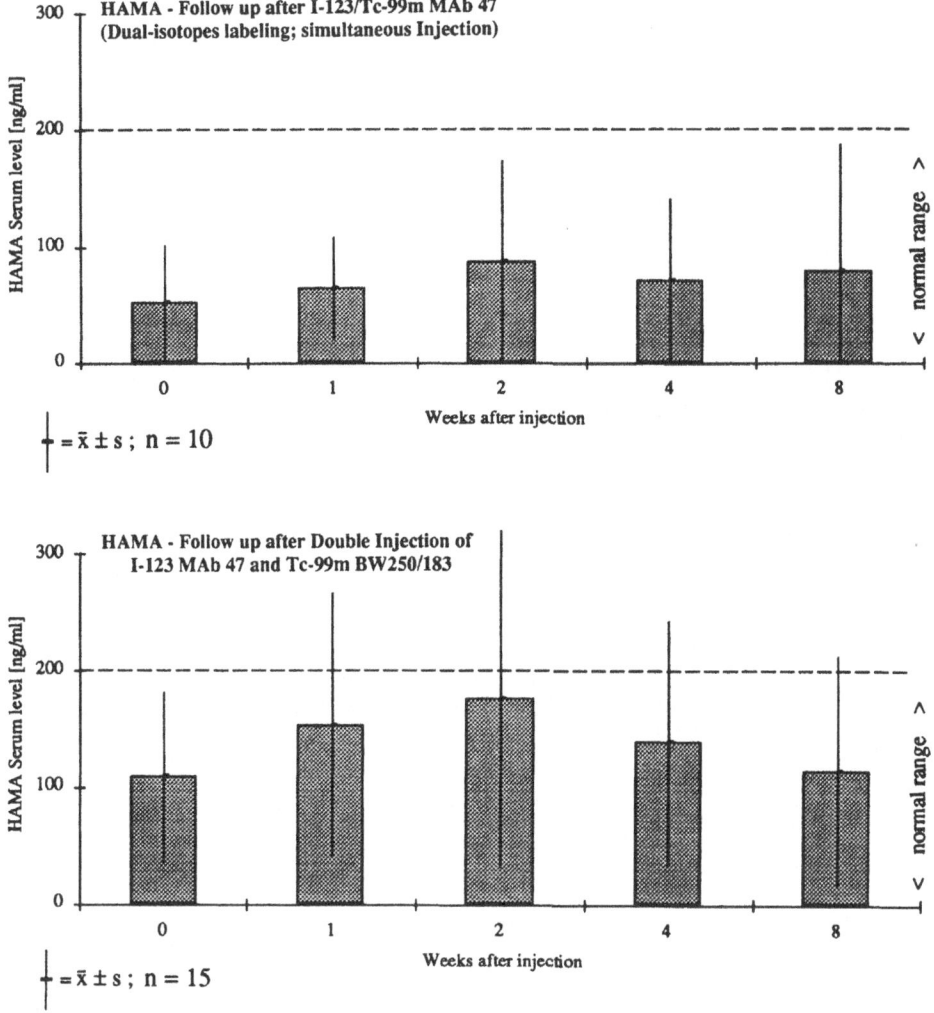

Figure 2. HAMA follow-up (mean values and standard deviations) in patients undergoing immunoscintigraphy of infection after simultaneous injection of 123I/99mTc MAb47 (above) and after repeated injection of 123I-MAb47 and 99mTc BW250/183 within a few days.

HAMA serum titers were determined before AGAb injection and 1, 2, 4 and 8 weeks thereafter by using an ELISA test system (ImmuSTRIP® HAMA, Immunomedics). This is a direct enzyme-linked immunosorbent assay for the detection and quantitation of human humoral antibodies (IgG, IgM, and IgE antibody classes) to mouse IgG (La Fontaine 1988). The test has been standardized against primate antimouse IgG serum and has a sensitivity of approximately 40ng/ml. Specific reagent formulation has eliminated the problem of background interference. HAMA serum levels below 200 ng/ml are considered to be normal.

RESULTS

In 23 of all 158 courses examined (15 %) we found elevated HAMA titers mostly

2 and 4 weeks after tracer injection and a normalization 8 weeks thereafter in most of the cases. In only 5/23 patients (with repeated injections) the HAMA titers remained elevated.

After a single dose administration of MAb elevated HAMA serum levels were seen in totally 8 % (10/114) of the courses (in 5 % (2/41) after 123I MAb47 and in 11 % (8/73) after 99mTc BW 250/183).

In figure 1, demonstrating the mean values and standard deviations of the HAMA follow-up in these two groups, there are seen no significant HAMA-changes after MAb 47 (above) but a temporary HAMA-elevation after the application of BW 250/183 with a three times higher protein amount (below).

Figure 2 shows the HAMA results of the dual isotopes-group (above) in comparison to the follow-up in patients after a repeated injection of MAb47 and BW 250/183. Though the protein amount in both groups was nearly the same, there was observed a stronger immunoreaction, if the two different antibodies were applied, than the MAb 47 with a dual isotopes labeling only. The reason for this observation still remains unexplained.

The overall pathological response after repeated or multiple injections of various antigranulocytes MAb was about 30 % (13/44) correlating well with an increase of the protein amount applied to the different groups.

No allergic or adverse reactions or side effects were observed in nearly all of the patients. Only one patient with strongly high HAMA titers after the 2nd and 3rd BW 250/183-injection showed an altered biodistribution of MAbs (low uptake in bone marrow due to a poor granulocytes labeling; high liver uptake; (Fritsche 1990, Hertel 1990, Leitha 1991, van Kroonenburgh 1988)) and a reduced imaging quality but no allergic reactions.

CONCLUSIONS

- After the administration of murine antigranulocytes antibodies the potential human immunoreaction, i.e. the HAMA-production seems to depend on the total Mab protein amount applied. Stronger immunoreactions can be seen especially after short time repetition.
- The maximum of the HAMA-response appears 2 and 4 weeks after MAb-injection, with a complete regression already after 8 weeks in most of the cases.
- In routine diagnostic work-up with a first administration of MAb the problem of HAMA is mostly neglectable regarding the imaging quality as well as allergic or adverse side effects.
- However, HAMA should be measured prior to repeated immunoscintigraphic studies, especially if using tracers with a higher MAb protein amount.

REFERENCES

Courtenay-Luck NS et al (1986). Developement of primary and secondary immunresponses to mouse monoclonal antibodies used in the diagnosis and therapy of malignant neoplassms. *Cancer Res* 46: 6489 - 6493.

Fritsche H (1990). Immunoscintographic follow-up studies with the 99m-Tc-marked monoclonal anti-CEA antibody BW 431/26. *Act Med Austriac* 17: 44 - 46.

Hertel A, Baum R P, Auerbach B, Herrmann A, Hoer G, (1990). The clinical relevance of human anti-mouse anti-body (HAMA) in immunoscintigraphy. *Nuklearmedizin* 29: 221 - 227.

Joseph K, Höffken H, Damann V (1987). In-vivo Markierung von Granulozyten mit 99mTc markierten monoklonalen Antikörpern: Erste klinische Ergebnisse. *Nuccompact* 18: 223 - 226

LaFontaine GS, Hansen HJ, Weiss BF, Goldenberg DM (1988). Enzyme immunoassay for the detection of circulating immunoglobulines in humans to mouse monoclonal antibody (HAMA). Presented at the Third International Conference of Monoclonal Antibody Immunoconjugates for Cancer: February 4 - 6.

Leitha T, Walter R, Schlick W, Dudczak R (1991). 99mTc-anti-CEA radioimmunoscintigraphy of lung adenocarcinoma. *Chest* 99: 14 - 19.

Lind P, Langsteger W, Koltringer P, Dimai HP, Passl R, Eber O (1990). Immunoscintigraphy of inflammatory processes with a technetium-99m-labeled monoclonal antigranulocyte antibody (MAb BW 250/183). *J Nucl Med* 31: 417 - 423.

Locher JT, Seybold K, Andres RY, Schubiger PA, Mach JP, Buchegger F (1986). Imaging of inflammatory lesions after injection of radioiodinated monoclonal anti-granulocytes antibodies. *Nucl Med Commun* 7: 695 - 670.

Pimm MW et al (1985). The characteristics of blood-borne radiolabels and the effect of anti-mouse IgG antibodies on localization of radiolabeled monoclonal antibody in cancer patients. *J Nucl Med* 26: 1011 - 1023.

Schroff RW et al (1985). Human anti-murine immunoglobulin responses in patients receiving monoclonal antibody therapy. *Cancer Res* 45: 879 - 885.

Seybold K, Locher JT, Coosemans C, Andres RY, Schubiger PA, Bläuenstein P (1988). Immunoscintigraphic localization of inflammatory lesions: Clinical experiences. *Eur J Nucl Med* 13: 587 - 593.

Van Kroonenburgh M J, Pauwels EK (1988). Human immunological response to mouse monoclonal antibodies in the treatment or diagnosis of malignant diseases. *Nucl Med Commun* 9: 919 - 930.

111IN-POLYCLONAL IgG AND 125I-LDL ACCUMULATION IN EXPERIMENTAL ARTERIAL WALL INJURY

L. Prat[1], I. Carrió[2], M. Roca[1], J. Blasi[1], V. Riambau[2], Ll. Berná[2],
G. Torres[2], D. Duncker[2] and M. Estorch[2]

[1]Ciudad Sanitaria Universitaria de Bellvitge
[2]Hospital de Sant Pau
Barcelona, Spain

INTRODUCTION

Atherosclerosis is a main cause of morbidity and mortality. Standard imaging techniques such as CT scanning, magnetic resonance imaging, ECO-DOPPLER, and angiography are inneffective to detect atheromatous plaques in early stages of developement, when the lesions are most metabolically active and medical interventions could be beneficial. There is therefore a clinical need to develop a noninvasive method that could assess the presence and the extension of atherosclerotic disease in patients in monitoring treatment.

We have studied human low density lipoproteins labeled with 125Iodine and human immunoglobulin G labeled with 111In as early markers of atheromatous plaques.

METHODS

Labeling Protocol

Low density lipoprotein (SIGMA) at a concentration of 6.4 mg/ml was labeled with 125I by the iodogen method. After dialysis, free Iodine was less than 1.6%. The injected dose was 200 uCi in 0.4 ml (containing 6.4 ug of LDL).

Intact human immunoglobulin G (ENDOBULIN) was labeled with 111In via the DTPA-antibody chelate method. After filtration labeling efficiency was 96%. The injected dose was 100 uCi in 0.2 ml (containing about 1 mg of immunoglobulin.)

Animals and Surgery

We performed balloon deendothelialization of carotid arteries, and balloon deendothelialization of abdominal aortas in two different animal experiments.

The first experiment was performed on a set of 14 New Zealand male rabbits in which balloon deendothelialization was performed over the right or left carotid artery at random.

The surgical procedure was as follows: Each animal was anaesthetized and after isolation of the carotid artery, a Fogarty embolectomy catheter was introduced through an arteriotomy. The balloon was inflated and three passes were made through the carotid artery to remove the endothelium.

After surgery the animals were fed with normal diet.

Six weeks later seven animals were injected with 200 uCi of labeled low density lipoprotein and seven animals were injected with 100 uCi of labeled immunoglobulin.

Fourty-eight hours after injection of tracers, 4 ml of 0.5% solution of Evans blue dye, were injected to each rabbit to stain areas of deendothelization. One hour later the animals were sacrificed and the carotid arteries were removed. Carotid arteries were washed with saline, and fixed with a 10% formalin. Each carotid artery was weighted, counted, opened, and covered with a plastic wrap, to perform macro-autoradiography. Light microscopy examination was also performed. Contralateral carotid arteries served as controls.

The second experiment was performed on a set of 5 New Zealand male rabbits with balloon deendothelialization performed over the abdominal aorta. Each animal was anaesthetized and after isolation of the right femoral artery, a Fogarty embolectomy catheter was introduced through an arteriotomy. The balloon was inflated and three passes were made through the abdominal aorta to remove the endothelium. After surgery the animals were fed with a 1% cholesterol supplemented diet.

Six weeks later the animals were injected with 200 uCi of labeled low density lipoprotein and 100 uCi of labeled immunoglobulin. Fourty-eight hours later, 4 ml of 0.5% solution of Evans blue dye, were injected to each rabbit, to stain areas of deendothelization. One hour later the animals were sacrificed. The aortas were removed, and divided in thoracic and abdominal regions. Each region was washed with saline, fixed with a 10% formalin, weighted, counted and fixed for autoradiography. Thoracic regions served as controls.

RESULTS

Light microscopy of carotid arteries revealed injured endothelium without active atheroma formation and without lipid accumulation.

The percentage of the injected dose/g of IgG-111In was significantly higher in injured carotid arteries as compared to the contralateral ones: 0.01885 ± 0.069 versus 0.005986 ± 0.003029, $p < 0.05$. No differences were observed in the values of %D.inj/g of LDL-125I between injured arteries and the contralateral ones: 0.001071 ± 0.0006369; contralateral 0.0014571 ± 0.0003735.

Autoradiography of the specimens revealed IgG-In111 uptake in the injured arteries, with localization mainly in the healing edges. Autoradiography of carotid artery after injection of LDL-I125 did not revealed tracer uptake in the injured carotid arteries.

The percentage of the injected dose /gram of IgG-111In was significantly higher in the abdominal aortas as compared to the thoracic regions: 0.00928 ± 0.00209 vs 0.02025 ± 0.00290, $p < 0.05$. Significant LDL-I125 uptake was also observed in the abdominal aortas: 0.001075 ± 0.000316 vs 0.002497 ± 0.000544, $p < 0.05$.

Autoradiography of the specimens revealed uptake of IgG and LDL in the abdominal aortas in comparison with the thoracic aortas, with the highest uptake corresponding to the healing edges of the lesions.

CONCLUSIONS

1. Administration of hipercholesterolemic diet after surgery is necessary to induce atheromatous lesions after balloon deendothelialization of the arterial wall.

2. 111In-IgG may accumulate in injured arteries without active atheroma formation.

3. 111In-IgG uptake is found both in arteries with injury alone and in arteries with atheromatous plaque formation after arterial wall injury.

4. Accumulation of IgG could be related to the inflammatory response after injury independently of atheromatous plaque formation.

REFERENCES

1. J.Rosen, P.Butler, G.Meinken, T.Wang, R.Ramakrishnan, S.Srivastava, P.Alderson, H.Ginsberg. Indium-111 labeled LDL: A potencial agent for imaging Atherosclerotic disease and lipoprotein biodistribution. *J.Nucl.Med.* 31: 343-350 (1990).
2. A.Fischman, R.Rubin, B.Khaw, P.Kramer, R.Wilkinson, M.Ahmad, M.Needelman, E.Locke, N.Nosull, W.Staruss. Radionuclide imaging f experimental atherosclerosis with nonspecific polyclonal immunoglobulin G. *J.Nucl.Med.* 30: 1095-1100 (1989).
3. I.Virgolini, P.Angelberger, J.O'Grady, H. Sinzinger. Low density lipoprotein labelling characterizes experimentally induced atherosclerotic lesions in rabbits in vivo as to presence of foam cells and endothelial coverage. *Eur.J.Nucl.Med.* 18: 944-947 (1991).
4. I.Virgolini, F.Rauscha, G.Lupatelli, A.Ventura, J.O'Grady, H.Sinzinger. Autologous low-density-lipoprotein labelling allows characterization of human atherosclerotic lesions in vivo as to presence of foam cells and endothelial coverage. *Eur.J.Nucl.Med* 18: 948-951 (1991).
5. F.Corstens, R.Claessens. Imaging inflammation with human polyclonal immunoglobulin: not looked for but discoverd. *Eur.J.Nucl.Med* 19: 155-158 (1992).
6. C.H.Paik K.Yokoyama, J.C.Reynolds, S.M.Quadri, C.Y. Min,S.Y.Shin, P.J.Maloney, S.M.Larson, R.C.Reba. Reduction of background activities by introduction of a Diester linkage between antibody and a chelate in radioimmunodetection of tumor. *J.Nucl.Med* 30: 1693-1701 (1989).
7. D.J.Hnatowich, R.L.Childs, D.Lanteigne, A.Najafi. The preparation of DTPA-coupled antibodies radiolabeled with metallic radionuclides: an improved method. *J.of Immunol. Methods.* 65: 147-157 (1983).
8. C.H.Paik, M.A.Ebbert, P.R.Murphy, C.R.Lassman, et col.Factors influencing DTPA conjugation with antibodies by ciclic DTPA anhidre. *J.Nucl.Med.* 24: 1158-1163 (1983).
9. C.H.Paik, J.J.Hong, M.A.Ebbert, S.C.Heald, R.C.Reba.W.C. Eckelman. Relative reactivity od DTPA,immunoreactive antibody-DTPA conjugates, and nonimmunoreactive antibody-DTPA conjugates toward Indium-111. *J.Nucl.Med* 26: 482-487 (1985).

RADIATION INDUCED CHROMOSOMAL DAMAGE TO LYMPHOCYTES IN USUAL 99mTc-HMPAO LEUKOCYTE PREPARATIONS

A. Furno[1], R. Gallo[2], M. Gambetti[2] and C. Basile[3]

[1]Dept. of Nuclear Medicine
[2]Dept. of Clinical Pathology
[3]Dept. of Immunohaematology
Ospedale Maggiore
Bologna, Italy

INTRODUCTION

99mTc-HMPAO leukocyte labeling (LL) was considered to result in a substantially "pure" granulocyte tagging because of the different elution rate of radioactivity from the blood elements.

Moreover, the use of 99mTc instead of 111In lowers the radiation burden to the cells.

However, elution from lymphocytes was shown not so fast as previously thought[1] and 99mTc also emits low energy electrons in its decay; therefore a significant self-irradiation of lymphocytes may be expected.

Aim of this study was to demonstrate and quantify chromosomal damage to lymphocytes in usual mixed leukocyte preparations.

METHODS

In 9 healthy donors (age 22-50, mean 33) 100 ml anticoagulated blood were withdrawn in two 50 ml separate aliquots. Both were processed according to the Hammersmith Hospital protocol, but only one underwent labeling with 740 MBq 99mTc-HMPAO.

After labeling lymphocytes from each aliquot were isolated by isopyknic centrifugation and the radioactivity distribution was evaluated in the labeled cell population.

After washing in plasma lymphocytes were resuspended in 10 ml RPMI-1640 with l-glutamine and then cultured.

From each subject 5 cultures were prepared, 2 from the not labeled lymphocytes, 3 from the labeled cell population.

For each culture 10 million lymphocytes were employed.

Culture medium was composed by RPMI-1640 with l-glutamine, fetal calf serum, antibiotics and phytohemagglutinin.

Culture were stopped after 70 h and processed.

One hundred metaphases/culture were examined.

RESULTS

A mean of 38 millions lymphocytes/subject were harvested and labeled.

Granulocyte bound radioactivity resulted significantly higher than limphocyte bound activity (Tab.1).

Table 1. Radioactivity distribution

Pt	Total Act.	Lymph.Act.	Gran.Act.	Labeled Lymph.x10^6
1	685	185	111	35
2	629	100	89	40
3	666	185	111	33
4	703	185	148	41
5	888	259	259	38
6	629	111	111	44
7	573	111	93	41
8	474	148	104	34
9	485	155	137	37
m=	637±124	129±52*	160±50*	38,1±3,7

* $p < 0,05$

Table 2. Abnormalities/100 metaphases

Pt	Unlabeled Lymph.	Labeled Lymph.
1	3	80
2	4	85
3	2	75
4	0	100
5	4	100
6	6	79
7	0	85
8	3	82
9	1	84

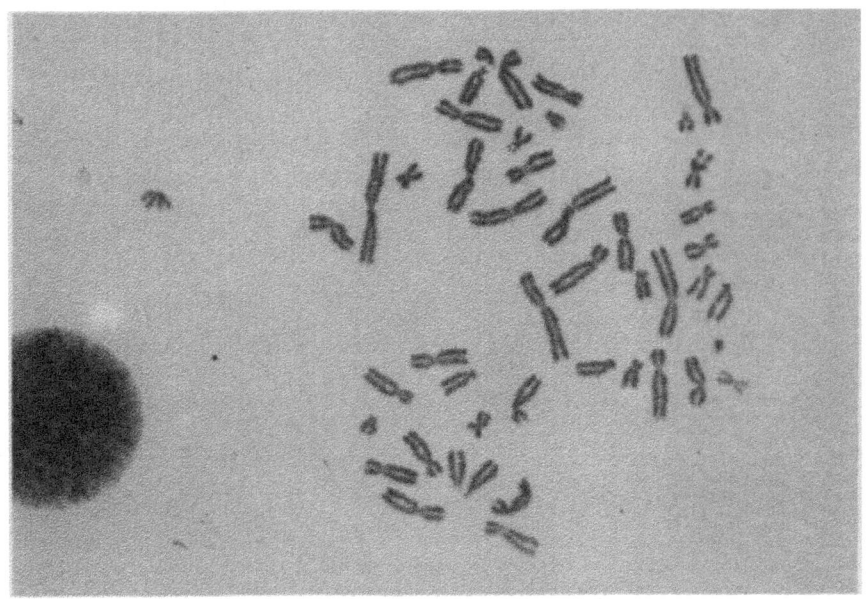

Figure 1. Metaphase from a not labeled lymphocyte culture: a chromosomal gap is present

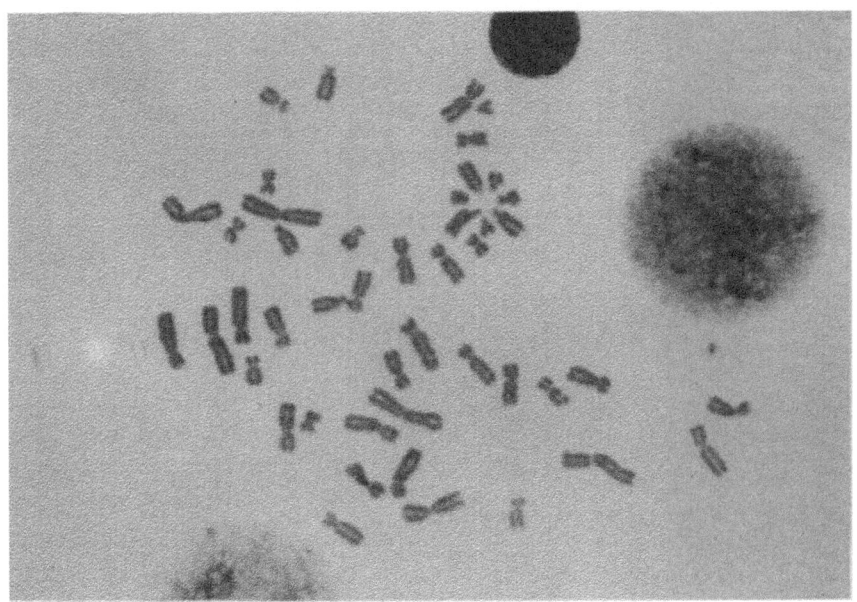

Figure 2

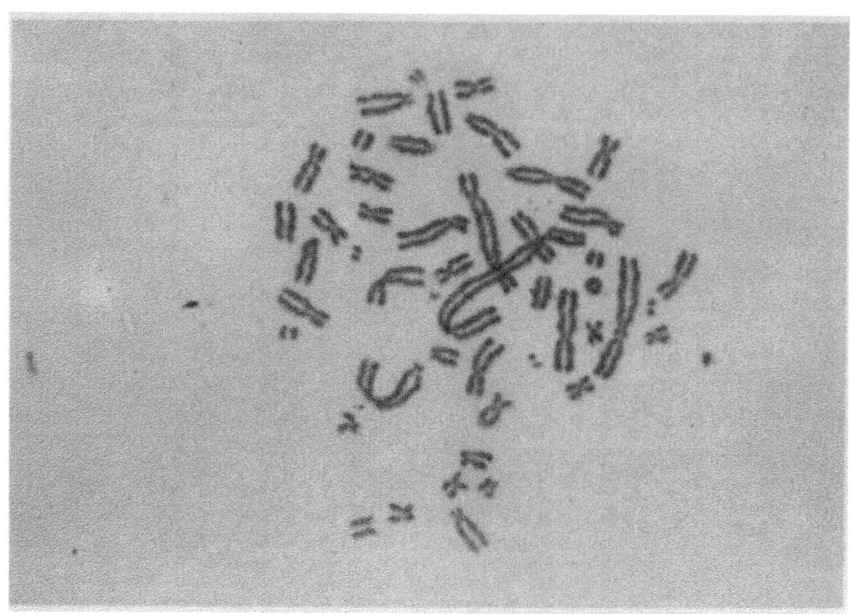

Figure 3

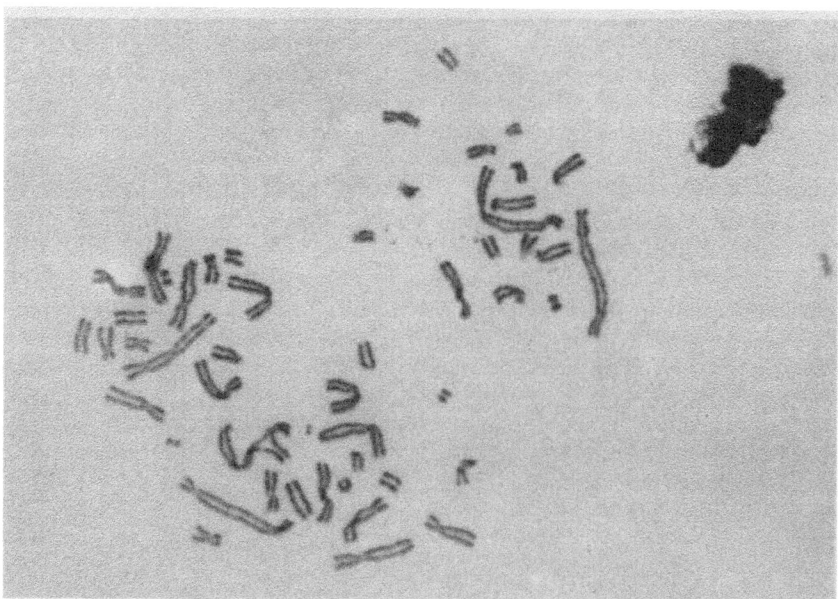

Figure 4. Figures 2-4 show various types of chromosome and chromatid damage in labeled lymphocyte cultures: chromatid gap (2), one ring, fragments, dicentrics (3), fragments, dicentrics and translocation (4)

For each subject 200 metaphases were examined, 100 from the labeled cells, 100 from the unlabeled population, and the number of aberrations scored (Table 2).

Labeled lymphocytes showed a mean of 20 aberrations/methapase with a chromatid/chromosome aberration ratio of 1:20.

Moreover, in 130/900 metaphases no significant aberrations were found, probably because of the not uniform distribution of the radioactivity into the cells[1].

In Fig.1 a methaphase from unlabeled cell culture is shown.

In Fig.2-4 various types of aberration in the labeled cell group are presented.

DISCUSSION

Among the circulating blood cells lymphocytes are the most susceptible to radiation damage and, as expected, we found a high number of metaphase abnormalities in lymphocytes obtained from mixed leukocyte preparations labeled with the usual dose of 740 MBq 99mTc-HMPAO.

Metaphase aberration were mainly of chromosomal type, but 5% were chromatid, indicating that radioactivity may induce lesions even in S and G2 stages of the cell cycle.

In a recent paper, Thierens et al. reported their experience on cultured lymphocytes obtained from 3 donors, studied after labeling with 99mTc-HMPAO[2].

With the usual dose of 740 MBq they observed an almost complete inhibition of the proliferative capacity of the labeled cells, so that a direct assessment of the radiation damage was not possible using the micronucleus assay.

For this reason they concluded that the risk for lymphoid malignancy at this high dose level can be regarded as small.

However, in our 9 cases the proliferative capacity of the labeled lymphocytes was strongly impaired, but not sufficiently to preclude a direct evaluation of the radiation damage by chromosomal analysis.

Moreover, in 130/900 metaphases (14.5%) we found no apparent aberration; although that may be explained by the not uniform distribution of radioactivity into the cells, we can't exclude a genic damage.

Therefore, in our opinion it is not possible to exclude the risk of malignancy only on the basis of a reduced proliferative capacity of labeled lymphocytes.

The clinical significance of chromosomal aberrations was elegantly discussed by Thakur and McAfee in 1984[3].

From experimental results and theoretical considerations they too concluded that the oncogenic risk due to different types of chromosomal damage can be considered small and we agree with this opinion.

CONCLUSIONS

Certainly, 99mTc-HMPAO LL causes significant genetic damage to the majority of lymphocytes, a fraction of which is not killed by radiation.

Regarding the ultimate destiny of irradiated lymphocytes in vivo, no conclusive data are available but, probably, their oncogenic potential is low.

But, small risk does not mean no risk, therefore we suggest to spend 30 minutes "extra time" to obtain "pure" granulocyte fractions for labeling procedures, mainly in young patients.

REFERENCES

1. De Labriolle-Vaylet C, Colas Linhart N, Petiet A, Bok B. Morphological and functional status of leukocytes labelled with 99mTc-HMPAO. In: Radiolabelled Cellular Blood Elements, Sinzinger H and Thakur ML Edts. Wiley-Liss New York 1990; 119-129
2. Thierens HMA, Vral AM, Van Haelst JP et al. Lymphocyte labeling with technetium-99m-HMPAO: a radiotoxicity study using the micronucleus assay. *J Nucl Med*; 33: 1167-74 (1992).
3. Thakur ML, McAfee JG. The significance of chromosomal aberrations in Indium-111-labeled lymphocytes. *J Nucl Med*; 25: 922-27 (1984).

RADIOBIOLOGIC STUDY OF 99mTc-HMPAO LABELLED LYMPHOCYTES

Cl. de Labriolle-Vaylet [1], M. Sala-Trepat [2], M.T. Doloy [3], A. Petiet [4] and N. Colas-Linhart [4]

[1]Service de Médecine Nucléaire, Hopital Saint-Antoine, Paris
[2]UA 1292 CNRS, Institut Curie, Section de Biologie, Paris
[3]Laboratoire de Radiopathologie, Commissariat à l'Energie Atomique Fontenay aux Roses
[4]Laboratoire de Biophysique des Traceurs, Faculté X. Bichat, Paris

INTRODUCTION

Labelling white blood cells with 99mTc-hexamethyl propylene amine oxime (HMPAO) is associated with the incorporation of radioactivity by granulocytes, but also by lymphocytes and monocytes[1,2]. Since 99mTechnetium emits low and moderate energy electrons (0,4 to 17 KeV) whose range is smaller than the cell dimensions, a significant cell irradiation may result from the presence of this radionuclide within the cells, and probably within their nucleus[3,4]. This is of major importance for lymphocytes, which are proliferating and very radiosensitive circulating cells. A study including physical and biological dosimetries, and the evaluation of the viability of the labelled lymphocyte was carried out to evaluate the consequences of this labelling on the lymphocyte survival.

LABELLING DATA

The leucocytes isolated from 60 ml of blood were incubated with 315 MBq (8,5 mCi) of 99mTc-HMPAO during 10 mn, and washed. The labelling efficiency was 37.7 +/- 9.7 % (n = 23, range 10-58%). Eleven per cent of the radioactivity was associated to mononuclear cells, including monocytes and lymphocytes (70 % to the PMN and 10 % to red blood cells). The final radioactive concentration was 325 KBq (8.75 μCi) per 10^6 lymphocytes. No significant elution was observed from mononuclear cells when they were kept in plasma at 37°C for two hours. When the cells were cultured in RPMI medium, the elution was 20% at the 4th hour and 50% at the 24th hour. The homogeneity of the labelling was studied using a microautoradiographic track method[2]. Four per cent of the labelled lymphocytes presented a high number of tracks (more than 50), while the others presented less than 10 tracks (fig 1). This non homogeneity of lymphocytes HMPAO labelling, previously described on mixed leucocytes[2], has been recently confirmed by ion microscopy[4].

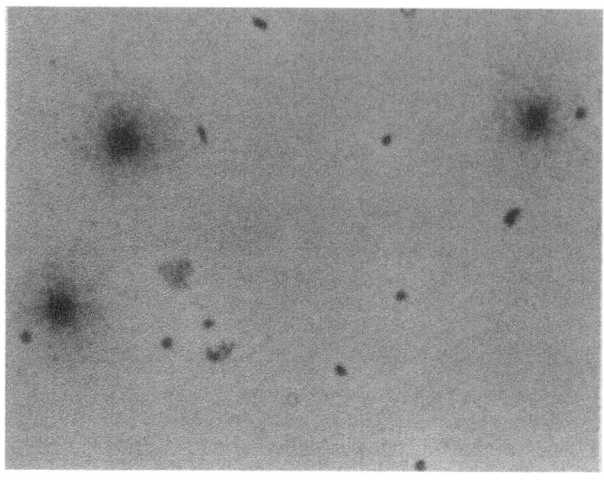

Figure 1. The microautoradiographic study demonstrates the non homogeneity of the 99mTc HMPAO labelling.

PHYSICAL DOSIMETRY

The mean cellular absorbed dose was calculated in two steps[5]. The external dose, which is the dose received by the cells during the incubation phase of labelling when the 99mTc atoms are outside the cells, was 0.13 Gy, as evaluated by classical methods[6]. The internal dose, i.e. the dose delivered by the 99mTc incorporated within the cells, calculated using Berger's scaled point kernels[7] with the assumption of an homogeneous distribution of the radionuclide in the cell, was 7.3 Gy in absence of elution and 5.5 Gy if the *in vivo* elution was supposed to be the same than in RPMI medium. Therefore, the total absorbed dose was comprised between 5.6 and 7.4 Gy.

BIOLOGICAL DOSIMETRY

The biological effects of the irradiation depend on the nucleus irradiation. As the intracellular distribution of 99mTc in the lymphocytes is not exactly known, the absorbed dose by the nucleus may be different from the mean cellular dose. The biological dosimetry was realized using chromosomal aberration counting[8]. No chromosomal aberrations were seen in the lymphocytes incubated in unlabelled HMPAO. Dicentrics and rings were present in the labelled lymphocytes. The chromosomal damages induced by the activity of 325 KBq (8.75 μCi) for 10^6 lymphocytes were equivalent to those observed after a irradiation of about 3 Gy delivered by 60Cobalt gamma rays at a high dose-rate.

LYMPHOCYTE VIABILITY

To evaluate the consequences of this irradiation on the viability of the labelled lymphocytes, T lymphocytes of two different donnors were grown in presence of

Phytohemaglutinin and Interleukin 2, for 3 weeks. For both donnors, the plating efficiencies of T lymphocytes labelled with a mean final activity approching nine microcuries are clearly different from zero (donnor n°1 : 11%, donnor n°2 : 6%).

CONCLUSION

Despite a high absorbed dose, delivered mostly when 99mTc decreases inside the cells, only a part of the lymphocytes labelled with 99mTc-HMPAO in routine conditions are dead, according to the radiobiological definition. A few T lymphocytes are still able to divide, and might carry stable mutations. The important variability of the final radioactive concentration on lymphocytes, due to the non homogeneity of the labelling and to the variability of the labelling efficiency from one patient to another, prevents the physicians to be sure that a higher radioactive concentration used for labelling will be suffisant to kill all the labelled lymphocytes. Therefore, it seems more prudent to avoid the presence of viable irradiated lymphocytes to be injected to the patient,by discarding the lymphocytes from the cell suspension before HMPAO labelling.

REFERENCES

1. Peters A.M., Osman S., Henderson .B.L., et al : Clinical experience with 99mTc-Hexamethyl prophylene amineoxime for labelling leucocytes and imaging inflammation. *Lancet*; 2 : 946-949 (1986).
2. Labriolle (de) - Vaylet Cl., Colas - Linhart N., Petiet A. et al. : Morphological and functionnal status of HMPAO labelled white blood cells. In "Radiolabelled cellular blood elements". Sinzinger (Ed.), Liss A. R. Inc, New York, 1990 ; p 119-129.
3. Costa D.C., Lui D. and P.J. Ell. White cells radiolabelled with 111In and 99mTc : a study of relative sensitivity and in vivo viability. *Nucl. Med. Comm.*; 9 : 725-731 (1988).
4. Fourré C., Clerc J., Halpern S. et al. Distribution du Technetium 99 dans les leucocytes : étude par microscopie ionique analytique (abstract). *J. Med. Nucl. Bioph.*, 3 : 238 (1992).
5. Bassano D.A. and McAfee J. Cellular radiation doses of labeled neutrophils and platelets. *J. Nucl. Med*; 20: 255-259 (1979).
6. Loevinger R., Berman M. A revised schema for calculating the absorbed dose from biologically distributed radionuclides. MIRD pamphlet N˚1, revised, New York, Society of Nuclear Medicine, 1976.
7. Berger M.J., Improved point kernels for electron and b ray dosimetry - Washington DC US Depart. of Commerce. National Bureau of Standards, 1973, 73-107.
8. Lloyd D.C., Purrot R.J. and Reeder E.J. The incidence of unstable chromosome aberrations in peripheral blood lymphocytes from unirradiated and occupationally exposed people. *Mutation. Res.*; 72, 523-532 (1980).

PEPTIDES AND PROTEINS IN RADIOLABELING OF BLOOD ELEMENTS

M.L. Thakur

Division of Nuclear Medicine
Department of Radiation Oncology & Nuclear Medecine
Tomas Jefferson University Hospital
Philadelphia, Pennsylvania

INTRODUCTION

111Indium was introduced as an efficient gamma emitting tracer to label cellular blood components nearly 17 years ago[1,2]. A year or so later, a report was published which described the feasibility of using 111In labeled antologous leukocytes to image inflammatory foci in humans[3].Today, this technique has become an established modality and a subject of numerous publications in diagnostic imaging and cell kinetic studies. Despite the succes this technique has enjoyed, there remains a compelling need to develop better agents which would eliminate some of the inherent drawbacks.

These stem primarily from; i) the lack of ready availability of 111In, ii) the less than adequate physical characteristics of the radionuclide, and above all, iii) the time consuming, in vitro procedure mandated by the mechanism by which cells are labeled with 111In oxine[4].

During the past few years, a considerable succes has been achieved in using, more desirable and readily available 99mTc. However, in this procedure too, the basic requirement for in vitro cell separation and subsequent labeling remains unchanged.

Advances in biotechnology have enabled researches to prepare, purify and identify biomolecules of unique receptor specificity that can selectively interact with targeted blood components in vivo[5-7]. Techniques have been developed to label these biomolecules with 123I, 111In or 99mTc[7-10]. As a result, an increased number of these molecules have emerged as potentially useful tools to radiolabed blood components. This receptor specifically permmits investigators to administer a desired agent directly, intravenously into a patient. The gent then binds to targeted blood component which in turn is expected to carry the radioactivity to the lesion under examination. This possibility generated by the merger of the two technologies has presaged an exiting period in the field of scintigraphic imaging.

In our laboratory, we have gained a limited experience using both peptides and monoclonal antibodies. These were labeled with 111In or 99mTc and evaluated for in vivo labeling of human neutrophils, platelets or lymphocytes. In this article, I shall briefly describe our procedures and outline impressions from the early experience.

Radiolabeled Blood Elements, Edited by J. Martin-Comin
Plenum Press, New York, 1994

MATERIALS, METHODS AND RESULTS

A. Labeling Human Neutrophils

i) With N-Formyl-Methionyl Leucyl Phenylalanine (FMLP): This peptide, originally identified as a product from bacteria that initiates chemotaxis migration of neutrophils. Upon contact FMLP was found to bind strongly to certain receptors on neotrophil (PMNs) membrane[11]. In 1978, we hypothesized that FMLP labeled with 111In and administered intravenously in small quantities, would selectively labed circulating PMNs in vivo and would thereby simplify the PMN labeling procedure.

FMLP was conjugated with human transferrin for it binds 111In with high stability[12]. The preparation was succesful but difficulties were encountered in achieving high specific activity for several FMLP molecules will bind to one transferrin molecule, the only binding site for 111In. Although the preparations labeled human neutrophils in high efficiency in vitro, it was considered that the quantity of FMLP required to label with 500 μCi 111In would be toxic. This was later confirmed that as little as 0.5 μg FMLP could induce severe neutropenia in rabbits[13]. The PMNs are activated by the peptide, and are quickly taken up by the lungs, liver and spleen. This induces transient neutropenia, in dogs, pigs, and primates. Since FMLP also activates human PMNs in vitro, it is very likely that the peptide may induce neutrophenia in humans.

Recently, A. Fischman and colleagues have labeled other analogs of FMLP with 111In via conjugation with cyclic anhydre of DTPA[14] and with 99mTc via conjugations with hydrazino nicotinamide derivative[15] and shown that the labeled peptide can be used to image experimental abscesses in the rat. No neutropenia in these animals was observed. Although, this is an excellent validation of our early hypothesis, caution in contemplating the application of chemotactic peptide in humans is warranted until a systematic data convincing a lack of neutropenia in humans are obtained.

ii) With radiolabeled, specific monoclonal antibodies, (MAbs): Several MAb specific for human neutrophils have been reported. We have evaluated ten of them, IgG and IgM in isotype[16]. These were labeled 111In using a c-DTPA as a bifunctional chelating agent and evaluated in vitro. Based on data obtained from Scatchard plot-analysis and in vitro human PMN binding assay, we have concluded that anti-stage specific embryonic antigen (α-SSEA-1) antibody was the agent of choice. It is an IgM antibody that recognizes lacto-N-fucopentoase glycoprotein on human PMN surface and has a Kd value of 1.6×10^{-11} M. It seems that the glycoprotein lacto-N-fucopentoase is available only on the membrane of human neutrophils. Presumably, as a result, the antibody does not interact with the PMNs in common laboratory animals. This has prevented us from using the antibody in experimental animal research.

Following extensive in vitro examinations, we have obtained approval from the U.S. Food Drug Administration to study the feasibility of using a-SSEA-1 (now Known as MCA-480 after the Wistar Institute cell line where the antibody was first produced[17]) in humans for imaging inflamatory foci[6].

For the human use, only 99mTc labeled MCA-480 was used. The labeling was achieved by two methods. In the first, antibody was first conjugated with c-DTPA and kept frozen until ready for labeling with reduced 99mTc. Reduction of 99mTc was accomplished with $Na_2S_2O_4$ at pH-11. In the second method, approximately one disulfide bridge from the MAb molecule was reduced with ascorbic acid (AA) to sulfhydryl groups[10] and 99mTc labeling was achieved as in the previous method. In either case, high labeling yields were obtained, but further purification was accomplished using Centricon-30 membrane filtration device. In each preparation, 100 μg MAb was used.

Clinical studies were carried out at UCLA-Harbor Medical Center in collaboration with Dr. Marcus. Patients with ongoing inflammatory processes signed a consent form and received i.v.approximately 10 mCi 99mTc preparations. Planar and occasionally SPECT imaging was performed for up to four hours post injection.

To date, five patients have been studied with 99mTc-c-DTPA-MCA-480 and 21 with 99mTc-AA-MCA-480. Although the degree of uptake in inflammatory foci varied, all lesions were correctly identified in all patients. The radioactivity bound to PMNs at 3-hours post injection varied between 14-51% and was dependent of the number PMNs in circulation. The radiactivity bound to lymphocytes averaged 8%, to platelets 3.0%, and to RBC approximately 1.3%.

The order of uptake of radioactivity in normal organs at two hours post injection was liver > red marrow (14 $\pm$ 1.8 %) > spleen > lungs > kidneys and bladder (1.3 $\pm$ 0.4 %). Although moderate bladder activity was detectable at 1 hour post injection, no intestinal uptake was seen within 4 hours. However, it was detectable 15 hours later.

All images were positive at 3 hours post injection and some were positive at as early as 10 minutes post injection. Several of these were the patient's with appendicitis and osteomyelitis. Anterior image of one patient with ascariasis in small bowel and abscess near the appendix is given in Figure 1. This condiction was confirmed by surgery.

No adverse reaction was noted in any patient.

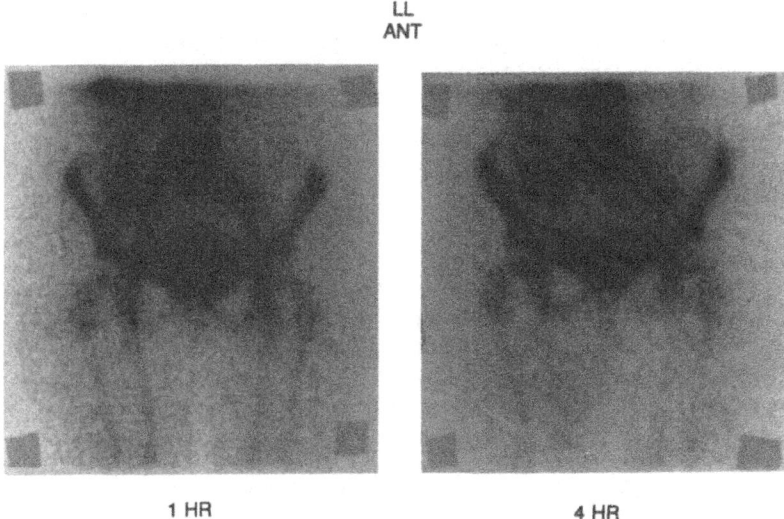

LL
ANT

1 HR   4 HR

Figure 1. Anterior images of 40 years old female who had received approximately 100 μg MCA-480 labeled with approximately 5 mCi 99mTc. The increased radioactivity uptake in the increased radiactivity uptake in the right pelvic area and resembling ascending colon was due to surgically seen asciriasis in the small bowel and absc near appendix. (Ref.6).

iii) Current Status: As can be noted elsewhere in this volume, there are three other antibody based agents being evaluated in humans. All of these are labeled with 99mTc and given intravenously to patients for imaging abscesses. All three of them are directed against NCA-95 glycoprotein on PMN surface and are labeled with 99mTc by the direct method in which sulfhydryls were generated by reduction with 2-mercapto ethanol (2-ME)[8]. Using this antibody labeled with 123I, Locher et al[7] were the first to validate the hypothesis that a radiolabeled neutrophil specific antibody could be injected directly for scintigraphic imaging of inflammatory foci.

All these agents appear to be excellent. However, they differ with 99mTc-MCA-480 by two important parameters. One is that the bone uptake with BW 250/183 for example, is as high as 70 % compared to that of only 14 % with MCA-480[5, 6]. Another is that with the use of BW 250/183, it is recommended that imaging be performed next day compared to that of within three hours post injection with 99mTc-MCA-480.

B. Labeling Platelets

i) **With monoclonal antibodies:** A large numbre of MAbs have been prepared against platelet membrane glycoprotein complex II.b.III.a. These have been labeled with 111In or 99mTc[18]. All 111In preparations were carried out using c-DTPA as a bifunctional chelating agent and all 99mTc preparations were accomplished by the 2-ME reduction method. Since human platelets have the survival time of 8 days, and radiolabeled platelets are frequently used for platelet survival studies, we considered that 99mTc tracer would be too short lived. This consideration was based on the assumption that the MAbs would selectively interact with normal healthy platelets and that after association with MAbs, their physiological charactirstics would remain unaltered.

We labeled with 111In two MAbs, B79.7 and B59.2, both specific for glycoprotein II,b.III.a.[19]. Antibodies labeled with 125I served as controls. The Kd values as determined by Scatchard plot for In-B79.7 and 125I-79.2 were 83.3×10^9 M and 113.3×10^9 M respectively. At saturation, the numbre of protein molecules bound per platelets was determined to be approximately 2×10^3. At this point, the aggregability of labeled platelets was reduced to approximately 50 % of the unlabeled control platelets. At 50 % antigen saturation, the platelet aggregability remained practically unchanged.

Canine platelets labeled at approximately 50 % saturation with 111In-B79.7 were administered intravenously to a dog bearing experimental venous thrombosis. The thrombus was easily detectable as early as 50 minutes post injection and had 15.8 times more radioactivity than in the corresponding weight of circulating blood at 2 hour post injection[19].

ii) **Current Status:** There have been several other MAbs examined with equally good or better in vitro and in vivo results. Perhaps the most studied anti-platelet antibody in humans is P.256 and P.256-F(ab')$_2$. It has been observed that nearly 75 % of the injected dose (1 mg MAb) binds to circulating platelets, yet the MAb does not reduce platelet aggregation. However, the clearance of radioactivity from circulation was very rapid[20].

Several other antibodies specific for blood components other than platelets have been evaluated as thrombus imaging agents[18]. Among these 99mTc labeled antifibrin antibody 59 D8-F(ab) has been most investigated in patients[21]. Details of this could be found elsewhere in this volume.

Peptides offer several advantages over monoclonal antibodies. Like MAb, they have the high specificity, but normally they do not induce immunologic reactions. This permits repeated studies without a serious risk to the patients. Furthermore, these molecules are relatively cheaper to produce, more robust than proteins and have faster blood clearance. All these qualities make them an excellent candidate as agents for in vivo labeling of blood agents.

On this subject, there are two reports in this monogram. One by Dr. Dean and the other by Dr. Coughlin. One describes synthetic peptides and the other, a molecular recognition unit (MRU).

Most clots are situated in high vascular region. For their early and unequivocal detection, low blood background becomes very helpful. Agents aimed at normal platelets may suffer from high blood background. Kloczewiak et al[22] have reported a 27 residue fragment of chain of fibrinogen that strongly and selectively interacts with activated platelets. The peptide inhibits fibrinogen from binding to platelets and prevents ADP activated platelets from aggregation. Modifications of the peptide that will permit us to label it with 99mTc are under progress. Studies must be performed carefully with the use of any receptor specific agent to ensure that the targeted cells are not activated and lost from circulation quickly and irreversibly.

C. Lymphocyte Labeling

Radiolabeled lymphocytes can facilitate scintigraphic detection of tumors, graft rejections, rheumatoid arthritis, other inflammatory lesions and organ specific autoimmune diseases. Surface specific tracers that may not internalize can offer added advantage of reduced radiation dose to these mononucleated, polifralating cells.

99mTc anti CD-3 and anti-CD-4 antibodies have been already evaluated in patients and promising results have been obtained[23]. We, in collaboration with Dr. Marcus and her collegues at Harbor UCLA Medical Center have labeled OKT3 with 99mTc and have performed feasibility studies in a limited number of patients with renal transplant and rheumatoid arthritis[24]. OKT3 is a murine monoclonal antibody directed to CD-3 glycoprotein with m.w. of approximately 20 KD on the surface of human T lymphocytes. OKT3 is IgG2a isotype an in therapeutic quantities functions as an immunosuppressive agent.

We labeled 20-30 μg of OKT3 with 5 mCi 99mTc by the ascorbic acid reduction method[6] and injected to only those renal transplant patients who were identified to receive OKT3. Institutional Review Board approved and informed consent forms were signed. In all patients, an intense uptake in transplanted kidneys, clinically determined to be being rejected was observed (Figure 2). In these patients, no immediate adverse reactions to OKT3 was apparent. Later, however, it was observed that even in kidneys with normal function was there relatively less but considerable uptake of radioactivity. This was discouraging.

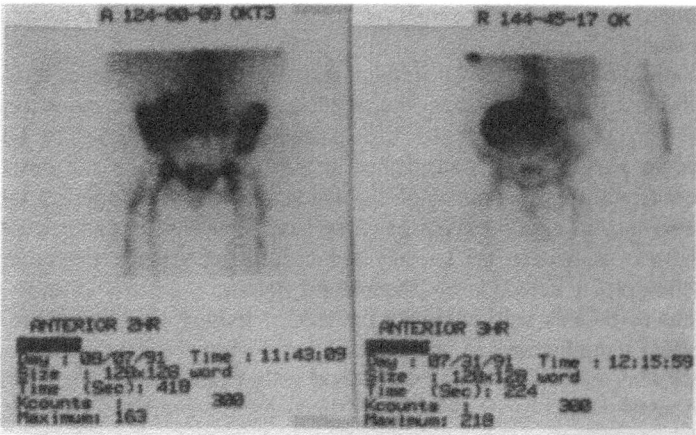

Figure 2. A composite of anterior gamma camera images of two patients with renal transplant, obtained two hours (left) and three hours (right) post injection of approximately 15 μg OKT3 labeled with 5 mCi 99mTc. Intense uptake in the transplanted kidneys in both patients is clearly visible. (Ref.24).

Seven patients with rheumatoid artritis and two patients with psoriatic arthritis were also examined. All lesions were correctly identified by scintigraphic imaging. However, in four of these patients, a mild immunologic reaction consistent with cytokine release syndrome was noted 50-60 minutes following administration of OKT3. Therefore, although these results are conceptually and practically interesting, the side effects even at the microgram levels limits its use in long term follow up of these patients.

DISCUSSION

The processes in which radioactive agents can be administered intravenously directly to the patients for specific radiolabeling of targeted blood components in vivo, are exciting and have already begun to generate promising results. This accomplishment presages an exiting time in the field of cell labeling not only because it simplifies the labeling procedure and eliminates many disadvantages associated with the in vitro labeling technique, but also because it emerges the fruitful combination of two technologies for improved management of certain life threatening diseases. It must be clear however, that the technique is still in its infancy and that the process has several disadvantages that must not be ignored.

At least three or four different types of 99mTc labeled monoclonal antibodies specific for human neutrophils (PMNs) have been examined and promising results have been obtained. Relatively fewer studies, however, have been performed to better understand the exact mechanism by which these agents accumulate in the inflammatory lesions. Determination of the proportion of the administered antibody binds to the neutrophils in circulation and to other blood components might indicated the role the labeled PMNs play in imaging. Other processes such as the binding of the labeled MAb molecules to the PMN membranes at the inflammation site may also be possible. Similarly, nonspecific accumulation of MAbs in the lesions by increased capillary permeability could not be eliminated. Also, lack at the present time are the studies comparing the efficacy of the MAb techniques with the established ones.

Determination of in vivo cell kenetics an their survival time, particularly in case of platelets, have been some of the major applications of 111In labeled platelets. With the use of shorter 99mTc as a tracer, the platelet survival studies would no longer be posible. Even the use of 111In labeled MAbs specific for platelets, the feasibility of this application has been doubtful, because of the rapid clearence of radioactivity from circulation[20]. This might be a major drawback.

Although the incidences of immunologic reaction have been relatively few or negligible in most first time studies, the risk has yet to be eliminated in repeated studies of patients who may have normal life expectancy. Antibodies like OKT3 may be administered to patients with transplanted organs, to determine the onset of rejection episodes because these patients may be the candidates for OKT3 therapy and the benefits they may receive, outweigh the risks they may face. However, in patients with rheumatoid arthritis, the use of 99mTc OKT3 may not be justified despite the promise the agent shows in scintigraphic detection of rheumatoid lesions.

The use of peptids may eliminate the risk of immunologic reactions and therefore permit repeated examinations in the same patients. However, the peptides, due to their high potency may induce severe loss of blood cells from circulation. Although this loss appears to sustain only for a very short time and is reversible, it must be carefully examined in an appropiate animal model. It should also be carefully determined that the cells that are lost from circulation are not those that were radiolabeled and if they were, then they too bounce back in circulation and make themselves available for accumulation in lesions under examination. Such studies in in vivo models together with Scatchard plot analyses and Ec-50 determinations would not only make the examinations scientifically sound but would also help to establish the intended applications of radiolabeled peptides at a rapid rate.

ACKNOWLEDGEMENT

The work described in part was supported by NIH Grant R01CA 51960. The author is thankful to Ms. Josita M. St. John for typing the manuscript.

REFERENCES

1. J.G. McAfee and M.L. Thakur. Survey of radioactive agents for in vitro labeling of phagocytic leukocytes. I. soluble agents *J Nucl Med* 17, 480 (1976).
2. M.L. Thakur, R.E. Coleman and M.J. Welch. Indium-111 labeled leukocytes for the localization of abscesses: Preparation, analysis, tissue distribution and comparision with Ga-67 citrate in dogs. *J Lab Clin Med* 89, 217 (1977).
3. M.L. Thakur, J.P. Lavender, R.N. Arnot et al. In-111 labeled autologous leukocytes in man. *J Nucl Med* 18, 1014 (1977).
4. M.L. Thakur, A.W. Segal, L.Louis et al. Indium-111 labeled cellular blood components: Mechanism of labeling and intracellular location in human neutrophils. *J Nucl Med* 18, 1020 (1977).
5. W. Becker, J. Marienhagen, D. Ordnung and F. Wolf. Kinetics of Tc-99m anti-CNA-95 Moab in vitro labeled and In-111-oxine labeled granulocytes. In "Radiolabeled Cellular Blood Elements" (Edited by H. Sinzinger and M.L. Thakur). Proceedings of the 5th Int. Symposium on Radioolabeled Cellular Blood Elements, Vienna, 1.989. Liss, New York (1990).
6. M.L. Thakur, C.S. Marcus, P. Hennemann et al. Imaging inflammatory diseases with neutrophil specific Tc-99m monoclonal antibody. *J Nucl Med* 32, 1836 (1991).
7. J.T. Locher, K. Seybold, R.Y. Andres, P.A. Schubiger, J.P. Mach and F. Buchegger. Imaging of inflammatory and infectious lesions after injection of radioiodinated monoclonal anti-granulocytes antibodies. *Nucl Med Commun* 7, 659 (1986).
8. A. Swarz, A. Steinstrabber. A novel approach to Tc-99m labeled monoclonal antibodies. *J Nucl Med* 28, 721 (1987).
9. S.J. Mather, D. Ellison. Reduction mediated Tc-99m labeling of monoclonal antibodies. *J Nucl Med* 31, 682 (1990).
10. M.L.Thakur, J. DeFulvio. Tc-99m labeled monoclonal antibodies for immunoscintigraphy. *J Immunol Methods* 237, 217 (1991).
11. H.J. Showell, R.J. Freer, S.H. Zigmond et al. The structure activity relations of synthetic peptides as chemotactic factors and endurance of lysomal enzymes secretion for neutrophils. *J Ep Med* 143 (1979).
12. S.S. Zoghbi, M.L. Thakur, A.Gottschalk et al. Selective cell labeling human neutrophils. *J Nucl Med* 22, 32 (1981).
13. J.G. McAfee, G. Subramanian and G. Gagne. Techniques for leukocyte harvesting and labeling: Problems and perspectives. *Seminars in Nuclear Medicine IXV*, 83 (1984).
14. A.J. Fishman, M.C. Pike, D. Kroon et al. Imaging focal sites of bacterial infection in rats with In-111 labeled chemostatic peptide analogs. *J Nucl Med* 32, 483 (1991).
15. M.J. Abrams, M. Juweid, C.I. Tenkate et al. Tc-99m human polyclonal IgG radiolabeled via hydrazino nicotinamide derivative for imaging focal sites of infection in rats. *J Nucl Med* 31, 2022 (1990).
16. M.L.Thakur, M.D. Richard, F.W.White. Monoclonal antibodies as agents for selective radiolabeling of human neutrophils. *J Nucl Med* 29, 1817 (1988).
17. D. Solter, B.V. Knowels. Monoclonal antibodies defining a stage-specific mouse in ionic antigen (SSEA-1). *Proc Natl Acad Science U.S.A.* 25, 5565 (1978).
18. M.L.Thakur. Scintigraphic imaging of venous thrombosis: the state of the art. *Thromb Haemorrh Disorders* 5, 29 (1992).
19. M.L.Thakur, P. Thiagrajan, W.F.W. White et al. Monoclonal antibodies as agents for specific cell labeling: Considerations, preparations and preliminary evaluation. *Nucl Med Biol* 14, 51 (1987).
20. A.J.W. Stuttle, A.M. Peters, I. Loutfi et al. Use of antiplatelet monoclonal antibody (F(ab')2 fragment for imaging thrombus. *Nucl Med Comm* 9, 647 (1988).
21. P. DeFaucal, P. Peltier, B. Planchon et al. Evaluation of In-111 labeled antifibrin monoclonal antibody for the diagnosis of venous thrombotic disease. *J Nucl med* 32, 785 (1991).

22. M. Kloczewiak, S. Timmons, M.A. Bednarek et al. Platelet receptor recognition domain on the gamma chain of human fibrinogin and its synthetic peptide analogues. *Biochemistry* 28, 2915 (1989).
23. W. Becker, F. Emmrich, G. Horneff et al. Imaging rheumatoid arthritis specifically with Tc-99m CD4-specific (T-helper lymphocytes) antibodies. *E J Nucl Med* 17, 156 (1990).
24. T.V. Huynh, C.S. Marcus, M.L. Thakur et al. Potential application of T-lymphocyte nuclear imaging in rheumatic joint diseases using anti-CD_3 monoclonal antibody OKT3. *Submitted to Rheumatology.*

PEPTIDES IN BIOMEDICAL SCIENCES: PRINCIPLES AND PRACTICE

R.T. Dean[1], J.L.- James[1], R.S. Lees[2], A.M. Lees[3], S. Vallabhajosula[4] and S.J. Goldsmith[4]

[1]Diatech, Inc., Londonderry, New Hampshire, USA
[2]Professor of Health Sciences and Technology, Harvard University and M.I.T., and President of Boston Heart Foundation
[3]Assistant Professor of Medicine, Harvard Medical School and Deaconess Hospital; Associate Director of Boston Heart Foundation (R.S.L. and A.M.L. have a direct financial interest in Diatech, Inc.)
[4]Mt. Sinai Medical Center, New York, NY

This review will discuss the evolution of radiopharmaceutical carriers and how peptides provide a new opportunity to develop highly specific carriers with desirable properties. The technical challenges in developing 99mtechnetium labeled peptides for imaging will also be discussed as well as the role this technology promises to play in the growth in imaging. Finally a specific example of the application of this technology to imaging unstable atherosclerotic plaque will be presented.

The development of new radiopharmaceutical products has depended on the ability of a radioisotope to reach and remain in a target area of interest long enough for the background to clear sufficiently to obtain a useful image. Many radioisotopes possess intrinsic properties which serve to carry the radioisotope to a desired target such as 131iodine and 201thallium. In these cases the radioisotope also serves as the carrier. New products have evolved from the search for and identification of new carriers. The carrier not only establishes the specific binding characteristics to a region of interest but also influences the biodistribution and clearance characteristics of the product. Carriers have evolved from the radioisotopes themselves to small non-radioactive molecules that bind to the desired target, and which can be easily attached to a radioisotope suitable for imaging. Good carriers in this class were often difficult to find and paralleled the intensive efforts typical of traditional drug discovery. Once found these carriers were relatively easy to manufacture and their small size usually presented favorable or easily modifiable clearance characteristics. With the advent of new technology to create monoclonal antibodies, it was quickly recognized that a wide variety of new carriers could be made available to bind specifically to a myriad of desirable targets. In a matter of months new antibody reagents could be prepared to serve as highly specific carriers, without the drawbacks of the expensive research programs to discover new small molecule drug leads. New labeling technology had to be developed to label antibodies and antibody fragments. In spite of the enthusiasm for these new reagents, certain limitations began to emerge during the development of products using antibodies . Compared to small molecules antibodies are more expensive to develop and manufacture. The manufacture of antibodies involves the hybridoma process itself, then large scale cell culture production, followed by a series of chromatographic purification steps. As these are cell derived products they must be controlled to minimize and test for virus and other microorganism contamination, and residual DNA content. These cumulatively add up to a substantial regulatory approval challenge. In addition since the preponderance of these products are murine derived they represent potential antigenic stimuli to the prospective patients[1]. The risk of a human anti-mouse antibody (HAMA) response appears to be greatest with whole immunoglobulins and progressively less with smaller fragments[2]. If the product produces a HAMA response it may compromise the patient for successive imaging or therapeutic uses. Since practically all these products are murine based, use of any one product can potentially interfere with future use of any other murine product. Nevertheless there may be overriding value for certain unique reagents produced within this class.

An additional limitation of these reagents derives from the fact that they are high molecular weight substances. Whole immunoglobulins have an approximate molecular weight of 150,000, (Fab)$_2$ fragments about 100,000 and Fab or Fab' fragments about 50,000 Daltons. For proteins in this size range clearance characteristics from the blood are dominated by the molecular weight. There has been relatively little success in favorably altering the clearance characteristics of these radiolabeled reagents by chemically modifying the carrier. Fast clearance from the blood is desirable in most cases in order to provide high target to background values within a short time after administration of the agent. This limitation has prompted the search for highly specific reagents, comparable to what can be achieved with monoclonal antibodies, but with faster blood clearance. Several years ago, several laboratories were able to demonstrate that short peptide sequences of about twenty amino acids were able to provide specific binding to target areas of interest. One such discovery was made by Lees and coworkers who were able to demonstrate that an 18 amino acid sequence of apoB-100 showed uptake properties in atherosclerotic lesions similar to that of LDL, but without the limitation of slow blood clearance. This discovery paved the way to exploring the possibility of using small peptides in place of large molecular weight protein substances as radiopharmaceutical carriers. It was quickly realized that peptide carriers offered other advantages. As they could be produced synthetically, they were more easily and inexpensively produced compared to monoclonal antibodies. There is no virus testing needed and there is a very low probability of an immune response since these are small molecules, given i.v. and cleared from the blood rapidly. Based on their properties it would appear that peptides are ideal carriers for radiopharmaceuticals. Because of the low cost and ready availability of 99mtechnetium one could conclude that the ideal new radiopharmaceutical is a 99mtechnetium labeled peptide.

The challenges of exploiting this technology rest on 1) developing peptides with desirable binding characteristics and 2) labeling the peptide with 99mtechnetium. Desirable binding characteristics of a peptide carrier include that it is specific to a given target, has a high binding affinity to the target and a low off rate, clears from the blood rapidly and has a favorable biodistribution. In considering the labeling of the peptide with 99mtechnetium, in the ideal case the label must be stable, the labeling must not interfere with peptide binding and must not adversely affect biodistribution of the agent. Given these considerations it is unlikely that previous technology that was developed to label monoclonal antibodies will be ideally suited for labeling peptides. A brief review of antibody labeling technology will serve to illustrate the point. Antibody labeling methods may be categorized into the following classes: 1) reaction of an activated acid-containing chelator with the antibody, 2) reaction of a sulfhydryl-specific chelator with the antibody, 3) reductive amination of an amine-containing chelator to the carbohydrate portion of an antibody and 4) direct labeling of a sulfhydryl-containing antibody with a reduced form of 99mtechnetium. In each of these cases there are multiple sites of reactivity on the antibody resulting in a distribution of reaction products. For example there can be as many as 10 or more lysines in the antibody to react with activated acid chelators and 4-10 sulfhydryls available for direct labeling. The reagents thus prepared are heterogeneous because the labeling chemistry does not produce a single specific product. Since antibodies are large molecules compared to the chelators attached to them, the effects on binding and biodistribution can be controlled so as to be minimal. For small peptides, however, the size of the chelator may be substantial compared to the peptide. For this reason new highly specific labeling technology is needed. The ideal characteristics of a peptide labeling technology are that it be precision labeling technology producing a single specific product, tailor-made for peptides, producing a high yield of product, with a stable label, in a fast and convenient manner for the clinical user.

The use of peptides to image atherosclerotic plaque serves as an example to illustrate the advantages of this technical approach. In 1983 Lees and coworkers demonstrated that LDL could be used to image atherosclerotic plaque in humans[3]. Though angiography is useful for the detection of arterial stenosis, this technology produces little information on the composition and character of the plaque. It has been pointed out frequently in the cardiology literature that plaques that produce mild-to-moderate stenosis angiographically often undergo abrupt disruption leading to acute events. What is needed is a method for detecting indicators of plaque instability. Following this course, Lees and coworkers reported in 1988 the results of imaging patients with carotid disease using 99mtechnetium labeled LDL[4]. Based on this study they concluded that the imaging of atherosclerotic plaque was feasible and may aid in differentiating quiescent from actively evolving plaque. Using radiolabeled LDL on a commercial basis is, however, impractical. LDL is too large a molecule to be produced commercially and suffers from extremely slow blood clearance. Lees and coworkers turned their attention toward peptides to solve these problems and in 1990 reported that an 18 amino acid peptide SP4 (Figure 1), which included residues 1000-1016 of apoB from LDL, was taken up specifically in arterial lesions of a rabbit model[5]. In 1991 Vallabhajosula and coworkers reported the ability to image atherosclerotic lesions in vivo in a cholesterol fed rabbit model with 123I SP4[6].

SP4

(Tyr and residues 1000-1016 of apoB)

TyrArgAlaLeuValAspThrLeuLys-

PheValThrGlnAlaGluGlyAlaLys-NH$_2$

Figure 1

Subsequently two different 99mtechnetium labeled analogs of SP4 were prepared, which have designated P199 and P215. Both have similar uptake and clearance characteristics in vivo. Figure 2 shows the blood clearance of 99mtechnetium P199 and P215 in both normal and hypercholesterolemic (HC) rabbits. The clearance of both compounds in the two types of animals is nearly identical. Both 99mtechnetium P199 and P215 clear faster than the 125I labeled SP4. Figure 3 shows the uptake of P199 in the arterial lesions created in the hypercholesterolemic rabbit. Rabbits were sacrificed at two hours post-injection and counts per pixel in regions of maximal uptake were compared to normal aorta. Uptake in the plaque was between 2.5 and 4.0 times that in normal aorta. Rabbits were imaged using a pinhole collimator at 15 min. and 2 hrs. post-injection of 99mtechnetium P199. Images show increased focal uptake of tracer in the region where lesions were verified after sacrifice, compared to normal. Analysis of data collected after sacrifice showed 49% of the counts from the image of the lesion containing aorta were due to uptake in the aorta, the remaining component was blood activity. The radioactivity in lesion-containing aorta plus contained in blood was 1.9 times greater than that in a similar volume of normal aorta plus blood (Figure 4). Based on these data we conclude that 99mtechnetium P199 and P215 are promising new candidates for clinical evaluation as agents for imaging atherosclerotic plaque and may provide information which differentiates actively evolving from quiescent plaque.

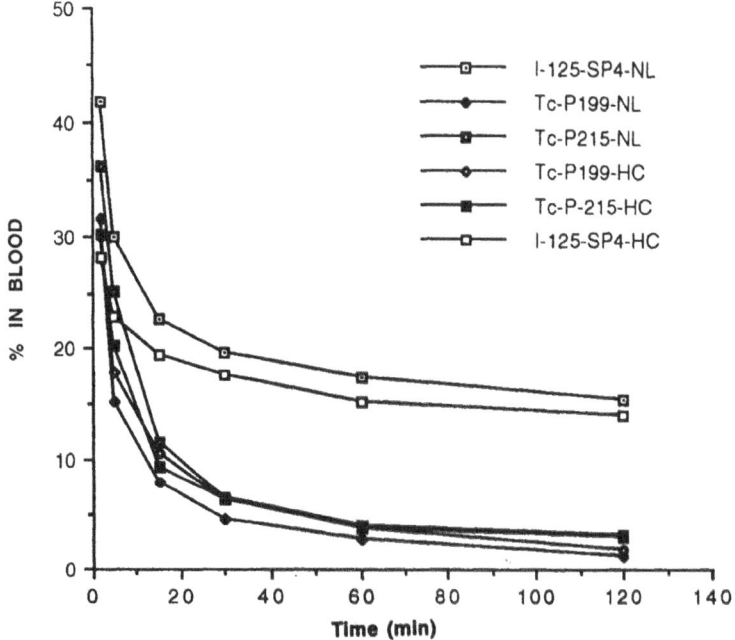

Figure 2. Blood clearance of radiolabeled peptides in normal and HC rabbits

Uptake of P199 in Arterial Fatty Lesions

in the Hypercholesterolemic Rabbit

Rabbit	1	2	3	4	Normal
Counts/ Pixel	6.6	8.6	7.7	10.5	2.6

Figure 3

Radioactivity in Aortic Wall of Hypercholesterolemic Rabbit

vs. Blood Contained in the Vessel Compared with Normal

Tc-99m P215

at 2 Hours Post-Injection (n=5)

Aorta % ID	Volume (mL)	Blood % ID	% of Counts from Aorta	(Lesion+Blood)/ (Normal+Blood)
0.0055	0.54	0.0058	49	1.9

Figure 4

CONCLUSION

In conclusion we believe that 99mtechnetium labeled peptides are a new advance in imaging that offer the opportunity to provide convenient, tissue specific imaging agents. These agents can in many cases replace antibodies and will expand the imaging market.

REFERENCES

1. Hoffman T. Anticipating, Recognizing, and Preventing Hazards Associated with In Vivo Use of Monoclonal Antibodies: Special Considerations Related to Human Anti-Mouse Antibodies. *Cancer Research (Suppl.)* 50, 1049s-1050s (1990)
2. Johnson L. L., Seldin D. W., Becker L. C., et al. Antimyosin Imaging in Acute Transmural Myocardial Infarctions: Results of a Multicenter Clinical Trial. *J. Am. Coll. Cardiol.* 13, 27-35 (1989).
3. Lees R. S., Lees A. M., Strauss H. W. External Imaging of Human Atherosclerosis. *J. Nucl. Med.* 24, 154-156 (1983)
4. Lees A. M., Lees R. S., Schoen F. J., Isaacsohn J. L., Fischman A. J., McKusick K. A., Strauss H. W. Imaging Human Atherosclerosis with 99mTc-labeled Low Density Lipoproteins. *Arteriosclerosis* 8, 461-470 (1988)
5. Shih I.-L., Lees R. S., Chang M. Y., Lees A. M. Focal Accumulation of an Apolipoprotein B-based Synthetic Oligopeptide in Healing Rabbit Arterial Wall. *Proc. Natl. Acad. Sci.* USA 87, 1436-1440 (1990)
6. Vallabhajosula S., Chinol M., Goldsmith S. J., Lister-James J., Dean R. T. Iodine-123 Labeled SP4 (Synthetic Oligopeptide): A New Radiopharmaceutical to Image Atherosclerotic Lesions In Vivo. *J. Nucl. Med. (Abstract)* 32, 1842 (1991)

MOLECULAR RECOGNITION UNITS (MRUs) AND THE IMAGING OF HUMAN DISEASE

D.J. Coughlin, V.L. Alvarez, R.D. Radcliffe, A.D. Lopes,
L.C. Knight[1] and J.D. Rodwell

CYTOGEN Corporation, 201 College Road East
Princeton NJ, 08540
[1]Department of Nuclear Medicine
Temple University School of Medicine
Philadelphia PA 19140

The use of monoclonal antibodies as *in-vivo* targeting vehicles for human imaging applications has gone from a research curiosity to wide clinical acceptance in the past several years. Monoclonal antibodies appear to be one of the best currently available targeting systems for a variety *in-vivo* delivery uses particularly for diagnostic and therapeutic radioisotopes[1]. While monoclonal antibodies represent an exquisite targeting vehicle for *in-vivo* use, they are not without drawbacks which may somewhat limit their use. For instance the use of murine monoclonals in humans may give rise to human-anti-mouse antibody response (HAMA). While the clinical manifestations of the HAMA response are still poorly understood, for some antibodies, this may be a problem for repeated *in-vivo* use.

Some potential problems of using murine monoclonal in humans have been addressed by a variety of methods. Using modern molecular biology techniques, researchers have developed engineered antibody structures such as chimeric and humanized antibodies to avoid some of the HAMA problems that may developed in patients from murine monoclonal antibodies. Other refinements of monoclonal antibodies as optimized *in-vivo* targeting agents have involved such constructs as single domain antibodies[2] and single chain antibodies[3] where a smaller protein construct is developed which contains the binding regions of the larger corresponding antibody, and thus antibody binding is reduced to a small protein unit. This reduction of antibody binding to smaller units may be particularly advantageous for pharmacokinetic reasons where rapid blood clearance of a smaller molecule, as opposed to a larger antibody, may be useful.

We have further refined this concept of reduction of antibody binding regions to very small peptides derived from the complimentary determining regions (CDRs) or binding regions of monoclonal antibodies and developed useful *in-vivo* targeting applications from these peptides. We call these small targeting peptides derived from the CDRs of monoclonal antibodies "molecular recognition units" or MRUs.

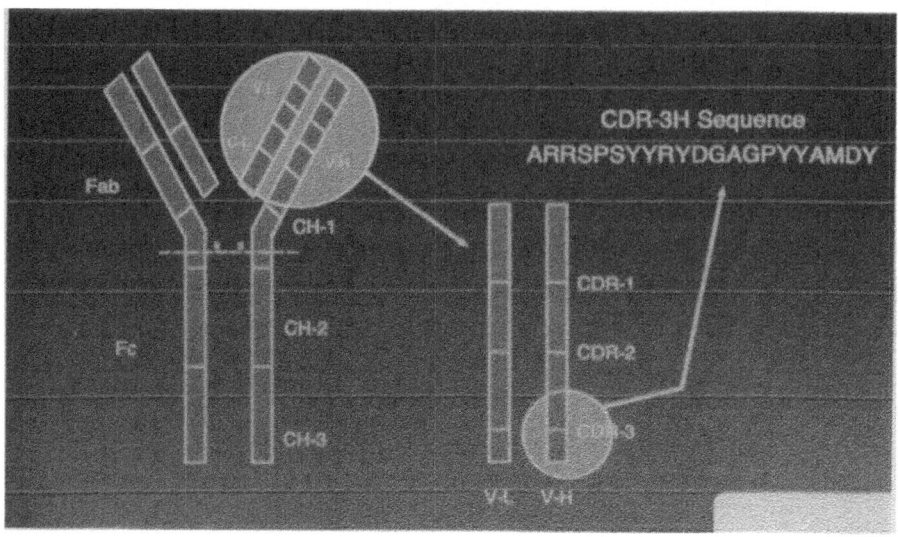

Figure 1. PAC 1.1 Antibody Structure with CDR-3H Sequence

The molecular recognition unit peptide that we first developed was derived from the third complementarity determining region of the heavy chain (CDR-3H) of the antibody PAC 1.1. PAC 1.1 is an IgM antibody to the fibrinogen receptor on activated blood platelets discovered by Shattil[4]. Upon sequencing, PAC 1.1 was discovered to contain a heavy chain CDR 3 with an unusually long, 21 amino acid sequence (Figure 1). This CDR-3H sequence contained an RYD triad in the 9-12 position. This RYD triad is similar to the RGD triad contained in several peptides which bind the same GPIIb/IIIa receptor on activated platelets. Shattil had shown[4] that the binding of PAC 1.1 to activated platelets could be inhibited by the small 21-mer peptide comprising the CDR-3H, and thus PAC 1.1 binding was mimicked by the small peptide derived from its CDR-3H. We reasoned that since PAC 1.1 binds to activated platelets, the antibody and peptides derived from PAC 1.1 may be useful for *in-vivo* targeting of activated platelets in human blood clots and with appropriate radioisotopes attached, would be useful for clot imaging. In order to make a useful platelet recognition and imaging construct from the PAC 1.1 CDR-3H peptide, several peptides derived from this sequence were designed and evaluated.

Table 1 shows the synthetic peptides derived from the CDR-3H region of PAC 1.1, that were evaluated for their binding to activated platelets using the inhibition of platelet aggregation as assay for the GPIIb/IIIa receptor binding on activated platelets. Peptide 1, the 21 amino acid sequence from PAC 1.1 showed an inhibition of platelet aggregation IC-50 value of 40 μM. A single amino acid change of Y to G in position 10 of this peptide lowered the IC-50 considerably. Thus substitution of a glycine for tyrosine in position 10 (Peptide 2) increases platelet binding in PAC 1.1 CDR-3H sequence. That the binding of the peptide to activated platelets was dependent on the RXD triad where X = Y or G was proven by the evaluation of the RYYD peptide (Peptide 3), where simple insertion of an extra tyrosine (Y) in the binding triad completely inhibited binding of the peptide to platelets. For comparison purposes two simple RGD peptides 5 and 6 were synthesized and evaluated in this assay system.

Table 1

PEPTIDE OPTIMIZATION FOR PAC 1.1 CDR-3H PEPTIDES AND FUSION PEPTIDES

Peptide	IC-50 μM
1. ARRSPSYY**RYD**GAPYYAMDY-NH$_2$	40
2. ARRSPSYY**RGD**GAPYYAMDY-NH$_2$	9
3. ARRSPSYY**RYYD**GAPYYAMDY-NH$_2$	500
4. **RGD**S	40
5. SY**RGD**SK-NH$_2$	34
6. ac-**RGD**VY-NH$_2$	49
7. ac-**RGD**V**RGD**VY-NH2	7.9
8. ac-**RGD**V**RGD**V**RDG**VY-NH$_2$	6.8
9. ac-PSYY**RGD**GA-NH$_2$	31
10. ac-PSYY**RGD**GAPSYY**RGD**GAPSYY**RGD**GA-NH$_2$	8.0
11. ac-PSYY**RGD**GAPSYY**RGD**GAPSYY**RGD**GA-NH$_2$	5.7
12. SGAYGS**RGD**GK**CTCCA**-NH$_2$	48
13. ac-SGAYGS**RGD**GK**CTCCA**-NH2	82
13. ac-SYG**RGD**V**RGD**FK**CTCCA**-NH$_2$	12

ac = acetyl

In order for small peptides to be useful for *in-vivo* targeting, they must have a reasonable half-life in the blood to allow reasonable localization. For imaging applications, the blood half-life should be balanced with the whole body clearance rate in order to optimize localization to target organs and deplete background to obtain the good image contrast. For small peptides, several methods are available to control degradation in blood from proteolysis and thus control blood half-life of the peptides. One method of reducing proteolytic degradation of peptides is the inclusion of an amino terminal acetyl group and a carboxy terminal amide group. These modifications were evaluated with the RGD peptide 6 where acetylation and amidation were shown to preserve good binding activity compared with similar RGD peptides 4 and 5. This method of blocking *in-vivo* peptide degradation was included in our subsequent peptide design. Peptides 7 and 8 show the effect of a "tandem repeat" RGD binding sequence incorporated into simple RGD peptides. The double tandem repeat in 7 increases binding activity considerably while inclusion of the triple tandem repeat binding sequence in 8 shows almost no more improvement. The double tandem repeat is probably optimal in this case when the complexity of synthesizing larger peptides is taken into consideration.

The concept of the tandem repeat RGD binding sequence was next applied to the two truncated peptides derived from the PAC 1.1 CDR-3H sequence, 10 and 11. As observed before, the double tandem repeat appeared optimal when one considers the increase in binding versus the complexity of a larger peptide. Because of this, a double tandem repeat of the RGD binding sequence was incorporated into our platelet targeting peptides.

The fusion of a platelet targeting sequence combined with a diagnostic radiometal binding sequence in a single peptide was examined, since such a fusion peptide would be an ideal MRU for *in-vivo* imaging of blood clots. The metal chelating hexapeptide KCTCCA, incorporated into the MRU peptides 12, 13 and 14, is derived from the carboxy terminal hexapeptide of the protein metallothionein. Metallothionein, a 62 amino acid protein, binds heavy metals, is cysteine rich, and contains seven metal bindings sites[5]. Thiophilic metals, particularly the useful diagnostic radioisotope 99mTc, are bound by metallothionein and its component peptides. Incorporating a KCTCCA sequence into a truncated PAC 1.1 CDR-3H derived peptide containing an RGD tandem repeat (14) preserved good platelet binding activity and this peptide was chosen as an optimized clinical candidate for *in-vivo* clot imaging studies. (Figure 2)

---

acetyl-SYGRGDVRGDFKCTCCA-amide

14

Figure 2. MRU Platelet Reactive Fusion Peptide

The preclinical evaluation of this MRU, fusion peptide 14 was performed in both a rabbit and dog model. Figure 3 shows the results of an imaging experiment in a rabbit using a blood clot model developed by Collen[6]. The MRU peptide 14 was labeled with 2.5 mCi of 99mTc by standard procedures and a 100 μg dose of the peptide administered to the animal. The clot in this rabbit model was induced in the left jugular vein and localization of the labelled peptide to the clot is shown by the area of bright intensity as indicated by the arrow. Localization and image quality improves with time as shown by the one hour and two hour rabbit image in Figure 3. The MRU fusion peptide 14 was highly effective for imaging blood clots in both rabbit and larger animal (dog) models.

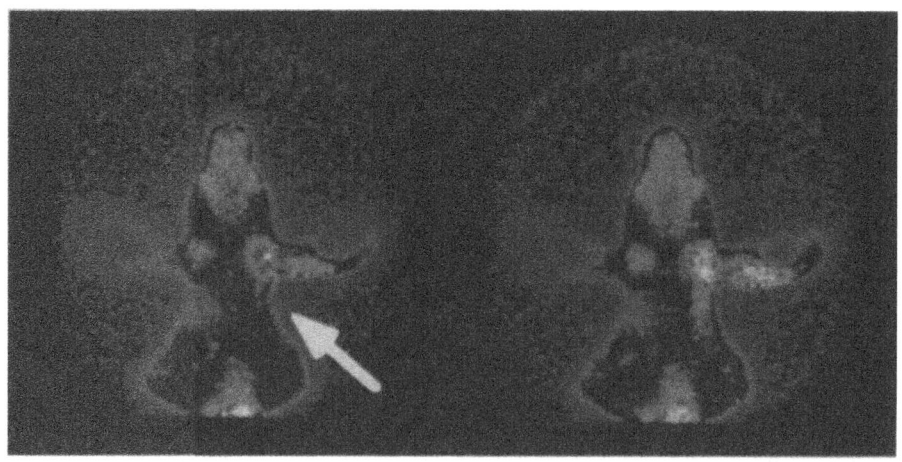

1 hr post inj   2 hr post inj

Figure 3. Rabbit Model Clot Imaging Using MRU 14

The demonstration of clinical efficacy in human blood clot imaging is shown in Figure 4. In this case a 1.0 mg dose of the MRU fusion peptide 14 was labelled with about 15-20 mCi of 99mTc and injected into a male patient. Localization of the peptide to a large, confirmed blood clot in the patient's right leg is shown by the dark band in the patient's right leg from the image in Figure 4. Further clinical evaluation of this MRU peptide is currently ongoing.

Post   Popliteal

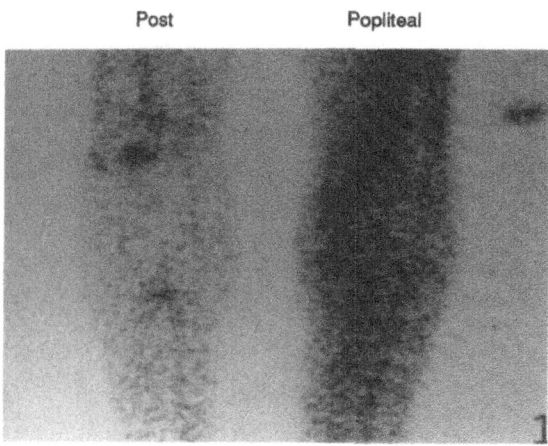

Figure 4. Post Poplireal Planar Image of MRU Peptide 14 in Human Patient

In conclusion, what we have demonstrated is that small peptides derived from antibody CDR binding regions, can be engineered and optimized to provide Molecular Recognition Units (MRUs), useful as *in-vivo* targeting agents. In this particular case, the small peptide MRU was derived from the CDR-3H of the activated platelet binding IgM antibody PAC 1.1. The PAC 1.1 CDR-3H peptide sequence was optimally engineered for platelet binding characteristics and combined with a metal binding peptide sequence to form a fusion peptide MRU.

This fusion peptide MRU serves as a useful construct for the imaging of blood clots in animal models as well as humans, and provides a useful construct for *in-vivo* targeting of radioisotopes for the imaging of human disease.

REFERENCES

1. a. Kuzel TM, and Duda RB; *Compr. Ther.* 18 (6): 16-20 (1992).
   b. Halpern SE; *Targeted Diagn. Ther.* 6: 1-22 (1992).
   c. Blend MJ; *Compr. Ther.* 17 (12): 5-11 (1991).
2. Ward ES, Güssow D, Griffiths AD, Jones PT, and Winter G. *Nature* 341: 544-546 (1989).
3. Skerra A, and Plückthun. *Science* 240: 1038-1041 (1988).
4. Taub R, Gould RJ, Garsky VM, Ciccarone TM, Hoxie J, Friedman PA, and Shattil SJ. *J.Biol. Chem.* 264: 259-265 (1989).
5. Hunziker PE and Kagi JHR; Metallothionein. In: Harrison P; ed.; Metalloproteins. Part 2: Metal Proteins with Non-Redox Roles; Verlag Chemie; Weinheim; p149 (1985).
6. Collen D, Stassen JM, and Verstraete M. *J.Clin. Invest* 71: 368 (1983).

TECHNIQUES FOR DIRECT RADIOLABELING OF MONOCLONAL ANTIBODIES

M.J. Marek, C.R. Lambert and B.A. Rhodes

RhoMed Incorporated
Albuquerque, New Mexico, U.S.A.

Regulated reduction, a controlled method for direct labeling of proteins, is defined. This procedure optimizes separate, but interdependent, parameters in the formulation of protein or peptide based radiopharmaceutical kits to increase radiochemical yields. Various analytical methods that can be used to establish radiochemical yields, radiochemical purity, and the immunoreactive fraction of the final labeled product will be summarized.

INTRODUCTION

Practical use of 99mtechnetium-labeled diagnostic or rhenium-186- or -188-labeled therapeutic radiopharmaceuticals demands a method of producing a clinically adaptable product that is efficacious, stable, easy to use and cost effective. Of the many methods which have been reported for labeling antibodies with various radionuclides, the technique that seems to be emerging as the method of choice is direct labeling of antibodies with 99mTc for diagnostic imaging and direct labeling with 186Re or 188Re for therapy (Crockford and Rhodes, 1978; Crockford and Rhodes, 1984; Reno and Bottino, 1989; Pak, 1988; Shochat, 1989, Griffiths, 1990; Hansen, 1991; Rhodes, 1992). 99mTechnetium, with its favorable physical characteristics (6.02 hr half life, 140 keV gamma photon), low cost and ready availability, is the radionuclide of choice for gamma scintigraphy. Generator produced 188rhenium (16.7 hr half life, 2.12 MeV beta photon, 155 keV gamma photon), with a chemistry similar to technetium, offers the added advantage of imaging during therapy (Griffiths et al., 1991).

Direct labeling of proteins refers to the labeling of proteins without using intermediates such as bifunctional chelates. A major advantage of the direct labeling method is that it can readily be reduced to a one-step labeling process, which is beneficial for making a marketable radiopharmaceutical kit. Another advantage of this method is that the bond formed between the reduced technetium and the protein is strong and thus resistant to transchelation. The technetium is unlikely to migrate to other molecules after it has been coupled to the protein. Direct labeling is site specific. By using groups that are distal to the antigen binding sites, interference by the labeling group with the antibody's immunoreactivity is avoided. Furthermore, the costs and complexities of synthesizing and purifying bifunctional reagents are avoided. Finally, metal binding groups introduced into proteins may act as haptens, potentially becoming immunogenic. Antibodies to DTPA, a common chelator group for binding radiometals to antibodies, have been made (Reardan et al., 1985). Direct labeling avoids this biological complication.

Macromolecules such as antibodies (and peptides) can provide a large number of binding sites for transition metals, including technetium and rhenium. Some of these sites are endogenous, while others can be "generated" by the use of reducing agents such as stannous ions and 2 mercaptoethanol, through reduction of cystine to cysteine. In highly complex protein molecules it should be expected that the primary, secondary, and tertiary structure can contribute to binding of 99mTc, and could result in 99mTc-protein bonds with slightly different bond strengths. This situation is distinct from low molecular weight complexing chelators which have a known and fixed number of donor atoms (Zamora and Rhodes, 1992).

The complexities of protein structures and the associated heterogeneity of metal binding sites poses unique considerations for both direct and indirect labeling procedures. Despite these complexities, a number of recent studies have shown that direct labeling methods provide very stable, high affinity-bonding between both technetium or rhenium and the labeled protein (Hawkins et al., 1990; Stray et al., submitted abstract; Thakur and Defulvio, 1991; Mather and Ellison, 1990; Griffiths et al., 1991; Becker et al., 1992).

Early attempts to label antibodies and proteins with 99mtechnetium met with considerable frustration. Bonding of the reduced technetium to the protein was unstable, and the bond quickly dissociated in vivo. It was observed that a fraction of the technetium was much more firmly bound to the protein (Rhodes et al., 1982; Paik et al., 1985). We and others concluded that reduced disulfide bridges in the protein provide sulfhydryl groups which strongly bond reduced technetium (Steigman et al., 1975; Rhodes et al., 1982). We have since developed a number of quality control methods to measure the relative amounts of weakly bound and strongly bound technetium (Rhodes, In preparation). By quantifying bonding, we are able to study the preparation and radiolabeling parameters to learn which are responsible for strong binding. This has enabled us to optimize radiopharmaceutical kit preparation of directly labeled proteins.

Direct radiolabeling of proteins with 99mTc comprises several steps, which can occur simultaneously or serially within the same reaction vial: (1) reduction of disulfide groups in the protein in such a way that the protein's biological characteristics are not altered; (2) preservation of the reactive sulfide groups created by the reduction of disulfide moieties; (3) reduction of pertechnetate ion to a redox state that is highly reactive with sulfide moieties; (4) preservation of 99mTc in the required redox state as a reactive intermediate by the presence of an appropriate complexing agent; and (5) incorporation of 99mTc into the protein by coordination of the reduced pertechnetate ion with available reactive sulfhydryl groups on the reduced protein in the presence of an appropriate complexing agent. The reactions are shown in figure 1. Steps 1 and 2 are given by equation (1); steps 3 and 4 are given by equation (2); and, step 5 is given by equation (3). Though each of these steps are interdependent and of equal importance in preparing a directly labeled, protein-based radiopharmaceutical of high radiochemical yield, it is critical to realize that each of these steps are separate and governed by unique parameters.

The purpose of this paper is to examine approaches to controlled reduction of disulfide groups in native proteins to provide sufficient sulfhydryl binding sites for technetium or rhenium labeling, and the subsequent stabilization of the modified protein to prepare one-step, direct-labeling radiopharmaceutical kits. We refer to this process as **"regulated reduction"**. Quality control methods used in evaluating and optimizing these parameters will also be discussed.

```
┌─────────────────────────────────────────────────────────┐
│              Chemical Reaction to Yield Tc-99m            │
│                   Strongly Bonded to Protein              │
│                                                           │
│    1.  R-S-S-R  +  SnX₂ ----->  2 R-S-Sn-X                │
│                                                           │
│    2.  TcO₄⁻ + SnX₂ + tartrate ----->  Tc[tartrate]       │
│                                                           │
│    3.  Tc[tartrate] + R-S-Sn-X ----->  R-S-TcX₂           │
│                                                           │
└─────────────────────────────────────────────────────────┘
```

Figure 1. Direct labeling reactions to form strongly bonded 99mTc-proteins.

THE PRETINNING METHOD OF THE ANTIBODY REDUCTION

Direct labeling of proteins with 99mTc to prepare a radiopharmaceutical requires careful consideration of at least two sets of variables. The first set is concerned with optimizing the reaction parameters involved in reduction of the native protein to provide sufficient, available reactive sulfhydryl binding sites for technetium or rhenium labeling. The objective is adequate reduction of disulfide bonds in the native protein without significant alteration of its physiologic properties. The second set is concerned with stabilizing the modified protein at sufficient concentration while preserving the reactive sulfhydryl donor ligands and avoiding side reactions that lead to undesirable reaction byproducts and radiochemical impurities.

A number of reductants are of practical use for protein reduction. One of the first methods of protein reduction applied to direct labeling of proteins was developed in 1979 and presented in December of that year at the First International Conference on the Radioimmunochemical Detection of Cancer (Rhodes et al., 1982). An "instant radiolabeling kit", developed from the basic methods, was presented at the 1980 annual meeting of the Society of Nuclear Medicine.

The use of stannous ion to both reduce cystine, the disulfide form of cysteine, and to protect the reduced bond is described by Harris (1922) and Andrews (1926). We have shown a time-dependent correlation between stannous incubation and antibody binding to thiol-binding gel (Rhodes, 1991). In this study, extrapolating from the measurements of the bound negative and positive controls, we estimated that only about 4% of the disulfide bridges were reduced. This observation is consistent with the findings of other investigators (Pak et al., 1989). With this low level of reduction, no change in HPLC profiles were observed.

Stannous ion has been widely used to reduce pertechnetate for forming 99mTc radiopharmaceuticals since it was first introduced by Alverez et al., (1967). The reaction of metal ions, including those of tin, with free sulfhydryl groups of proteins to form reversible co-ordination complexes is well studied (Gurd and Wilcox, 1956; Cecil and McPhee, 1959). The use of stannous both to reduce disulfide bonds and to convert them into reversible coordination complexes preparatory to 99mTc labeling was introduced in 1979 (Rhodes et al., 1982). This method of reducing antibodies with stannous ions was named "pretinning", because it was assumed that the tin fulfills three roles: reduction of disulfides, coordination with free sulfhydryl groups, and reduction of the pertechnetate.

As a result of the complex size and structure of macromolecular proteins, metal binding sites in both the native and modified protein are very heterogeneous. We have experimentally determined that, unlike the pretinning process where stannous ion acts at a specific concentration to reduce disulfides, to protect free sulfhydryl groups, and to reduce pertechnetate, regulated reduction, in which each of these parameters is separately controlled, allows us increased control for optimizing labeling parameters in the final formulation of the radiopharmaceutical kit.

We routinely perform stannous reductions on antibodies. Batches of 500 mg of human polyclonal human gamma globulin are pretinned to prepare control labeling kits for routine use in quality control procedures. Antibody is reduced at 5 mg/ml in nitrogen-purged, 40 mM potassium hydrogen phthalate, 10 mM potassium sodium tartrate in 2 mM stannous tartrate, at pH 5.6. Maltose 5 % in 0.3 M Glycine are added to stabilize the protein. The antibody is reduced at 21° C for 21 hours under nitrogen. The reduced Sn(II) protected antibody can then be directly labeled with 99mTc or rhenium at an antibody concentration of 1 mg/ml.

Two parameters of immunoreactivity as a function of stannous reduction have been studied: (1) the affinity of the antibody and (2) the immunoreactive fraction. The ELISA data given in figure 2 show no alteration of the affinity of antibody to purified antigen after stannous reduction. The immunoreactive fraction of radiolabeled antibody is measured using a solid phase antigen (Rhodes et al., 1990).

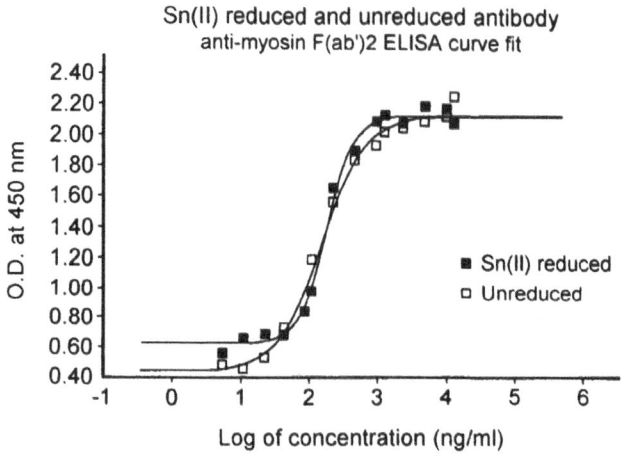

Figure 2. Binding curve showing substantially similar immunoreactivity with Sn(II) reduced and unreduced antibody.

REGULATED REDUCTION

Regulated reduction generally necessitates removal of the stannous or other reducing agent at an experimentally predetermined time or degree of protein reduction optimal for radiolabeling. Reduction is completed either by neutralizing the reducing agent or, as in the case of stannous, removal by gel filtration. Pertechnetate reduction buffer, which contains less total stannous than that required for disulfide bond reduction, is added to the reduced, protected protein in the final kit formulation. Specifically, following the stannous reduction of HgG, the reduced protein is placed on a Sephadex G-25, medium size exclusion column and eluted with 0.15 M NaCl 40 mM phthalate, 10 mM tartrate, in 4 mg/ml inositol and 4 mg/ml glycine, at pH 5.6. The reduced HgG is stored under nitrogen at 4° C during the subsequent protein assay. The extent of reduction can be determined at this step with Ellman's reagent assay for free thiols. The reduced HgG may also be stored long term under nitrogen at -70° C for later kit preparation. Once the protein concentration is determined, the reduced HgG is diluted to 2 mg/ml with elution buffer. Sodium pertechnetate reducing solution is added as 1 part 10 mM phthalate and 10 mM tartrate buffer with 0.75 mM stannous tartrate, pH 5.6 to 1 part reduced HgG at 2 mg/ml. The bulk labeling kit solution is immediately dispensed in 0.5 ml fill volumes into chilled vials and lyophilized under argon. Control HgG kits labeled with 1 to 20 mCi 99mTc or 2 mCi 186Re typically give percentage yields of radiolabeled antibody of greater than 95% by HPLC analysis with less than 3% colloid and no free pertechnetate by ITLC analysis. Hawkins et al., 1990, tested the stability of the technetium-sulfide bond by challenging 99mTc-labeled antibodies with various competing ligands and found that no exchange occurred even between reduced IgG and IgM antibodies.

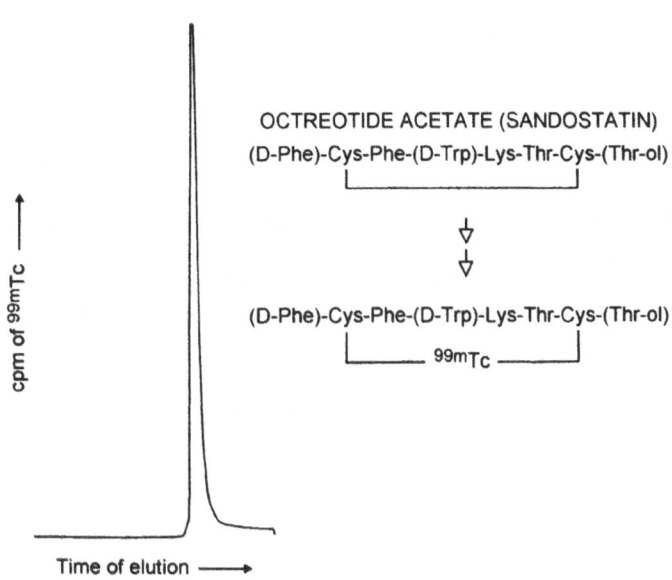

Figure 3. HPLC profile of 99mTc direct-labeled ocreotide (Sandostatin', Sandoz Ltd).

Recently, direct labeling by regulated reduction was used to prepare instant labeling kits for A6H (anti-renal cell carcinoma) and B72.3 (anti-human colon carcinoma) monoclonal antibodies labeled with 99mTc and 186Rhenium (Stray et al., abstract submitted). We have successfully labeled cysteine-containing peptides including octeotide, a synthetic somatostatin analogue, by this procedure (figure 3).

The formation of a stannous metallosulfur-coordinate intermediate may be important for subsequent, high efficiency labeling with technetium. Free sulfhydryl groups are vulnerable to oxidation which results in the reformation of the disulfide bridges.

Sulfhydryl group oxidation occurs by the action of dissolved oxygen and is promoted by traces of metal ions such as Cu(II) and Fe(III) and by alkaline pH (Gurd and Wilcox, 1956; Cecil and McPhee, 1959). The kinetics of sulfhydryl oxidation are also time and temperature dependent (Petersen and Dorrington, 1974). Reno and coworkers (Reno and Bottino, 1987; Reno et al., 1989) have used a metallosulfur-coordinate intermediate to protect the free sulfhydryl groups that they generate by reducing antibodies with dithiothreitol. They add Zn(II) to protect sulfhydryl reactivity during the period following reduction and prior to combining the reduced antibodies with technetium, and report the preparation of stable, reduced Zn-protein complexes. These intermediates appear to be similar, with respect to their reactivity with technetium, to the reduced Sn-protein complexes prepared by pretinning. Reduced proteins, in the presence or absence of stannous, are protected during regulated reduction by maintaining low oxygen tension, low pH and low temperature in all buffers used following protein reduction. The presence of trace reductants, such as stannous ion or 2-mercaptoethanol, can also act as thiol protectants, increasing labeling yields (Rhodes, 1991; Mather and Ellison, 1990; Pimm et al., 1991).

Disulfides are easily and specifically reduced by thiols, which are the most widely used reagents for this purpose (Jocelyn, 1987). Cleland (1964) describes a protective reagent for thiol groups. Because of its low redox potential (0.33 volts at pH 7), dithiothreitol (DTT) is capable of maintaining monothiols in a reduced state and of reducing disulfides quantitatively. DTT has an additional advantage over other thiols, in that its oxidation reaction is intramolecular resulting in a sterically favored cyclic disulfide. These circumstances favor the oxidation equilibrium of this dithiol, particularly in dilute solutions.

The use of DTT allows controlled, disulfide-specific reduction of antibodies at near physiologic pH. The reduction is easily slowed or stopped by pH reduction and subsequent removal of the reductant by gel filtration. Final kit formulation is completed by the addition of pertechnetate reducing solution.

Specifically, MCA-480, an IgM antibody directed against stage-specific embryonic antigen, is reduced in 0.5 mM DTT, at 5 mg/ml in 5% maltose, 0.3 M glycine in nitrogen-purged glycylglycine and phthalate buffer pH 8.0. The antibody is reduced for 30 minutes at 21° C under nitrogen. Reduction is stopped by adjusting the pH with 1 N HCl to pH 5.6, followed by gel filtration on cellulose size exclusion columns. The reduced antibody at pH 5.6 is eluted from the column with chilled, nitrogen-purged 5% maltose, 0.3 M glycine, 5 mM potassium hydrogen phthalate with 0.01 % Tween 80, pH 5.6 and is maintained under nitrogen, at 4° C, while being assayed for protein concentration. The extent of antibody reduction can, at this point be assayed by Ellman's assay for thiol groups. The final formulation is completed by the addition of 1 part nitrogen-purged sodium pertechnetate reducing solution containing 5 mM phthalate, 10 mM tartrate with 1 mM stannous tartrate in 0.15 M NaCl (pH 5.6) to 1 part reduced MCA-480 at 2 mg/ml. This final bulk formulation is dispensed in 0.25 ml fractions into chilled vials and is immediately lyophilized under argon. Radiochemical yields are typically 95% by HPLC analysis with less than 5% colloid and no free pertechnetate by ITLC analysis.

COORDINATION OF TECHNETIUM IN PROTEIN

Data accumulated on labeling of reduced antibodies suggest that although the reaction goes to completion within a few minutes, it is not instantaneous. It has been proposed that the reduced technetium species formed by pertechnetate reduction are immediately complexed to an intermediate. The complexed 99mTc is then transferred to the reactive protein binding sites (Rhodes, 1974). Complexes of reduced technetium formed by the reduction of pertechnetate with polyhydric alcohols and acids, as they are applied to the formulation of radiopharmaceuticals, were studied by Richards and Steigman (1975). A number of chelates or ligands have proven useful in the stabilization of metals as metal ion buffers (Perrin and Dempsey, 1974). Chelates or complexing agents have also been used to stabilize reduced technetium, when binding technetium to reactive sulfhydryl groups of reduced proteins. For the pretinning method (Rhodes et al., 1980), the complexing agent is tartrate. Schwartz and Steinstraber (1987) used methylene diphosphonate as the complexing agent. Pak et al., (1989) have used a D-glucarate ligand in the presence of stannous chloride and a DTT-reduced IgG fragment. We have found that, to achieve high radiolabeling yields, it is necessary to reduce the pertechnetate ion in the presence of ligand and adequately reduced protein at sufficient concentration. HPLC profiles of 99mTc-labeled human gamma globulin (figure 4) show a quantitative increase in labeling yield over increasing concentrations of sufficiently reduced antibody at labeling concentrations of 1 mg/ml. Percent yields are shown in table 1.

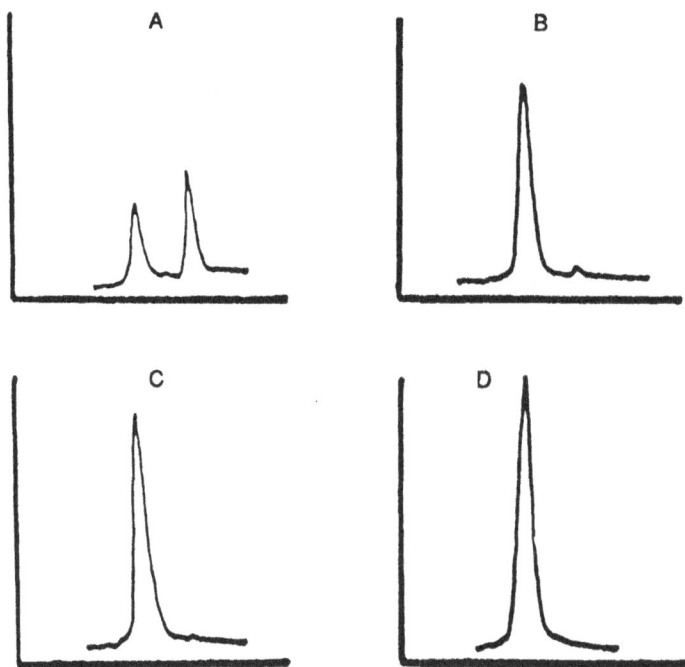

Figure 4. HPLC profiles of increasing concentrations of reduced HgG direct-labeled with 99mTc at a labeling concentration of 1 mg/ml total HgG. A. 1000 μg unreduced HgG. B. 800 μg unreduced HgG/200 μg reduced HgG. C. 400 μg unreduced HgG/600 μg reduced HgG. D. 1000μg reduced HgG.

RADIOCHEMICAL ANALYSIS OF THE LABELED PROTEIN

The final labeled product is composed of technetium strongly bound to a protein that has retained its full biologic activity and is free of radiochemical impurities. Unbound or free technetium may also be present as a result of incomplete reduction of the pertechnetate or oxidation of reduced technetium to reform pertechnetate. In addition, soluble forms of technetium other than pertechnetate may be present. The latter result from contamination of the original sodium pertechnetate solution with technetium having an oxidation state other than +7. Soluble technetium may also be bound to components or impurities of the buffer or protein solutions.

When 99mTc sodium pertechnetate is reduced in the presence of stannous and protein, peptized 99mTc colloid may occur. Such colloids are difficult to detect because they are very small colloid particles, which are disbursed by and weakly attached to the protein and are detected with or as protein in some analytical systems. Eckelman and Steigman (1991) discuss the role of this problem in complicating the development of protein labeling methods. Table 2 lists the various classes of known radiochemical impurities.

Table 1

Reduced HgG / Native HgG	HPLC % Yield	ITLC % TcO_4-
IgG control Kit	93.86	0.47
0.0 ug / 1000 ug	19.60	58.13
200 ug / 800 ug	76.43	17.80
600 ug / 400 ug	88.87	6.08
100 ug / 0.0 ug	104.15	2.22

Table 2

1.	99mTc-labeled colloids
2.	Free pertechnetate
3.	99mTc-labeled small molecules
4.	99mTc weakly bonded to protein
5.	99mTc-labeled, size-altered proteins due to aggregation or cross-linking, refolding of fragments, or chain splitting
6.	99mTc-labeled, biologically altered protein

Methods which have been shown to be useful for determining the radiochemical impurities present in solutions of 99mTc labeled proteins, especially antibody proteins, are high pressure liquid chromatography (HPLC) and instant thin layer chromatography (ITLC). HPLC is done using size exclusion chromatography columns. ITLC is done using silica gel coated strips. HPLC is carried out using two detectors; one measures the optical density and is used to determine the relative amounts and the transit times of proteins of different sizes; the other measures radiation and is used to determine the relative amounts and transit times of different 99mTc species. Colloidal materials and 99mTc loosely bound to proteins are trapped in the HPLC column and thus must be quantitated by other means. ITLC on a protein-coated silica gel strip is used to determine colloidal 99mTc. Protein bound 99mTc and free technetium migrate with the solvent while the colloids remain at the origin. ITLC on an uncoated silica gel strip separates free technetium (i.e. soluble species), which migrates with the solvent, from colloids and proteins which remain at the origin. 99mTc loosely bound to proteins is quantitated by measuring the percentage of radioactivity injected into the HPLC that is collected in the eluate. With this combination of measurements, the full spectrum of radiochemical species in a 99mTc-labeled antibody-based radiopharmaceutical can be established.

The radiochemical impurity that requires special analysis is 99mTc strongly bonded to a protein that has the same molecular weight as the immunoreactive antibody. This impurity can either be antibody which is not immunoreactive or another protein that contaminates the immunoreactive antibody preparation. To determine the immunoreactive fraction of a radiolabeled antibody, binding of the radiolabeled antibody to solid phase antigen is determined under conditions of antigen excess. This is accomplished by using RhoChek™ (RhoMed, Albuquerque, N.M.), a solid-phase antigen mixture containing determinants that are bound by several important antibodies including those reactive with CEA, TAG-72, CSAp, tumor necrosis factor, and SSEA-1. Alternative methods for measuring the immunoreactive fraction of radiolabeled antibody employ RhoChek II™, an affinity thin layer chromatography system, or in the case of anti-SSEA-1 antibodies, binding to human granulocytes.

HPLC PROCEDURE FOR DETERMINING ANTIBODY COMPOSITION

The protein composition is determined simultaneously with the determination of the different 99mTc species. An HPLC system equipped with a TSK-G3000 size exclusion column and a TSK-pre column and a gamma radiation detector is used for this assay. The first sample to be analyzed is a set of molecular weight standards, (Bio-Rad Gel Filtration Standard, Catalog No. 151-1901). The standard, which is a mixture of 5 proteins with molecular weights ranging from 1,350 to 670,000, is prepared according to the manufacturer's instructions. These proteins are separated as they move through the size exclusion column of the HPLC and are detected by reading the optical density at OD_{280}. A tracing of the elution profile which gives the transit time in minutes of each peak is provided. A plot, on semi-log paper, of molecular weights is created using the known molecular weights of each of the protein components of the standard versus their respective transit times. Given the transit time, which is determined from the elution profiles of individual samples, the molecular weights of unknown proteins can be read from this graph. Alternately, the molecular weight of an unknown protein can be calculated by using a least square method for determining the straight line of the log of the molecular weight versus the transit times of each of the protein components of the standard. Identification of the antibody protein, i.e., whole antibody, $F(ab')_2$, Fab', or minor fragment is made using historically established values for each of the components together with their order of elution.

Molecular weight determinations by size exclusion chromatography are not absolute measures, but rather reflect both the size and the shape of the protein molecules. Thus, these estimates of molecular weight are not used to precisely define the molecular weight of a protein; they are used to identify the protein fractions when the protein being analyzed is already known. The data for the molecular weight standards are used to assure that the currently measured transit times can be compared to previously measured transit times of a known antibody and its fragments.

HPLC PROCEDURE FOR RADIOCHEMICAL COMPOSITION

After a 30-minute incubation, the radiolabeled sample to be tested is passed through a 3 mm, HPLC-certified, 0.45 micron Acrodisc filter to assure that no particulates are injected into the HPLC system. One 20-μl sample of the 99mTc-radiolabeled antibody solution is added to a 50 ml tube containing 21 ml of 0.5% bovine serum albumin in phosphate buffered saline (pH 7.0) and mixed well. This is the HPLC "Control". A 20 μl sample is then injected into the HPLC system which contains a 20 μl sample loop. The column is eluted with phosphate buffered saline (pH 7.0) at a flow rate of 1 ml/min, with a run time of 20 minutes. The HPLC eluate (20 ml) is collected in a 50 ml tube containing 1 ml of a 105 mg/ml bovine serum albumin in phosphate buffered saline (pH 7.0) solution. This solution is the HPLC "Eluate". After careful mixing, a 0.5 ml aliquot of the HPLC "Control" and of the HPLC "Eluate" are counted to measure the net radioactivity of each, and the overall HPLC Recovery is calculated:

$$\frac{\text{net CPM "Eluate"}}{\text{net CPM "Control"}} \times 100 = \% \text{ HPLC Recovery}$$

The integrated net radioactivity of each peak (% Protein Peak Bound) in the HPLC profile is determined by making a photocopy of the profile, then cutting out each peak and weighing it. The weight of the peak relative to the weight of the total corresponding area under the 99mTc curve is calculated. The molecular weight of each peak is determined by comparing its elution time to a curve of elution times plotted against the set of molecular weight standards.

The percent radiochemical yield of high affinity bonded 99mTc antibody (or antibody fragment) is calculated:

$$\% \text{ Protein Peak Bound} \times \% \text{ HPLC Recovery} = \% \text{ Radiochemical Yield}$$

The 99mTc which does not elute from the HPLC column is assumed to be primarily 99mTc weakly bound to the proteins. Other 99mTc impurities can also be determined from the analysis of the HPLC elution profile.

ITLC PROCEDURE FOR DETERMINING FREE TECHNETIUM

ITLC-SG paper [Gelman Sciences, Catalog No. 61886], cut into 1.5 x 10 cm strips, is activated by baking in a dry oven for 30 minutes at 110° C. The strips are stored at room temperature until used.

Five microliters of the 99mTc-labeled sample is spotted 2 cm (origin) from the bottom of the heat-activated strip and allowed to absorb into the strip. The strip is then immediately developed in a 50 ml centrifuge tube containing 5 ml of 85% methanol. The chromatogram is allowed to develop until the solvent front migrates to 1-2 cm from the top of the strip (5-10 minutes). The strip is removed using forceps and allowed to dry. After drying, the strip is cut into ten, 1-cm segments. The segments are placed in numbered counting tubes and counted for 1 minute in a gamma scintillation detector.

The percentage of the radioactivity migrating to the top half of the strip corresponds to the fraction of the radioactivity present as free technetium. Free technetium includes pertechnetate and other methanol soluble species. Protein-bound 99mTc and colloidal 99mTc do not migrate in this system.

Percent free 99mTc is determined as:

$$\frac{\text{Total cpm for segments 2 thru 5 } - \text{ 4 x background}}{\text{Total cpm for segments 1 thru 10 } - \text{ 10 x background}} \times 100 = \% \text{ Free 99mTc}$$

ITLC PROCEDURE FOR DETERMINING 99mTc COLLOIDS

This is the Swanson method, first reported by Thrall, et al. (1978). ITLC-SG paper [Gelman Sciences, Catalog No. 61886], cut into 1.5 x 10 cm strips, is activated by baking in a dry oven for 30 minutes at 110° C. The strips are then soaked for 30 minutes in a solution of Bovine Serum Albumin diluted to 5 mg/ml with 0.9% NaCl solution. The strips are rinsed in distilled water for 5 seconds, allowed to dry overnight at room temperature, then are stored at 4 degrees C until used.

Five microliters of the 99mTc sample is spotted 2 cm from the bottom of the BSA-treated ITLC Strip. The strip is then developed in a 50 ml centrifuge tube containing 5 ml of ethanol:ammonia:water (2:1:5). The strip is dried, cut and counted as above.

Percent colloid 99mTc is determined as:

$$\frac{\text{Total cpm for segments 2 thru 5 - 4 x background}}{\text{Total cpm for segments 1 thru 10 - 10 x background}} \times 100 = \% \text{ Colloid 99mTc}$$

STANDARDS

Sodium pertechnetate injection, USP, is purchased as needed from a commercial radiopharmacy. This radioactive solution is used for labeling instant 99mTc labeling kits and as a standard for both the HPLC and the ITLC analytical tests. The solution is diluted to 1 mCi per ml with 0.15 M NaCl and analysed by HPLC and ITLC.

Instant kits (Gamma-G™ Kits) for labeling human gamma globulin with 99mTc are manufactured at RhoMed Inc., Albuquerque, New Mexico. These kits contain 0.5 mg of human gamma globulin (Cutter Gamimune-N™) prepared for instant radiolabeling with sodium pertechnetate 99mTc. The kits are labeled with 0.5 mCi 99mTc in a final volume of 0.5 ml. The sample is tested 0.5 hours after the addition of the radioactivity.

PROCEDURES

The two standards, sodium pertechnetate 99mTc and 99mTc-human gamma globulin, are tested first, followed by the protein-based radiopharmaceutical. Samples are labeled according to the manufacturer's instruction, or to the above protocol, and are tested 30 minutes after the radioactivity has been added to the vial.

After the analysis has been completed, different protein fractions are identified and the relative percentages of each are calculated. These calculations are also made for the two standards. A running tabulation of means and standard deviations of the standards is maintained and current results for the standards are compared to the historical values to validate that the current analytical results are within expected ranges.

In addition to calculating the values of the different components determined by ITLC, the ITLC profiles are plotted and compared visually to historical profiles of the standards. For the analytical results to be acceptable, the profiles of the standards must not be significantly different from their expected appearance.

The performance characteristics of the HPLC size exclusion chromatography column may change with use. Thus each column use is given a serial number to permit the determination of changing column performance.

RESULTS

Figure 5 shows the ITLC results obtained for a lyophilized HgG direct label kit (Gamma-G™ RhoMed, Albuquerque, N.M.) labeled with 99mTc. No unbound 99mTc is seen. Colloidal 99mTc is an acceptable 4%. Figure 6 shows the HPLC profile for the same labeled kit with 96 % yield of labeled antibody.

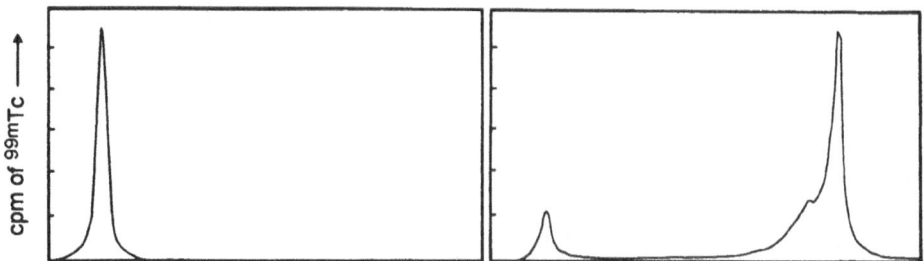

Figure 5. A. ITLC for percent free pertechnetate, HgG control Tc-labeling kit (Gamma-G™, RhoMed Inc., Albuerque, NM). B. ITLC for percent coloid, HgG control Tc-labeling kit (Gamma-G™, RhoMed Inc., Albuquerque, NM).

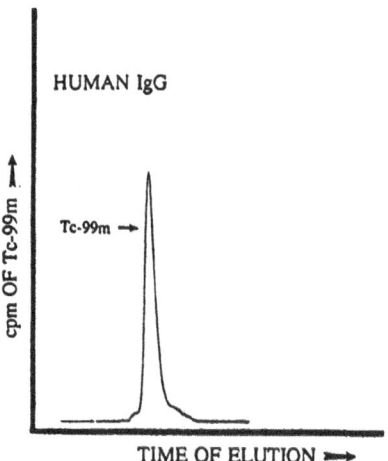

Figure 6. HPLC profile of 99mTc direct-labeled HgG control kits (Gamma-G™ RhoMed., Albuquerque, NM).

CONCLUSION

One-step, 99mTc labeling kits for preparing 99mTc-labeled antibody, peptide or other proteins are rapidly being introduced for use in clinical nuclear medicine. These direct labeling methods employ a common sequence of separate, but interdependent, chemical reactions. The reducing agent used to reduce both the protein and the 99mTc sodium pertechnetate may vary. Different complexing agents may be used, but all complexing agents must form weak to moderately strong complexes with reduced technetium. High radiochemical yields of technetium-labeled proteins are attained when technetium is reduced in the presence of a weak complexing agent and sufficient reactive sulfhydryl donor ligands provided by appropriately reduced proteins. Direct labeling of proteins by regulated reduction provides a controlled method for optimizing the sequence of events in the direct labeling process necessary for the formulation of high radiochemical yield protein-based or peptide-based radiopharmaceutical kits. Strict quality control through radiochemical analysis enables reproducible, cost effective radiopharmaceutical kit manufacture.

REFERENCES

Alvarez J., Maas R. and da Arriaga C. (1967) Reunion Annual d la Sociedas Mexicana Nuclear, San Jose de Vista Hermose, 7-8 April 1967. Cited by Maas R., Alvarez J. and da Arriaga C. (1967) On a new tracer for liver scanning. *Int. J. Appl. Radiat. Isot.* 18: 653-654.

Andrews J. C. (1926) The optical activity of cysteine. *J. Biol. Chem.* 69: 209-217.

Becker W., Kinne R. *et al.* (1992) Experiences in immunoscintigraphy of blood cells. *Revista Espanola de Medicina Nuclear* 11, 146 (Abstract).

Cecil R. and McPhee J. R. (1959) The sulfur chemistry of proteins. *Adv. Protein Chem.* 24: 255-389.

Cleland W. W. (1964) Dithiothreitol, a new protective reagent for SH groups. *Biochemistry* 3, 480-482.

Crockford D. R., and Rhodes B. A. (1978) Tc-99m labeled antigens and antibodies for cancer detection in humans. U.S. Patent No. 908,568.

Crockford D. R. and Rhodes B. A. (1984) Method for radiolabeling proteins with Tc-99m. U.S. Patent No. 4,424,200.

Eckelman W.C. and Steigman J. (1991) Direct labeling with Tc-99m. *Nucl. Med. Biol.* 18: 3-7.

Griffiths G. L. (1990) Method for technetium/rhenium labeling proteins. International Patent Application No. PCT/US90/03142.

Griffiths G. L., Goldenberg D. M. *et al.* (1991) Direct radiolabeling of monoclonal antibodies with generator-produced rhenium-188 for radioimmunotherapy: Labeling and animal biodistribution studies. *Cancer Res.* 51: 4594-4602.

Gurd F. R. N. and Wilcox P. E. (1956) Complex formation between metallic cations and proteins, peptides, and amino acids. *Adv. Protein Chem.* 11: 311-427.

Hansen H. J. (1991) Method for rapidly radiolabeling monovalent antibody fragments with technetium. International Patent Application No. PCT/US90/05196.

Harris L. J. (1922) On a series of metallo-cysteine derivatives. *I. Biochem. J.* 16: 739-746.

Hawkins E. B., Pant K. D., Rhodes B. A. (1990) Resistance of direct Tc-99m-protein to transchelation. *Antibody Immunoconjugates, And Radiopharmaceuticals* 3: 17.

Jocelyn P. C. (1987) Chemical reduction of disulfides. *Methods Enzymol.* 46: 246-256.

Mather S. J. and Ellison D. (1990) Reduction-mediated technetium-99m labeling of monoclonal antibodies. *J. Nucl. Med.* 31: 692-697.

Paik C. H., Phan L. N. B., Hong J. J. *et al.* (1985) The labeling of high affinity sites of antibodies with Tc-99m. *Int. Nucl. Med. Biol.* 12: 3-8.

Pak K. Y. (1988) Method for labeling antibodies with a metal ion. International Application Patent No. PCT/US88/01048.

Pak K. Y., Nedelman M. A. *et al.* (1989) A rapid and efficient method for labeling IgG antibodies with Tc-99m and comparison to Tc-99m Fab' antibody fragments. *J. Nucl. Med.* 30: 793 No. 268 (Abstract).

Perrin D. D. and Dempsey B.(1974) Metal ion buffers. In *Buffers for pH and Metal Ion Control* 1974 (Edited by Perrin D. D. and Dempsey B.), pp.94-108. Chapman and Hall, New York.

Petersen J. G. L. and Dorrington K. J. (1974) An in vitro system for studying the kinetics of interchain disulfide bond formation in immunoglobulin G. *J. Biological Chemistry* 249: 5633-5641.

Pimm M. V., Rajput R. S. *et al.* (1991) Anomalies in reduction-mediated technetium-99m labeling of monoclonal antibody. *Eur. J. Nucl. Med.* 18: 973-976.

Reardan D. T., Meares C. F., Goodwin D. A. *et al.* (1985) Antibodies against metal chelates. *Nature (Lond.)* 316: 265-268.

Reno J. M. and Bottino B. J. (1987) Improved radionuclide antibody coupling. European Patent Office Application EP 0 237 150 A2.

Reno J. M., Bottino B. J. and Wilbur D. S. (1989) Radionuclide antibody coupling. U.S. Patent No. 4,877,868.

Reno J. M. and Bottino B. J. (1989) Radionuclide Antibody Coupling. U.S. Patent No. 4,877,868.

Richards P. and Steigman J. (1975) Chemistry of technetium as applied to radiopharmaceuticals. In *Radiopharm. Int. Symp.* 1974 (edited by Subramanian G., Rhodes B. A., Cooper J F. and Saad V. J.), pp. 23-35. The Society of nuclear Medicine, New York.

Rhodes B. A. (1974) Considerations in the radiolabeling of albumin. *Semin. Nucl. Med.* 4: 281-293.

Rhodes B. A., Torvestad D. A., Breslow K. et al. (1980) A kit for direct labeling of antibody and antibody fragments with Tc-99m. *J. Nucl. Med.* 21, P54 (Abstract).

Rhodes B. A., Torvestad D. A., Breslow K. *et al.* (1982) Tc-99m labeling and acceptance testing of radiolabeled antibodies and antibody fragments. In *Tumor Imaging* (Edited by Burchiel S.W. and Rhodes B.A.), pp.111-123. Proceedings of the Conference "The Radioimmunochemical Detection of Cancer" 5-6 Dec. 1979, Albuquerque, N.M., Masson, New York.

Rhodes B. A., Zamora P. O., Newell K. D. *et al.* (1986) Technetium-99m labeling of murine monoclonal antibody fragments. *J. Nucl. Med.* 27: 685.

Rhodes B. A., Buckelew J. M., Pant K. D., *et al.* (1990) Quality control test for immunoreactivity of radiolabeled antibody. *BioTechniques* 8: 70-74.

Rhodes B. A. (1991) Direct labeling of proteins with Tc-99m. *Nucl. Med. Biol.* 18: 667-676.

Rhodes, B.A. Radiochemical analysis of Tc-99m-proteins by high pressure liquid chromatography and instant thin layer chromatography. In preparation.

Rhodes, B.A. (1992) Radiolabeling antibodies and other proteins with technetium or rhenium by regulated reduction. U.S. Patent No. 5,078,985.

Shochat D. (1989) Method for radiolabeling proteins. European Patent No. 89303270.6.

Schwartz A. and Steinstraber A. (1987) a novel approach to Tc-99m labeled monoclonal antibodies. *J. Nucl. Med.* 28: 721.

Steigman J., Williams H. P., and Soloman N. A. (1975) The importance of the protein sulfhydryl group in HSA labeling with technetium-99m. *J. Nucl. Med.* 16: 573.

Stray J. E., Vassella R. L. *et al.* (submitted abstract) Direct labeling of the anti-renal cell carcinoma antibody A6H with rhenium-186: Targeting of human renal cell carcinoma xenografts.

Thakur M. L. and DeFulvio J. D. (1991) Technetium-99m labeled monoclonal antibodies for immunoscintigraphy. *J. Immunological Methods* 137: 217-224.

Thrall J. H. *et al.* (1978) Clinical comparison of cardiac blood pool visualization with technetium-99m human serum albumin. *J. Nucl. Med.* 19: 796-803.

Zamora, P.O., and Rhodes, B.A. (1992) Imidazoles as well as thiolates in proteins bind Technetium-99m. *Bioconj. Chem.* 3: 493-498.

LIPOPROTEIN LABELING AND ANALYSIS TECHNIQUES

P. Angelberger

Austrian Research Center Seibersdorf
Austria

INTRODUCTION

In human plasma Low Density Lipoprotein (LDL) is the major transport protein for endogenous cholesterol being transferred between body tissues. It is a spheric macromolecule (d 2160 nm, MW 2600 kD) with a lipid core consisting mainly of cholesterol esters (42 % w/w of LDL), phospholipids (22 %), free cholesterol (8 %) and triglycerides (6 %). The particle surface is formed by a protein helix (22 %), in case of LDL apoprotein B-100 (MW 500 kD) which is recognized by specific receptors located on the surface of liver cells and other tissue cells whereas vascular cells contain only very few LDL receptors. This leads to receptor binding of LDL followed by cellular uptake and lysosomal degradation of about 2/3 of LDL particles thereby maintaining cholesterol homeostasis[1]. Reduced numbers or reduced activity of LDL receptors cause elevated plasma cholesterol levels that are associated with progression of atherosclerosis. Localized endothelial damage promotes increased uptake (not yet proven to be LDL-receptor-mediated) and degradation of LDL by vascular smooth-muscle cells and macrophage foam cells of the intima. These are the earliest detectable events that can develop into an atherosclerotic plaque[2, 3]. Thus high interest is evident in radiolabeled LDL as tracer and receptor ligand to study these processes.

123IODINE LABELED LDL (123I-LDL)

Since many in-vitro studies had been performed with 125I-LDL[4], the cyclotron-produced radionuclide 123I was chosen to label LDL for in-vivo studies and potential scintigraphic applications[2, 3, 5]. 125I-LDL had been labeled mostly by the Iodine monochloride (ICl)-method[6, 5] but also by the Iodogen (IG)-method[7] with equally good results, both methods being established for electrophilic radioiodination of proteins with minimal damage. Thus both IG and ICl were applied in an optimized mode for labeling 123I-LDL and each was combined with purification by size-exclusion-chromatography (SEC) or equilibrium dialysis (D)[8].

IG labeling: in a microvial 500 μl $CHCl_3$-solution of 30 μg IG was evaporated with a stream of N_2, redissolved and blown dry again to produce an even surface coating. To the IG-coated vial was added 1-2 mg (protein, 2-4 nmol) LDL in pH 7.5 phosphate buffered saline (PBS), about 1 mCi (0.05 nmol) 123I-NaI and 1 nmol NaI carrier to establish a constant molar ratio I/protein of 0.5-0.25. After 10 minutes reaction time the mixture (500 μl) was applied to a Sephadex G25M column (9x100 mm, preeluted with identical unlabeled LDL) and eluted with PBS. The first radioactive protein peak was collected by means of UV- and radioactivity-detectors and filtered through a sterile 0.2 μm membrane (Fig.1). Alternatively the reaction mixture was sterile filtered into a dialysis

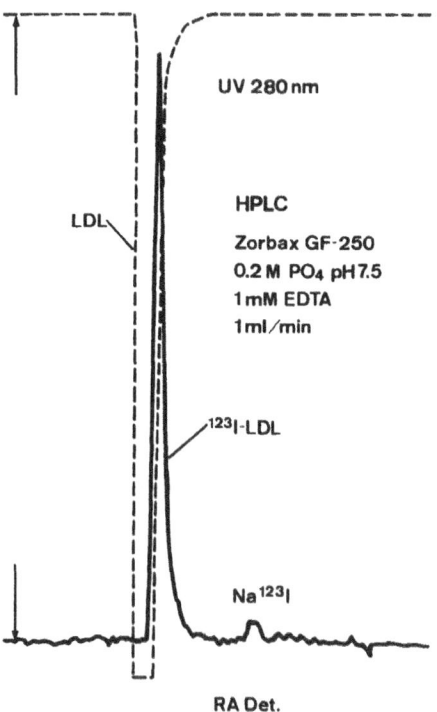

Figure 1. Preparative HPLC of 123I-LDL (IG or ICl reaction mixture). Column: Zorbax GF250. Eluent: aqu. 0.2 M PO$_4$ pH 7.5, 1mM EDTA. Flow: 1 ml/min. Detectors: NaI(Tl); scintillation and UV (280 nm) in series.

tube that was kept in dialysis buffer (PBS with 0.2 mM EDTA) until use of 123I-LDL. ICl labeling: to a microvial was added 1-2 mg (protein, 2-4 nmol) LDL in PBS, 1M glycine buffer pH 10, about 1 mCi (0.05 nmol) I123-NaI and 3-7 μg ICl freshly diluted in 2M NaCl (1:100) from stock (34 mM in 6M HCl, purified by extraction with CHCl$_3$) to give a molar ratio ICL/LDL protein of 10/1. The reaction mixture (500 μl) was stirred for 10 minutes at 4 and purified by dialysis or SEC as described.

Iodine/LDL molar ratios used for labeling, typical radiochemical yields and specific activities of isolated products are summarized for the 4 labeling-purification method combinations in Table 1.

Table 1. Comparison of labeling and purification methods for 123I-LDL

| Method | | Molar Ratio | Radiochem. | Specific Activity |
Labeling	Purification	I/LDL	Yield, %	mCi/mg
Iodogen	SEC	0.5	88	0.98
Iodogen	Dialysis	0.5	92	1.02
ICl	SEC	10	69	0.77
ICl	Dialysis	10	72	0.80

Radiochemical purity was determined by:

a) trichloroacetic acid (TCA) protein precipitation at 10 % final TCA concentration.
b) cellulose acetate electrophoresis (CA-EP): 0.05M barbital buffer pH 8.6, containing 1mM EDTA and 1 % HSA, horizontal zone electrophoresis at 300 V for 10 minutes (Fig.2).
c) polyacrylamide gel electrophoresis (PAGE): gradient gel, T=8-18; gel buffer 0.12M Tris, 0.12M acetate and 0.1 % SDS, pH 6.4; 200 V/25 mA for 20 minutes, then 600 V/25 mA for 60 minutes (Fig.3).
d) In order to determine the percentage of total radioactivity bound to lipoprotein of identical density, aliquots of labeled LDL were added to unlabeled LDL and analysed by ultracentrifugation at a KBr-density of 1.063 g/ml. The radioactivity found amounted to 92±4 % for 123I-LDL in the LDL-specific fraction (supernatant, d 1.019-1.063) indicating that nearly all of the radioactivity bound to a product with the density of native LDL.

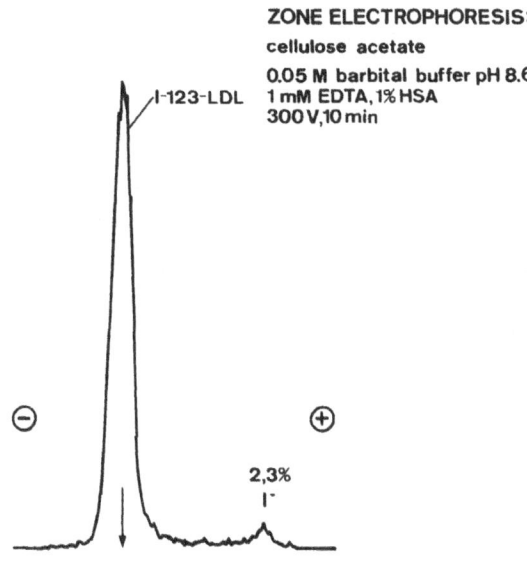

ZONE ELECTROPHORESIS:

cellulose acetate

0.05 M barbital buffer pH 8.6
1 mM EDTA, 1% HSA
300 V, 10 min

I-123-LDL

⊖   ⊕

2,3%
I⁻

Figure 2. Zone electrophoresis of 123I-LDL. Stationary phase: cellulose acetate. Electrolyte: 0.05 M barbital pH 8.6, 1 mM EDTA, 1 % HSA. Field: 300 V. Run time: 10 min.

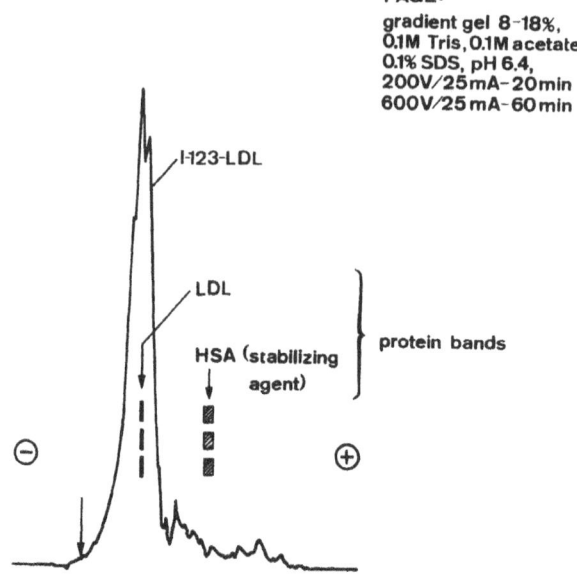

PAGE:

gradient gel 8-18%,
0.1M Tris, 0.1M acetate
0.1% SDS, pH 6.4,
200V/25mA-20min
600V/25mA-60min

I-123-LDL

LDL

HSA (stabilizing agent)

protein bands

⊖   ⊕

Figure 3. SDS-PAGE of 123I-LDL. Gradient gel, T = 8-18 %. Non-reducing SDS-buffer: 0.1 % SDS, 0.12 M Tris, 0.12 M acetate, pH 6.4. Run: 200V/25 mA for 20 min, then 600 V/25 mA for 60 min. LDL aproprotein band (Ag staining) coincides with 123I-radioactivity peak.

Radiochemical purity values of the four 123I-LDL preparations at 5 minutes and 2 hours after purification are summarized in Table 2:

Table 2. Radiochemical purity and stability of 123I-LDL

Method Labeling	Purification	TCA % precipitate		Electrophoresis % iodide	
		5 min	2 hours	5 min	2 hours
			after purification		
Iodogen	SEC	90 ± 6	79 ± 5	3.4 ± 2.3	9.6 ± 4.2
Iodogen	Dialysis	91 ± 4	80 ± 5	2.5 ± 1.3	6.0 ± 2.3
ICl	SEC	95 ± 2	86 ± 3	1.1 ± 0.2	4.9 ± 2.2
ICl	Dialysis	96 ± 3	85 ± 5	0.7 ± 0.1	3.2 ± 2.2
				$x\pm$s.d., n=6	

The differences in radiochemical purity and in-vitro stability between the 4 labeling-purification methods were rather small, however, ICl-labeling consistently produced a slightly higher purity and stability. Most of the kinetic studies with 125I-LDL in animals and almost all in-vitro receptor binding studies have utilized LDL labeled with the ICl-method[5, 6]. On the other hand IG has been well established as a mild labeling method suitable even for sensitive proteins. Since IG is not soluble in the aqueous reaction medium, it does not expose LDL to an excess of oxidising agent and has been shown not to alter in-vivo catabolism and plasma clearance of LDL compared to ICl-labeling[7]. Thus it was of interest to compare ICl and IG with regard to in-vitro receptor binding properties of labeled LDL: specific binding (~95 %) to human liver plasma membranes, concentration of unlabeled LDL causing half-maximum inhibition (IC_{50} range 7.7 - 9.3 μg LDL/ml), dissociation constant (K_d 0.9-1.4 μg LDL/ml) and receptor concentration (Bmax 141-163 ng LDL/mg membrane protein) were all not significantly different for the 4 labeling-purification methods[8].

99m Tc-LDL

For scintigraphic imaging of LDL influx into atherosclerotic lesions and of hepatic LDL receptor concentration 99mTc would be the ideal radionuclide due to its physical properties. Moreover it may obviate the problem of in-vivo dehalogenation of 123I-LDL which is also useful for imaging. 99mTc-labeling of LDL was first developed by Lees et al.[9] and subsequently investigated by our group with the aim of optimizing radiochemical purity and stability[10, 11, 12].

99m Tc-labeling: into a microvial was added 2-3 mg (protein, 4-6 nmol) LDL in PBS, 40-60 mCi $99mTcO_4^-$ in saline and about 100 μl 0.2M $NaHCO_3$ for a reaction pH of 8 or alternatively additional 0.01M NaOH to adjust the pH to 9. $Na_2S_2O_4$ was added either freshly dissolved in a minimal volume of 0.01M NaOH to a concentration of 0.05-0.03M in the reaction mixture or in solid form to achieve a concentration of 0.3M. The reaction mixture was slowly stirred for 30-60 minutes and injected into a SEC HPLC-column Zorbax GF-250 which had been preeluted with identical unlabeled LDL using 0.2M $NaHCO_3$, 0.2 mM EDTA as eluent at 1 ml/min. The 99mTc-LDL peak was isolated by means of radioactivity- and UV-detectors in series and further purified as needed by dialysis in PBS containing 1 mM EDTA.

A typical preparative HPLC isolation of 99mTc-LDL is shown in Fig.4: Compared to SW-250 column, which revealed only the 99mTc-LDL product peak and the unreacted $99mTcO_4$, the GF-250 column with improved resolution separated additionally 1 or 2 peaks of reduced 99mTc not bound to LDL ("Tc red.") containing about 30 % of injected 99mTc.

The quantitative relation of Tc red.- and TcO_4-peaks varied widely between different LDL-preparations and there was an inverse relation of TcO_4- and Tc-LDL-peaks. Studying labeling parameters it was discovered that 0.03M $Na_2S_2O_4$ left more than 50 % of TcO_4 unreduced. Subsequently employed 0.3M $Na_2S_2O_4$ had a positive effect on radiochemical yield, purity and stability of 99mTc-LDL (Table 3).

Table 3. Influence of $Na_2S_2O_4$-concentration

$Na_2S_2O_4$		99mTc-LDL	Radiochem. purity	
0 mM	(n=1)	1.5 % yield	-	% TCA ppt
30	(n=10)	31 ± 13	72 ± 14	
300	(n=20)	45 ± 15	84 ± 12	

Radiochemical purity was determined by:

a)   paper chromatography (PC): Whatman 3MM; acetone.

b)   paper electrophoresis (PE): Whatman No. 1; 0.05M barbital buffer pH 8.6, 1 mM

EDTA, 1 % HSA; 300 V, 10 min.
c)   TCA protein precipitation: 10 % final TCA concentration.
d) $CHCl_3$: MeOH (2:1) extraction
e)   analytical HPLC: size exclusion column Zorbax GF 250; 0.2M PO_4 pH 7.5, 1 mM EDTA; 1 ml/min.

a) and b) separate only free TcO_4 from Tc-LDL, whereas c) and d) separate Tc-LDL from TcO_4 and reduced Tc-species; e) detected 2 species of reduced Tc not bound to LDL, and TcO_4 which increased considerably with time (Fig.5a), (Table 4).

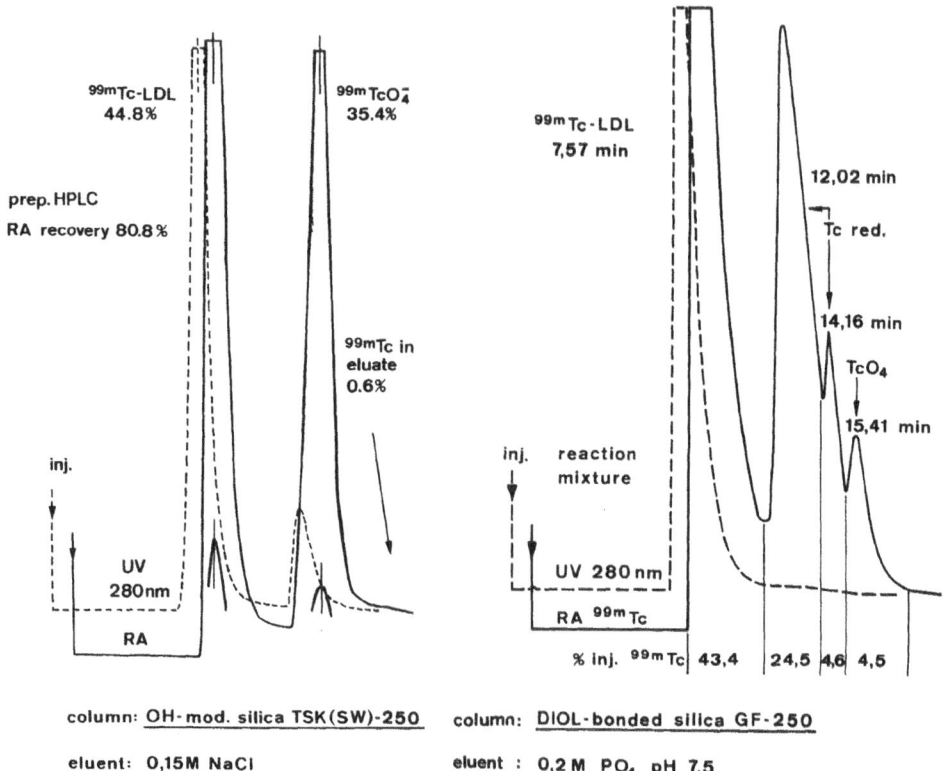

Figure 4. Preparative HPLC of 99mTc-LDL on SEC-columns, left: hydroxyl-modified silica TSK SW-250 eluted with PBS, 1mM EDTA; right: diol-bonded silica Zorbax GF-250 eluted with 0.2 M PO_4 pH 7.5, 1 mM EDTA. Flow: 1 ml/min. Detectors: NaI(Tl) scintillation and UV (280 nm) in series.

Table 4. Radiochemical impurities in isolated 99mTc-LDL

after prep. HPLC hours	PC, PE % TcO4	TCA ppt % (TcO_4 + Tc red)	anal.HPLC % TcO_4	%Tc red
0.5	3.8 ± 1.6 (n=15)			
2	8.4 ± 3.0 (15)	15.1 ± 5.3 (12)		
4	20.9 ± 4.6 (10)	31.3 ± 6.9 (8)	22 ± 5 (8)	9 ± 3 (8)

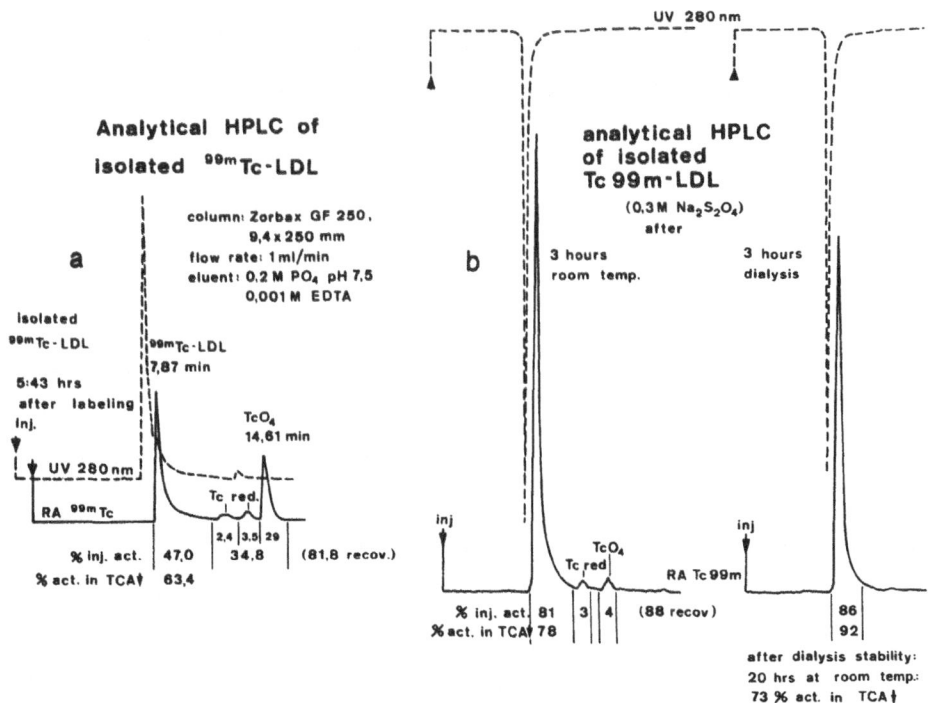

Figure 5. Analytical HPLC of 99mTc-LDL. Column: Zorbax GF-250. Eluent: 0.2 M PO₄ pH 7.5, 1 mM EDTA. Flow: 1 ml/min. a) 6 hrs after prep. HPLC b) left: after 3 hrs at r.t.; right: after 3 hrs in dialysis.

Obviously the in-vitro stability at room temperature was rather low: after 4 hours about 20 % TcO_4^- and 10 % reduced Tc not bound to LDL were determined with a satisfactory correlation between analytical methods.

Since in-vitro stability could not be improved by modifications of labeling parameters, dialysis against PBS plus 1 mM EDTA was studied as separation and purification method.

Using dialysis alone for separation and purification, after 10 hours dialysis radiochemical purity was only about 80 % TCA ppt. When however prep. HPLC was performed first and followed by dialysis, only about 3 hours dialysis increased purity to more than 90 %. The improvement in purity and stability of HPLC plus dialysis versus HPLC alone is summarized in Table 5 and shown in Fig.5b.

Table 5. 99mTc-LDL in-vitro stability after purification

purification	hours after purification		
	0,5	3	19
HPLC (n=20)	84 ± 12	78 ± 10	- % TCA ppt
HPLC <u>and</u> Dialysis (n =15)	94 ± 5	88 ± 7	72 ± 14

In vitro receptor binding was studied with human hepatoma cells and fibroblasts: in both cell types endocytosis of 99mTc-LDL and 125I-LDL was equally supressed to less than 30 % (of the uptake of each labeled LDL alone) by a 20-fold excess of cold LDL, thereby demonstrating competitive recognition of 99mTc-LDL by high affinity binding sites[12].

111In-(DTPA)-LDL

Recently Rosen et al. reported studies with 111In(DTPA)LDL suggesting that it might act as an intracellularly trapped ligand[13]. However in-vitro receptor binding displayed an increased non-saturable component compared to 125I-LDL. Consequently it was of interest to investigate the receptor binding of 111In-LDL in the same system already used for different 123I-LDL preparations[8].

LDL-DTPA conjugation: to 1 mg (protein, 2 nmol) LDL in PBS was added 0.5M NaHCO$_3$ buffer pH 8 and dropwise 36 μg (100 nmol) cyclic DTPA anhydride (cDTPAa) in dry DMSO. The reaction mixture was stirred at room temperature for 1 hour and applied to a Sephadex G50 column (5 x 70 mm) in metal-free acetate buffered saline (ABS) pH 5.5.

111In-labeling: to the protein fraction (DTPA-LDL) eluted from the first column in ABS was added about 600 μCi 111InCl$_3$ (<0.5 nmol In/mCi). After 1 hour incubation the mixture was applied to a second identical column in ABS. The protein fraction (111In-DTPA-LDL) was eluted in ABS and formulated in PBS, 1 mM DTPA.

The number of DTPA-groups per LDL molecule was determined by 111In-labeling of the conjugation mixture without prior separation of unbound DTPA. The bound fraction (111In-DTPA-LDL) and unbound fraction (111In-DTPA) was quantified by TLC (Fig.6) and allowed to calculate the desired number from the known molar quantities of reactants: using cDTPAa and LDL in a molar ratio of 50:1, about 5 (range 3-9) DTPA-groups were conjugated per LDL molecule. Isolated radiochemical yield of 111In(DTPA)LDL was 72$\pm$9 % (n=30) with a specific activity of 160 - 240 μCi/mg LDL protein.

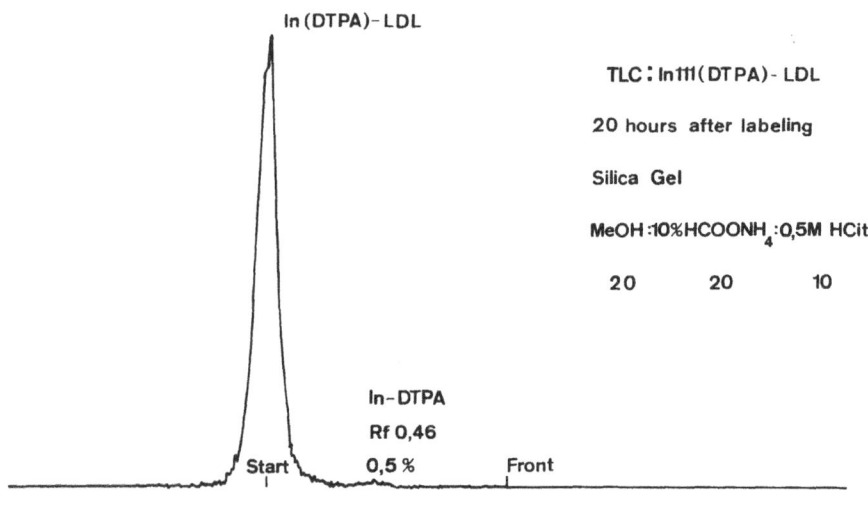

Figure 6. TLC of 111In(DTPA) LDL. Adsorbent: silica gel. Eluent: MeOH: aqu. 10 % HCOONH$_4$: 0.5 M HCit (20:20:10). Radioactivity distribution measured by Thin Layer Analyzer.

Radiochemical purity was determined by

a) TLC on silica gel (Merck) developed in MeOH : 10 % $HCOONH_4$: 0.5M Citric acid (20 : 20 : 10). (Fig.6)
b) Cellulose acetate electrophoresis in 0.05M barbital buffer pH 8.6 containing 1 mM EDTA and 1 % HSA, at 300 V for 20 min. 111In-LDL migrates only about 5 mm, while In^{3+} and In-DTPA migrate 25 and 40 mm respectively.
c) Ultracentrifuge as described for 123I-LDL.
d) PAGE: gradient gel (T = 8 - 18 %); gel buffer 0.12M Tris, 0.12M acetate, 0.1 % SDS, pH 6.4; 50 mA, 200 - 600 V for 60 min.

111In(DTPA)LDL contained less than 1 % In^{3+} and In-DTPA and this high purity remained stable for more than 18 hours (Table 6). Native LDL and 111In(DTPA)LDL exhibited identical protein bands in PAGE demonstrating no damage to the apoprotein by DTPA-conjugation.

Table 6. 111In(DTPA)LDL radiochemical purity and stability

Electrophoresis		TLC		Ultracentrifuge	
2	18	2	18	20 hrs	after purification
0.3 ± 0.1	0.7 ± 0.3	99.5 ± 0.2	99.2 ± 0.3	94 ± 3	(x $\pm$ s.d.,n=6)
	% (In^{3+} + In-DTPA)		% In(DTPA)LDL		% LDL (d 1.019-1.063)

In-vitro binding studies with human liver plasma membranes containing the LDL-apoB-receptor revealed a significantly higher binding affinity of 111In(DTPA)LDL (K_d 0.6 ± 0.2 μg LDL protein/ml (n=6)) compared to 123I-LDL (K_d 1.2 ± 0.7). Specific saturable binding capacity was also higher for 111In(DTPA)LDL (B_{max} 239 ± 26 ng LDL protein / mg membrane protein) than for 123I-LDL (B_{max} 148 ± 18), while inhibition of binding by native LDL (IC_{50} 1.7 ± 0.7 μg LDL protein/ml) was more pronounced than for 123I-LDL (IC_{50} 7.7 ± 1.0)[14].

In conclusion the data presented should illustrate the role of the diverse radiochemistry of different radionuclides and of the molecular structur of the substrate in radiolabeling a biologically relevant molecule. Consideration of these aspects and specific method development are required to obtain high quality labeled LDL.

REFERENCES

1. J.L. Goldstein, T.Kita, M.S. Brown, N. Engl. J. Med. 309: 288-296 (1983).
2. H. Sinzinger, H. Bergmann, J. Kaliman, P. Angelberger: Imaging of human atherosclerotic lesions using 123I-Low-Density-Liporoteins. *Eur. J. Nucl. Med.* 12: 291-2 (1985).
3. H. Sinzinger, P. Angelberger, H. Pesl, J. Flores: Further insights into lipid lesion imaging by means of 123I-labeled autologous LDL. In: G. Crepaldi et al, Eds. Atherosclerosis VIII. Excerpta Medica 1989: 645-653.

4. M.S. Brown, J.L. Goldstein: Familial hypercholesterolemia: defective binding of lipoproteins to cultured fibroblasts associated with impaired regulation of 3-hydroxy-3-methylglutaryl coenzyme A reductase activity. *Proc. Natl. Acad. Sci. USA* 71: 788-792 (1974).

5. M. Hüttinger, J.M. Corbett, W.J. Schneider, J.T. Willerson, M.S. Brown, J.L. Goldstein: Imaging of hepatic low-density liproprotein receptors by radionuclide scintiscanning in vivo. *Proc. Natl. Acad. Sci. USA* 81: 7599-7603 (1984).

6. T.Langer, W. Strober, R.I. Levy: The metabolism of LDL in familial type II hyperlipoproteinemia. *J. Clin. Invest.* 51: 1528-1536 (1972).

7. R.C. Pittman, T.E. Carew, C.K. Glass, S.R. Green, C.A. Taylor, A.D. Attie: A radioiodinated intracellularly trapped ligand for determining the sites of plasma protein degradation in vivo. *Biochem. J.* 212: 791-800 (1983).

8. I. Virgolini, P. Angelberger, J. Pidlich, G. Lupattelli, E. Molinar, H. Sinzinger: Comparison of different methods for LDL-isolation and radioiodine labeling on liver receptor binding. *Int. J. Nucl. Med. Biol.* 78: 513-517 (1991).

9. R.S. Lees, H.D. Garabedian, A.M. Lees, J Schumacher, A. Miller, J.L. Jsaacsohn, A. Derksen, H.W. Strauss: Technetium-99m low density lipoproteins: preparation and biodistribution. *J. Nucl. Med.* 26: 1056-1062 (1985).

10. P. Angelberger, M. Hüttinger, R. Dudczak: Comparative study of 123I- and 99mTc-Low Density Leprrproteins (LDL). *J. Lab. Compd. Radiopharm.* 23: 1309-1311 (1986).

11. P. Angelberger, M. Hüttinger, R. Dudczak, T. Leitha: Development of 99mTc-Low Density Lipoprotein (LDL) with high radiochemical purity at tracer application. *J. Lab. Compd. Radiopharm.* 26: 271-273 (1989).

12. T. Leitha, M. Hüttinger, P. Angelberger, R. Dudczak: 99mTc-LDL as tracer for quantitative LDL scintigraphy. I) tracer purification, in vitro validation and biodistribution. *Eur. J. Nucl. Med (in press).*

13. J.M. Rosen, S.P. Butler, G.E. Meinken, T.S. Wang, R. Ramakrishnan, S.C. Srivastava, P.O. Alderson, H.N. Ginsberg: 111In-labeled LDL: a potential agent for imaging atherosclerotic disease and lipoprotein biodistribution. *J. Nucl. Med.* 31: 343-350 (1990).

14. I. Virgolini, P. Angelberger, S.R. Li, F. Koller, E. Koller, J. Pidlich, G. Lupatelli, H. Sinzinger: 111In-labeled Low-Density Lipoprotein binds with higher affinity to the human liver as compared to 123I-labeled LDL. *J. Nucl. Med.* 32: 2132-2138 (1991).

111In ANTIFIBRIN MONOCLONAL ANTIBODIES IN THE EVALUATION OF THE DEEP VENOUS THROMBOSIS OF THE LOWER LIMBS: AN ITALIAN MULTICENTER STUDY

L. Lusiani[1], P. Zanco[2], E. Brianzoni[3], L. Feggi[4], M. Gallazzo[5], P. Rossini[6] and R. Spaziante[7]

[1]Dept. of Internal Medicine, University of Padova
[2]Dept. of Nuclear Medicine of Castelfranco Veneto
[3]Dept. of Nuclear Medicine of Macerata
[4]Dept. of Nuclear Medicine of Ferrara
[5]Dept. of Nuclear Medicine of Milano
[6]Dept. of Nuclear Medicine of Brescia
[7]Dept. of Nuclear Medicine of Pordenone
Italy

INTRODUCTION

From January 1987 and December 1988, a multicenter study has been conducted in Italy by six Nuclear Medicine Departments, in order to establish the value of 111In-labeled antifibrin monoclonal antibody 59D8 (Fibriscint, Centocor) for the diagnosis of deep venous thrombosis (DVT) of the lower limbs. This antibody (a Fab fragment obtained by a murine hybridoma) is highly specific for a defined epitope of the beta chain of human fibrin, and does not cross-react with fibrinogen[1].

This study was interrupted for two reasons: 1. the 111In-labeled product became unavailable; 2. diagnosing a DVT was no longer considered as a problem, after the improvement of ultrasonic techniques (namely, duplex scanning and color-Doppler). Ultrasounds permit a quick, safe, accurate diagnosis of proximal venous thrombosis (that is, from popliteal vein up) and have made phlebography unecessary in most cases; in particular, their negative predictive value attains 100%[2]. However, they do not allow us to assess whether a thrombus is actively growing or not. From this standpoint, scintigraphic techniques are still of interest and deserve attention.

We reviewed our past experience with 111In-labeled antifibrin monoclonal antibodies, with this specific question in mind.

MATERIAL AND METHOD

We investigated 86 consecutive patients (55 M, 33 F; age range 24-84 years), of whom 68 had a DVT of the lower limbs (63 acute, 5 chronic), while the remaining 18 had neigther clinical nor instrumental signs of leg involvement and were considered as controls. The 63 acute DVT were studied within 15 days from the onset of symptoms; the 5 chronic DVT had had recurrent episodes, and were studied within 15 days from the most recent one. Of the 18 controls, 8 had pulmonary embolism. Sixty-eight patients were been treated with heparin, when investigated.

The definitive diagnosis of DVT was made through ultrasonic duplex scanning (in all patients) and phlebography (in 57); we did not require a phlebography to exclude DVT.

All patients received 111In antifibrin at the dose of 74 MBq i.v. and were scanned with a total body automatic device at a speed of 10 cm/min both in anterior and posterior projections, with a large field-of-view gamma camera, coupled with a medium energy, parallel-hole collimator. Scintigraphic images of the lower limbs were obtained at 30 min, 3, 6 and 24 hours, and were interpreted by three indipendent observers. Although positive images (abnormal uptake along the course of the deep veins in either leg) could be observed as early as three hours post-injection, only the persistence of the uptake up to 24 hours was considered specific for diagnosis. This requirement prevented false positive results and the misinterpretation of any abnormal uptake due to stasis and varicose veins.

RESULTS

The examination was positive in all 63 patients with acute DVT (true positive), in 3 (true positive) out of 5 patients with chronic DVT and in 5 (false positive) out of 18 controls; it was negative in the remaining 2 chronic DVT (false negative) and 13 controls (true negative) [tab. 1]. Thus, the sensitivity was 100% for acute DVT, and 97% for all DVT (chronic DVT included); the specificity was 72%; the overall accuracy was 92%. The false negative results were interpreted as due to the chronicity of the process, while the false positive as due to venous stasis.

Table 1 . Results of 111In-labeled antifibrin monoclonal antibodies in patients with deep venous thrombosis of the lower limbs.

	111In ANTIFIBRIN		
	NEGATIVE	POSITIVE	TOTAL
ACUTE DEEP VENOUS THROMBOSIS	0	63	63
CHRONIC DEEP VENOUS THROMBOSIS	2	3	5
CONTROLS	13	5	18

Most DVT (as viewed through phlebography and/or duplex scanning) were massive, and involved all the deep venous system from the popliteal veins up to the femoro-iliac tracts; in spite of this, the scintigraphic images almost invariably showed an abnormal uptake restricted to the most proximal portion of the thrombi, and not all along their lenght.

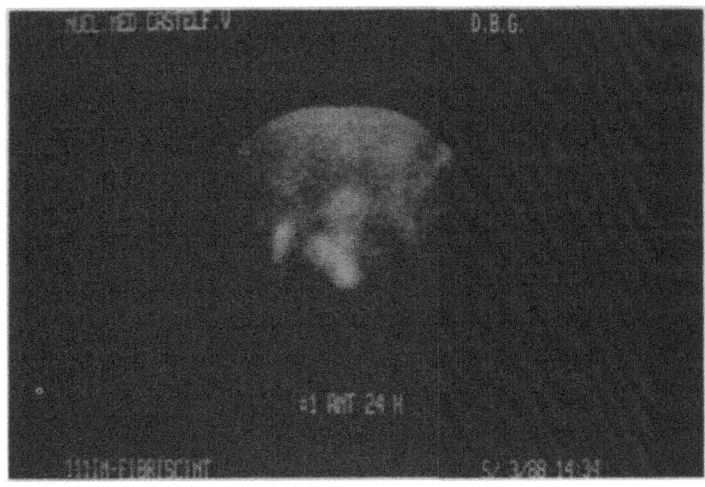

Figure 1 . Deep venous thrombosis of the right femoro-iliac vein. Anterior view. An abnormal uptake is clearly visible along the right side.

COMMENTS

Many radionuclide tests for DVT have been developed in the past, with various degree of success, in order to find a non-invasive alternative to phlebography. After the advent of the ultrasonic duplex scanning, which is an excellent diagnostic tool, the challenge for Nuclear Medicine techniques is to add functional informations, and specifically (and most relevantly) to assess whether a thrombus is actively growing or not.

Our results show that 111In antifibrin scintigraphy is extremely sensitive for acute venous thrombosis. Although we cannot exclude that a more intense uptake might be obtained without heparin, apparently such therapy did not adversely affect sensitivity in our series. These data compare well with other studies conducted with 111In-labeled monoclonal antifibrin antibody[3, 4, 5].

Due to the risk of a high number of false positive results in early images, we based the final diagnosis on the inspection of late (24 hours) images, when a better signal-to-background ratio and a satisfactory clearance of the venous pooling could be obtained. However, a 24 hour delay before a reliable diagnosis can be achieved may not be acceptable in most clinical settings.

We obtained poor results in the five patients with a chronic DVT, who had a history of several episodes. Since we had very few such patients, the overall accuracy of the examination was not affected; but the indication is there, that monoclonal antifibrin antibodies may not react with old thrombi (which is resonably acceptable), and that the apposition of newly formed clot may be too small to be detected (and yet be sufficient for symptoms to recur).

The sensitivity of antifibrin for DVT has been confirmed by more recent studies, using 99mTc labeled antibodies[6].

The fact that antifibrin visualized only the most proximal portion of large thrombi can be interpreted in various ways. It may reflect the inability of the antibodies to reach the bulk of the thrombus, but, altenatively, it may indicate an actively growing end. This hypothesis needs purposedly oriented studies to be clarified.

REFERENCES

1. Hui KJ, Haber E, Matsueda GR. Monoclonal anibodies to a specific fibrin-like peptide bind to human fibrin but not fibrinogen. *Science*; 222:1129-1132 (1983).
2. Cronan JJ, Dorfman GS. Advances in ultrasound imaging of venous thrombosis. *Semin Nucl Med*; 21:297-312 (1991).
3. Jung M, Kletter K, Dudczak R, et al. Deep vein thrombosis: scintigraphic diagnosis with In-111 labeled monoclonal antifibrin antibodies. *Radiology*; 173:469-475 (1989).
4. Alavi A, Palevsky HI, Gupta N, et al. Radiolabeled antifibrin antibody in the detection of venous thrombosis: Preliminary results. *Radiology*; 174:79-85 (1990).
5. De Faucal P, Peltier P, Planchon B, et al.: Evaluation of In-111 labeled antifibrin monoclonal antibody for the diagnosis of venous thromboembolic disease. *J Nucl Med*; 32:785-795 (1991).
6. Schaible TF, Alavi A. Antifibrin scintigraphy in the diagnostic evaluation of acute deep venous thrombosis. *Semin Nucl Med*; 21:313-324 (1991).

INTERACTIONS OF BLOOD CELLS WITH THE VESSEL WALL

J.L. Gordon and A.J.H. Gearing

British Bio-technology
Watlington Road, Cowley
Oxford, OX4 5LY, U.K.

INTRODUCTION: ADHESION MOLECULES

Blood leucocytes undergo regulated trafficking from the circulation into lymphoid organs and into sites of inflamation. The vascular endothelium lining the vessel walls plays a central role in controlling this leucocyte emigration. The interactions between the leucocyte and endothelium are mediated by cell adhesion molecules (CAMs) which have been identified using a combination of monoclonal antibodies which block adhesion and by direct expression cloning of cDNAs (for review see Simmons and Needham 1991). The vascular endothelial adhesins include: [1]E and P-selectins, which bind to complex saccharides on the leucocyte; [2]Intercellular adhesion molecules-1 and-2 (ICAM-1 and ICAM-2) which bind to the leucocyte $\beta2$ integrins LFA-1 and MAC-1; [3]vascular cell adhesion molecule-1 (VCAM-1), which binds to the leucocyte $\beta1$ integrin VLA-4 (Springer 1991). Leucocytes also express L-selectin (LAM-1) which binds to carbohydrate ligands on the endothelium. Studies on the binding of isolated leucocytes to cell lines transfected with cDNAs for individual CAMs have shown that different leucocyte subclasses use particular adhesins. For example, all lymphocytes can bind to ICAM-1 and VCAM-1 whereas only the CD45RO positive T cells can bind to E-selectin (Shimizu et al 1991). The expression of CD45 isoforms distinguishes subpopulations of T lymphocytes. Memory Tcells express CD45RO, whilst naive T cells express CD45RA (Beverley 1992). The carbohydrate ligand for E-selectin, which is expressed on CD45RO cells, is carried on the cutaneous lymphocyte antigen (CLA), and is immunologically distinct from the neutrophil ligands for E-selectin (Berg et al 1991). CD45RO cells express higher levels of LFA-1 and VLA-4 than CD45RA cells and they preferentially accumulate at inflammatory sites (Thornhill and Haskard 1991).

Cell biological studies have indicated that the selectins are involved in the initial capture of leucocytes from the circulation, an interaction which results in the so called "rolling" response (Lawrence and Springer 1991). The rolling contacts allow activation of leucocytes by endothelial-derived chemoattractants such as PAF or GMCSF. A rapid consequence of this activation is upregulation of the lymphocyte integrins for their endothelial ligands (ICAMs and VCAM). The integrin-mediated adhesion then allows the formation of tighter contacts between the lymphocyte and the endothelium, and thus arrests rolling and facilitates subsequent extravasation.

IMMUNOHISTOLOGICAL STUDIES

The precise roles of individual adhesins in the rolling, flattening and extravasation of lymphocytes *in vivo* remain to be clarified. Several CAMs can be expressed on the endothelium in inflamed tissues (Adams 1989; Rice 1991; Leung 1991) and CAM expression is differentially regulated, both temporally and spatially, within the developing inflammatory site.

The control of CAM expression on endothelium in human volunteers has been studied using intradermal provocation with inflammatory stimuli such as endotoxin, TNF, IFNγ, purified protein derivative of tuberculin, specific allergen or ultraviolet light (Munro 1989; Norris 1991). Whilst biopsies of normal skin show little or no endothelial expression of ICAM-1, VCAM-1 or E-selectin, intradermal provocation can cause the induction of all three CAMs. The kinetics of CAM appearance are similar (2-6 hours) to those observed *in vitro* with human umbilical vein endothelial cells in culture, but the CAMs can remain elevated for up to a week. As with *in vitro* studies, the nature of the stimulus can affect the expression of adhesins. Thus, following UV challenge, E-selectin and ICAM but not VCAM-1 were induced on dermal EC, whereas VCAM was also induced on EC following PPD injections (Norris 1991). Lymphocyte infiltration into tissues was particularly associated with expression of ICAM and VCAM but not with E-selectin.

We have studied CAM expression in pathological tissues using monoclonal antibodies specific for ICAM-1, VCAM-1, and E-selectin which were produced as described in Pigott et al (1991) by immunising mice with cytokine-activated human umbilical vein endothelial cells. Specificity was confirmed by binding to Cos or CHO cells transfected with cDNA for ICAM-1, VCAM-1 or E-selectin (Simmons and Needham, 1991). These studies demonstrated differential expression of CAMs in conditions characterised by cellular infiltration with leucocytes, such as graft rejection, acute and chronic inflammation, and lymphoid malignancies. For example, in cardiac allograft rejection, in which the infiltrate is predominantly lymphocytes and monocytes, ICAM-1 and VCAM-1 appear to be upregulated on the endothelium of venules, arterioles and endocardium, whereas E-selectin is not (Taylor et al 1992). ICAM-1, VCAM-1 and E-selectin were all upregulated in the microcirculation of rejecting hearts. The donor hearts before transplantation also show some evidence of endothelial expression of ICAM-1, VCAM-1 and E-selectin, suggesting that the pre-transplant handling procedures may have stimulated this expression. This may predispose the organ to early rejection crises.

In lymphoid malignancies and reactive lymph nodes, adhesion molecules can be detected on the endothelium of involved tissues (Ruco and Gearing 1991). One explanation is that secretion of cytokines at sites of tumour deposition could lead to activation of endothelium and prime that site for recruitment of more tumour cells and reactive leucocytes. In support of this, immunohistological studies suggest that the presence of cells secreting IL-1 or TNF is the critical factor determining E-selectin and VCAM-1 expression in lymph nodes (Ruco et al 1990). In contrast to the nodular sclerosis variant of Hodgkin's disease, the mixed cellularity variant shows weak expression of VCAM-1 and E-selectin. The enhanced E-selectin expression in nodular sclerosis correlates with infiltration of the lymph nodes with neutrophils (Ruco et al 1992). The pattern of CAM expression varies with the type of disease. In general, diseases such as granulomatosis, Hodgkin's disease and T cell non-Hodgkin's lymphomas (in which lymph nodes are infiltrated with T cells or macrophages) show strong staining for VCAM-1 and E-selectin. In contrast, those diseases characterised by B cell infiltration, such as Castleman's disease and B cell non-Hodgkin's lymphoma, are characterised by weak expression of VCAM-1 and E-selectin (Ruco et al 1992). In summary, CAM expression on lymphoid tumours and on the endhotelium within sites of tumour deposition may control the cellular content of the tumours, and therefore the pattern of CAM expression may provide information useful in tumour typing.

SOLUBLE ADHESION MOLECULES

Although immunohistological studies such as the ones described above can provide valuable information on the localisation of CAMs, the limited number and size of biopsies which can be taken from most tissues makes it difficult to correlate CAM expression accurately with changes in disease progression. Working on the hypothesis that endothelial cells may release CAMs from their cell surface, we developed specific two-site ELISAs to detect soluble forms of ICAM-1, VCAM-1 or E-selectin (Pigott et al 1992). The assays were calibrated with standard preparations of recombinant soluble adhesins. We have shown that cytokine-activated endothelial cells in culture can release soluble forms of ICAM-1, VCAM-1 and E-selectin (Pigott et al 1992), although the mechanism of release is unclear. So far, we have found no evidence for alternatively spliced soluble or Pi-linked variants of these adhesins, suggesting that proteolytic cleavange from the cell surface is the most likely mechanism of release.

Samples of human serum from healthy volunteers were found to contain soluble CAMs (Gearing et al 1992). In a sample of 62 individuals, mean levels of ICAM-1 were 56 U/ml, VCAM-1 54 U/ml and E-selectin 10 U/ml. We also examined serum samples from 32 patients with diabetes mellitus, 9 on chronic ambulatory peritoneal dialysis (CAPD) and 10 with hypertension. Although mean levels of soluble ICAM-1, VCAM-1 and E-selectin were higher than mean control levels in each of the patient groups, only patients on CAPD had significantly elevated levels of ICAM-1 (141 U/ml) and VCAM-1 (118 U/ml). Diabetics only had significantly elevated levels of E-Selectin (23 U/ml). The finding of detectable ICAM-1, VCAM-1 and E-Selectin in normal serum is surprising given the relative lack of E-Selectin, VCAM-1 and even ICAM-1 on normal tissue sections, but may reflect release from organs such as lung which suffer minor inflammatory insults on a daily basis. The differential release of soluble adhesins in conditions such as CAPD and diabetes presumably reflects differences in the underlying pathology.

Preliminary studies of soluble adhesins in serum of patients following renal allograft have shown that levels of ICAM-1, VCAM-1 and E-selectin vary with time, and that levels increase coincident with clinical signs of rejection such as increases in serum creatinine. Futher longitudinal studies are in progress to investigate the prognostic significance of measuring soluble adhesins in transplant rejection and inflammatory disease.

ANIMAL MODELS

Further evidence of CAM involvement in pathology has come from animal models of disease (see, for example, Harlan et al 1992; Mulligan 1991; Wegner 1990). Monoclonal antibodies which block the interaction of LFA-1 or MAC-1 with ICAM-1 have shown benefit in models of septic and hypovolemic shock, myocardial reperfusion injury, airway eosinophilia, and renal or cardiac transplantation. Blockade of VLA-4 has been beneficial in rat models of experimental autoimmune encephalomyelitis, rheumatoid arthritis and cutaneous inflammation, and blockade of E-selectin has been shown to reduce immune complex mediated vascular injury in rats and late phase airway obstruction in monkeys.

DEVELOPMENT OF DRUGS TO BLOCK ADHESION

Experiments such as these support the concept of adhesion blockade as a therapeutic strategy. Monoclonal antibodies similar to those used in the animal models described above are entering clinical trials for life-threatening conditions. However, several problems are associated with the use of protein drugs. These include antigenicity, the need for delivery by injection, and the cost of production, all of which restrict the scope for the therapeutic use of monoclonal antibodies. Wider applications of adhesion blockade will therefore require the development of orally available low molecular weight drugs. These will come from the applications of medicinal chemistry to leads emerging from screening programmes, from ligand based analogues and from structural studies of binding sites.

In the case of E-Selectin, for example, soluble forms of the molecule can be used for high throughput screens of chemical libraries or natural products, seeking antagonists. The ligand for E-selectin, sialylated Lewis x (a complex tetrasaccharide), can be used as the starting point for analogue chemistry. The complementarity determining regions from anti-E-selectin monoclonal antibodies can also be used as the basis for peptidomimetic chemistry.

In order to identify the key binding determinants of E-Selectin, we have used a combination of domain deletion analysis and site directed mutagenesis to identify the functional components. We have found that our blocking monoclonal antibodies to E-selectin all bind to the lectin domain but that their binding is dependent on the presence of the EGF domain; that the minimal structure which retains adhesion for leucocytes is the lectin/EGF pair; and that point mutations within the lectin domain can result in loss of adhesion (Pigott et al. 1991). As our results indicate that the lectin/EGF pair is the minimal ligand-binding portion of the molecule, we are working towards a solution NMR structure for the lectin/EGF pair. Such structural information is valuable in refining drug leads.

ACKNOWLEDGEMENTS

We would like to acknowledge the invaluable contributions made to the work presented in this manuscript by Prof. Andy Rees, Royal Postgraduate Medical School, Hammersmith Hospital, Dr. Marlene Rose, Harefields Hospital and Dr. Luigi Ruco, University of Rome.

REFERENCES

Adams D.H., Hubscher S.G., Shaw J., Rothlein R. & Neuberger J.M. (1989). ICAM-1 on liver allografts during rejection. *Lancet* 2: 1122-1125.

Berg E.L., Yoshino T., Rott L.S., Robinson M.K., Warnock R.A. Kishimoto T.K., Picker L.J., Butcher EC. (1991).The cutaneous Lymphocyte antigen is a skin homing receptor for the vascular lectin ELAM-1. *J. Exp. Med.* 174: 1461-1466.

Beverley P.C.L. (1992). Functional analysis of human T cell substs defined by CD45 isoform expression. *Seminars in Immunology* 35-41.

Gearing A.J.H. Hemingway i., Pigott R., Hughes J., Rees A. & Cashman S.J. (1992). Soluble forms of Vascular Adhesions Molecules, E-Selectin, ICAM-1 and VCAM-1 : Pathological significance. Annals NYAcad.Sci. 667:324-331.

Harlan J.M., Winn R.K., Vedder N.B., Doerschuk C.M., Rice C.L. In vivo models of leucocyte adherence to endothelium. In Eds. Harlan JM & Liu DY, Adhesion: Its role in inflamatory disease. WH Freeman, New York.

Lawrence M.B., Springer T.A. (1991). Leucocytes roll on a selectin at physiological flow rates: Distinction from and prerequisite for adhesion through integrins. Cell:859-873.

Leung D.Y., Pober J.S. & Cotran R.S. (1991). Expression of ELAM-1 in elicited late phase allergic reactions. *J. Clin. Invest.* 87:1805-1809.

Mulligan M.S., Varani J., Dame M.K., Lane C.L., Smith C.W., Anderson D.C. & WARD P.A. (1991). Role of ELAM-1 in neutrophil mediated lung injury in rats. *J. Clin. Invest.* 88: 1396-1406.

Munro J.M., Pober J.S. & Cotran R.S., (1989). Tumour necrosis factor and interferon γ induce distinct patterns of endtothelial activation and associated leucoyte accumulation in skin of Papio anubis. *Am. J. Pathol.* 135: 121-133.

Norris P., Poston R.N., Thomas D.S., Thornill M., Hawk J. & Haskard D.O. (1991). The expression of ELAM-1, ICAM-1 and VCAM-1 in experimental cutaneous inflammation: a comparision of UVb erythema and delayed hypertensitivity. *J. Invest. Dermatol.* 96:763-770.

Picker L.J., Kishimoto T.K., Smith C.W. Warnock R.A. Butcher E.C. (1991). ELAM-1 is an adhesion molecule for skin-homing T cells. *Nature* 349: 796-799.

Pigott R., Needham L.A., Edwards R.M., Walker C.A. & Power C. (1991). Structural and functional studies of the activation antigen ELAM-1 using a panel of monoclonal antibodies. *J. Immunol.* 147: 130-135.

Pigott R., Dillon L.P., Hemingway I.H. & Gearing A.J.H. (1992). Soluble forms of E-selectin, ICAM-1 and VCAM-1 are present in the supernatants of cytokine activated cultured endothelial cells. *Biochem. Biophys. Res. Comm.* 187: 584-589.

Rice G.E., Munro J.M., Corless C. & Bevilacqua. (1991) Vascular and non-vascular expression of INCAM-110. *Am. J. Pathol.* 138: 385-393.

Ruco L.P., Pomponi D., Piggot R., Stoppacciaro A., Monardo F., Uccini S., Boraschi D., Tagliabue A., Santoni A., Dejana E. & Baroni C.D. (1990). Cytokine production (IL-1a, IL-1b, and TNFa) and endothelial cell activation (ELAM-1 and HLADr) in reactive lymphadenitis, Hodgkins disease, and in non-Hodgkins lymphoma: an immunochemical study. *Am. J. Pathol.* 137: 1163-1171.

Ruco L.P., Pomponi D., Pigott R., Gearing A.J.H., Baicchini A. & Baroni C.D. (1992). Expression and cell distribution of the adhesion molecules ICAM-1, VCAM-1, ELAM-1 and endoCAM (CD31) in reactive human lymph nodes and in Hodkins disease. In Press *Am. J. Pathol.*

Ruco L.P. & Gearing A.J.H. EALM-1 expression in human malignancies.(1991). In ED. Gordon J.L. Vascular endothelium: Interactions with circulating cells. Elsevier Science publishers B.V.

Ruco. L.P., Gearing A.J.H., Pigott R., Pomponi D., Burgiov L., Cafolla A.A., Baiocchini A. & Baroni C.D. (1992). Expression of ICAM-1, VCAM-1 and ELAM-1 in angiofollicular lymph node hyperplasia (Castlemans disease) evidence for dysplasia of follicular dendritic reticulum cells. *Histopathology* 19:523-528.

Shimizu Y., Shaw S., Graber N., Gopal T.V., Horgan K.J., Van Seventer G.A. & Newman W. (1991). Activation-independent binding of human memory T cells to adhesion molecule ELAM-1. *Nature* 349: 799-802.

Simmons D.L., & Needham L.A. (1991). Cloning cell surface molecules using monoclonal antibodies. In Ed. Gordon J.L. Vascular endothelium: Interactions with circulating cells. Elsevier Science publishers B.V.

Springer T.A. (1991) Adhesion receptors of the immune system. *Nature* 364:425-434.

Taylor P.M., Rose M.L., Yacoub M.H. & Pigott R. (1992). Induction of vascular adhesion molecules during rejection of human cardiac allografts. *Transplantation.* 54:451-457.

Thornhill M.H. & Haskard D.O. (1991). Lymphocyte adhesion in inflammation In J.L. Gordon Ed. Vascular Endothelium: Interactions with Circulating cells. Elsevier Science Publishers B.V.

Wegner C.D., Gundel R.H., Reilly P., Haynes L.G. & Rothelin R. (1990). ICAM-1 in the pathogenesis of asthma. *Science.* 274: 456-459.

IS 111In-LEUCOCYTE SCINTIGRAPHY USEFUL IN THE EVALUATION OF PATIENTS WITH PROLONGED FEVER OF UNKNOWN ORIGIN?

K. Schmidt, I.M. Wedebye, B. Haastrup, J.W. Rasmussen and P.B. Frederiksen

Department of Nuclear Medicine
Odense University Hospital
DK-5000 Odense C, Denmark

A substantial proportion of the patients referred for 111In white blood cell scanning (111In WBCS) have been febrile for prolonged periods with no or only vague symptoms or signs to suggest the cause of the fever. The paucity of 111In WBCS-data in this clinical setting thus seems surprising.

The present paper reviews the results of published 111In WBCS-studies in patients with prolonged fever of unknown origin (FUO). It is a prerequisite that the patients fulfill (or are very close to fulfill) the FUO criteria originally defined by Petersdorf and Beeson[1], i.e. at least 3 weeks' illness with a temperature exceeding 38.3° C on several occasions, and no established diagnosis after at least 1 week's evaluation in a hospital. Updated results of our own 111In WBC-studies of FUO patients will also be presented.

The results of 111In WBCS from refs. 2-5 are shown in Table 1. It is suggested that a truely positive scintigraphic finding corresponds to an infective cause of FUO. It can be seen that most studies show a low predictive value of a positive test, and a somewhat higher predictive value of a negative test. Another important finding is the wide confidence limits encompassing almost all numerical terms of diagnostic probabilities, reflecting in particular the small number of patients in most studies.

Specific comments: Syrjälä et al[2] injected pure granulocyte suspensions. Scintigraphy was postponed to the following day. FUO corresponded to at least 2 weeks' fever > 38.0°C. The final diagnoses were not stated. Postoperative patients were not included. Schmidt et al[3] injected granulocyte-enriched leucocytes. FUO was strictly defined. Postoperative patients and patients with focal symptoms or signs which in retrospect could be connected with the final diagnosis or should have directed an alternative diagnostic approach were not included. MacSweeney et al[4] injected pure granulocyte suspensions. FUO was strictly defined. Repeat scans were included in the calculations (25 patients, 30 scans). The study included 11 postoperative scans. Davies and Garvie[5] injected mixed WBC. FUO corresponded to > 3 weeks' fever (> 38.0° C) in 25 patients, and to 2-3 weeks' fever in 3 patients. The final diagnoses were not stated (18% infections?). Postoperative patients were not included.

Table 1. Results of four 111In-WBC studies of patients with FUO

	Ref. 2	Ref. 3	Ref. 4	Ref. 5
No. of patients	68	32	30	28
Sensitivity	90% (70-99%)	70% (35-93%)	55% (23-83%)	60%(15-95%)
Specificity	85% (72-94%)	82% (60-95%)	74% (49-91%)	78%(56-93%)
Accuracy	87% (76-94%)	78% (60-91%)	67% (47-83%)	75%(55-89%)
PVPT	73% (52-88%)	64% (31-89%)	55% (23-83%)	38% (9-76%)
PVNT	95% (84-99%)	86% (64-97%)	74% (49-91%)	90%(68-99%)

$$Sensitivity = \frac{TP}{TP+FN} \qquad Specificity = \frac{TN}{TN+FP}$$

$$Accuracy = \frac{TP+TN}{TP+FP+TN+FN}$$

$$PVPT \ (predictive \ value \ of \ a \ pos. \ test) = \frac{TP}{TP+FP}$$

$$PVNT \ (predictive \ value \ of \ a \ neg. \ test) = \frac{TN}{TN+FN}$$

TP = true-positive   FP = false-positive
TN = true-negative   FN = false-negative

95%-confidence limits are shown in brackets

Factors that may affect the result of 111In WBC scintigraphy in FUO: 111In WBCS is considered a specific and sensitive method for the detection and exclusion of focal inflammatory and infectious processes[6-8]. There are some shortcomings and pitfalls, however, which should be kept in mind in the study of FUO patients. Longstanding osseus infections, particularly in the spine, may go undetected[9,10]. The lesions of subacute endocarditis very rarely take up 111In-leucocytes[11,12]. Malignant tumours have shown 111In-leucocyte uptake in several studies[13-15]. Non-infected renal transplants that function normally can accumulate 111In-leucocytes[16,17]. Upper abdominal infections may be difficult to show because of the normal radioactivity in the spleen and liver. There is reason to suggest that longstanding infections take up 111In WBC less avidly than do infections of shorter duration[18,19], a view that is not supported by all studies[20,21], however. A phenomenon that can make the interpretation of WBC scans difficult is "non-specific" colonic activity, which we have seen in particular in viral infections and in patients with connective tissue diseases. Imaging of the head and neck allows identification of upper

Table 2. Results of 111In-granulocyte scintigraphy (111In GS) in 112 patients with FUO. The diagnostic probabilities (with 95%-confidence limits) using 6 different criteria of interpretation of an 111In GS-study are shown.

			All abnormal tracer accumulations are considered positive	Only distinctly abnormal tracer accumulations are considered positive
True pos. 111InGS corresponds to an inf./infl. process		false negative		
		Sensitivity	A1 74% (57-88%)	A2 74% (57-88%)
		Specificity	61% (49-72%)	79% (68-88%)
		Accuracy	65% (56-74%)	78% (70-86%)
		Pred. value pos.111InGS	46% (33-60%)	62% (46-76%)
		pred. value neg.111InGS	84% (72-92%)	87% (77-94%)
	A neg.111InGS-study in endocarditis is considered	true negative		
		Sensitivity	B1 90% (73-98%)	B2 90% (73-98%)
		Specificity	64% (53-74%)	81% (71-89%)
		Accuracy	71% (63-79%)	83% (76-90%)
		Pred. value pos.111InGS	46% (33-60%)	62% (46-76%)
		pred. value neg.111InGS	95% (85-99%)	96% (88-99%)
True pos. 111InGS corresponds to an inf./infl./neopl.proce ss		false negative		
		Sensitivity	C1 74% (60-85%)	C2 67% (53-79%)
		Specificity	72% (59-83%)	90% (79-96%)
		Accuracy	73% (65-81%)	79% (71-87%)
		Pred. value pos.111InGS	71% (58-83%)	86% (71-95%)
		pred. value neg.111InGS	75% (62-86%)	74% (62-84%)
	A neg.111InGS-study in endocarditis is considered	true negative		
		Sensitivity	D1 83% (70-93%)	D2 75% (60-86%)
		Specificity	75% (63-85%)	91% (81-96%)
		Accuracy	79% (71-87%)	84% (76-91%)
		Pred. value pos.111InGS	71% (58-83%)	86% (71-95%)
		pred. value neg.111InGS	86% (74-94%)	83% (72-91%)

airway infections and makes possible the identification of swallowed radioactivity which shows up as bowel activity on late scintigrams. Early scanning facilitates the interpretation of abdominal tracer accumulations because of the transport of intraluminal intestinal radioactivity during the scanning period.

The considerations above relate to the pattern of patient referral for 111In WBCS and to the definition of a positive and a negative scintigram. The latter issue is illustrated in Table 2 which gives an account of our results of 111In-granulocyte scintigraphy in 112 patients with FUO defined as in ref. 3. Various criteria of a true-positive and a true-negative scintigram have been applied. Specifically, as we often find tumours to accumulate 111In-granulocytes[14], and never have seen a positive 111In-granulocyte scintigram in a case of endocarditis, we have exploited the impact of changing the criteria of interpretation in accordance with the clinical findings. These criteria should be influenced by the composition of the patient population, which will vary between institutions and with time[22]. The 112 FUO patients studied by us comprised 39 patients with infectious diseases, 19 patients with malignant tumours, 26 patients with connective tissue disorders, 3 with miscellaneous diseases, and 25 patients who remained undiagnosed. Apart from a somewhat declining proportion of patients with connective tissue diseases, and an increasing fraction of undiagnosed patients during the 10-year study period, the referral pattern did not change. In the light of a constant 15-20% proportion of patients with neoplastic diseases which in our hands often accumulate 111In-granulocytes[14], we prefer criterion D1 for a positive scintigram. By defining weak tracer accumulations as positive it is possible to prescribe supplementary studies, in particular CT, which diagnosed malignant tumours in 2 patients with weak tumour accumulation of 111In. Three malignant tumours went undetected by 111In GS. CT was not required in a large proportion of the 36 patients in whom 111In GS yielded decisive diagnostic information.

In conclusion, our results indicate that 111In GS is useful for the evaluation of patients with FUO. Around 40% of our patients were subjected to abdominal CT, which should be preceded by 111In GS for optimal diagnostic benefit in our population of FUO patients.

REFERENCES

1. Petersdorf RG, Beeson PB. Fever of unexplained origin: report of 100 cases. *Medicine*;40:1-30 (1961).
2. Syrjälä MT, Valtonen V, Liewendahl K, Myllylä G. Diagnostic significance of indium-111 granulocyte scintigraphy in febrile patients. *J Nucl Med*;28:155-60 (1987).
3. Schmidt KG, Rasmussen JW, Sørensen PG, Wedebye IM. Indium-111-granulocyte scintigraphy in the evaluation of patients with fever of undetermined origin. *Scand J Inf Dis*;19:339-45 (1987).
4. MacSweeney JE, Peters AM, Lavender JP. Indium labelled leucocyte scanning in pyrexia of unknown origin. *Clin Radiol*;42:414-7 (1990).
5. Davies SG, Garvie NW. The role of indium-labelled leukocyte imaging in pyrexia of unknown origin. *Br J Radiol*;63:850-4 (1990).
6. Peters AM, Saverymuttu SH, Reavy HJ, Danpure HJ, Osman S, Lavender JP. Imaging of inflammation with indium-111 tropolonate labeled leukocytes. *J Nucl Med* 24: 39-44 (1983).
7. Becker W, Fischbach W, Reiners C, Börner W. Three-phase white blood cell scan: diagnostic validity in abdominal inflammatory diseases. *J Nucl Med*; 27:1109-15 (1986).
8. Schmidt KG, Rasmussen JW, Wedebye IM, Frederiksen PB. Speed of accumulation of 111In-labelled granulocytes in focal non-osseous inflammatory processes. *Nucl Med Commun*;8:623-30 (1987).
9. Palestro CJ, Kim CK, Swyer AJ, Vallabhajosula S, Goldsmith SJ. Radionuclide diagnosis of vertebral osteomyelitis: indium-111-leukocyte and technetium-99m-methylene diphosphonate bone scintigraphy. *J Nucl Med*;32:1861-5 (1991).
10. Whalen JL, Brown ML, McLeod R, Fitzgerald RH. Limitations of indium leukocyte imaging for the diagnosis of spine infections. *Spine*;16:193-7 (1991).
11. McAfee JG, Samin A. In-111 labeled leukocytes: a review of problems in image interpretation. *Radiology*; 155:221-9 (1985).

12. Riba AL, Thakur ML, Gottschalk A, Andriole VT, Zaret BL. Imaging experimental infective endocarditis with indium-111-labeled blood cellular components. *Circulation*; 59:336-43 (1979).

13. Fortner A, Datz FL, Taylor A, Alazraki N. Uptake of 111In-labeled leukocytes by tumor. *AJR*; 146:621-5 (1986).

14. Schmidt KG, Rasmussen JW, Wedebye IM, Frederiksen PB, Pedersen NT. Accumulation of indium-111-labeled granulocytes in malignant tumors. *J Nucl Med*;29:479-84 (1988).

15. Lamki LM, Kasi LP, Haynie TP. Localization of indium-111 leukocytes in noninfected neoplasms. *J Nucl Med*; 29:1921-6 (1988).

16. Collier BD, Isitman AT, Kaufman HM, Rao SA, Knobel J, Hellman RS, Zielonka JS, Pelc L. Concentration of In-111-oxine-labeled autologous leukocytes in noninfected and nonrejecting renal allografts: concise communication. *J Nucl Med*; 25:156-9 (1984).

17. Sebrechts C, Biberstein M, Klein JL, Witztum KF. Limitation of indium-111 leukocyte scanning in febrile renal transplant patients. *AJR*; 146:823-9 (1986).

18. Sfakianakis GN, Al-Sheikh W, Heal A, Rodman G, Zeppa R, Serafini A. Comparisons of scintigraphy with In-111 leukocytes and Ga-67 in the diagnosis of occult sepsis. *J Nucl Med*; 23:618-26 (1982).

19. Bitar RA, Scheffel U, Murphy PA, Bartlett JG. Accumulation of indium-111-labeled neutrophils and gallium-67 citrate in rabbit abscesses. *J Nucl Med*; 27:1883-9 (1986).

20. Datz FL. Thorne DA. Effect of chronicity of infection on the sensitivity of the In-111-labeled leukocyte scan. *AJR*; 147:809-12 (1986).

21. Schmidt KG, Rasmussen JW, Wedebye IM, Frederiksen PB. Analysis of factors that may affect the speed of accumulation of 111In-labelled granulocytes at sites of inflammation. *Nucl Med Commun*; 9:97-103 (1988).

22. Knockaert DC, Vanneste LJ, Vanneste SB, Bobbaers HJ. Fever of unknown origin in the 1980s. *Arch Intern Med*; 152:51-5 (1992).

DIAGNOSIS OF INFLAMMATORY BONE AND JOINT DISEASES WITH MONOCLONAL ANTIBODIES (BW 250/183)

A. Kroiss[1], F. Böck[3], G. Perneczky[3], Ch. Auinger[1], G. Weidlich[2] and A. Neumayr[4]

[1]Institute of Nuclear Medicine
[2]1st Med. Department
[3]Neurosurgical Department
[4]Ludwig Boltzmann Forschungsst für Klin Geriatrie
KA Rudolfstiftung, Vienna, Austria

The localisation of infectious diseases has become a challenge for the physicians specialised in nuclear medicine[7]. Years ago we used Ga-67 for the diagnosis of inflammatory diseases and achieved good results. A major disadvantage of this isotope consists in the fact that colon excretion may be found therefore the interpretation of higher bowel uptake is often problematic. Moreover, the radiation dose is very high[4]. Since Thakur and other groups have reported the possibility of labeling leucocytes with 111Indium-oxine this method has won a dominating place in imaging inflammatory processes[10]. The introduction of anti-granulocyte antibodies has offered a new possibility of coping with this diagnostic problem[1,5,9]. We have used 99mTc labeled antibodies.

Patients with diabetes mellitus are predisposed to a variety of inflammatroy processes, among which infections account for major morbidity. Bone scanning using technetium-99m phosphonates is a very sensitive tool in detecting various skeletal abnormalities. Its greater sensitivity over radiographs plays an important role, especially in the early diagnosis of osteomyelitis. Radiographs provide information about the structures of foot bones involved with diabetic osteoarthropathy, but are insensitive in early diagnosis of osteomyelitis[6,11].

Preoperative exclusion or confirmation of periprosthetic infection is essential for correct surgical management of patients with suspected hip prostheses[2,3].

A number of diagnostic modalities including conventional x-rays, lumbar computed tomography (CT), nuclear magnetic resonance (NMR) and planar bone scintigraphy have been used to evaluate patients to determine the cause of persistence of back pain. However, with the introduction of SPECT scanning of the spine the image contrast has been improved, but it was not possible to differentiate between a post operative transformation or local inflammatory disease.

The aim of this study was to prove the clinical relevance of monoclonal granulocytes antibody in combination with bone scintigraphy with 99mTc disphosphonat in different bone and joint diseases.

PATIENT AND METHOD

After information and formal consent 119 patients (56 female, 63 male, age from 18 - 81; mean 31 ± 20 years) have been studied.

The antibody (Ab) we used was the BW 250/183 from the Behringwerke, FRG. This is an immunoglobulin IgG1 isotype and binds to an epitope of NCA 95. In a simple labeling procedure 1.0 - 0.5 mg of this monoclonal Ab is labeled with 10 mCi (370 MBq) 99mTc - in SPECT studies 20mCi (740 MBq). There is no further purification necessary and the percentage of free Tc-pertechnetate is less than 1%.

After slow intravenous injection of the labeled Ab without premedication - except blockade of the thyroid with perchlorate - the imaging was done by rotating digital camera (Elscint, APEX 409 A). We performed images 4 - 6 hours and 24 hours planar (256x256 matrix) and mostly SPECT (64x64 matrix), especially in patients with diseases of the spine. Three dimensional reconstructions were done in a thickness of the slices of 13.6mm.

The three phase bone scintigraphy was done by a bolus injection.

15 - 20mCi (740 MBq) 99mTc-MDP we injected intravenously by positioning the area of interest in the field of view of the scintillation camera. Serial images were done, 10min after application a planar picture was done and 2 - 3 hrs after injection a late picture was performed.

RESULTS

After application of the 99mTc labeled Ab (BW 250/183) the whole body imaging after 6 and 24 hours showed the distribution of the Ab: high uptake in the spine, pelvis ribs and especially in liver and spleen. Although the uptake in the bone marrow was very high infectious lesions of bones and joints could be demonstrated very clearly. For the demonstration of processes in the spine and hip prosthesis SPECT imaging is absolutely necessary because sensitivity is considerable improved thereby and the extent of the infection is better demonstrated. The lesions were already visualized within 4 to six hours, but 24 hour pictures are desireable becaue localization is easier.

The investigation was performed in 26 patients with infections diabetic foot, 25 pts. with osteomyelitis, 12 pts. with septic hip prosthesis, 25 pts. with loosening hip prosthesis, 9 pts. with spondylitis and 22 pts. with postoperative spondylodiscitis (table 1).

Table 1

Diagnosis	
Infectious diabetic foot	26
Osteomyelitis	25
Septic hip prosthesis	12
Loosening hip prosthesis	25
Spondylitis	9
Spondylodiscitis - postop.	22

We found in 61 pts a true positive result, in 43 pts a true negative result, in 9 pts a false negative result and in 6 pts a false positive result.

This would mean a sensitivity of 87% and a specificity of 88%.

The results were proved by surgery (56 %), by biopsy (25%) and clinical indices, conventioneal x-rays, CT, MRI, myelography (19%).

CONCLUSION

This method developed by Schwarz et al[8] for the 99mTc labeling of Ab's is very efficient, kit preparation is easy, and the imaging is less time-consuming compared to other tracers (111In, 123I). This Ab labeling technique makes the time-consuming procedure of cell isolation superfluous. The quality of the images is excellent and in hip prosthesis and diseases of the spine SPECT images are necessary. We found a good binding of the 99mTc to the Ab and the investigation is always available.

We observed no side-effects or signs of allergic or adverse reactions.

Granulocyte antibody imaging combined with bone scans have been useful tools solving important diagnostic questions. This Ab method is helpful for localisation and extent of a septic process in bone and joint diseases. Therefore those therapeutically strategies can be pursued systematically and more consequently.

REFERENCES

1. Hotze AL, Briele B, Overbeck B, Kropp J, Gruenwald F, Mekkawy MA, von Smekal A, Moeller F,Biersack HJ. Technetium-99m-labeled anti-granulocyte antibodies in suspected bone infections. *J Nucl Med* 33:526-531 (1992).
2. Kroiss A, Böck F, Perneczky G, Auinger Ch, Weidlich G, Kleinpeter G, Brenner H.Immunszintigraphie zur Aufdeckung von Entzündungsherden bei Knochen- und Gelenkserkrankungen. *Wien Klin Wochenschr* 102:713-717 (1990).
3. Kroiss A, Kölbl Ch, Tuchmann A, Auinger Ch, Weidlich G, Weiss W, Neumayr A.Immunszintigraphie (IS) bei entzündlichen Erkrankungen mit Tc-99m-MAK BW 250/183. *Acta Med Austriaca* 16:11-16 (1989).
4. Kroiss A, Weiss W, Kahn P, Neumayr A. Untersuchungen von Oberbaucherkrankungen mittels Gallium-67-Zitrat. In:"Nuklearmedizin", Schmidt HAE, Woldring M Hrsg, Schattauer, Stuttgart New York (1977).
5. Lind P, Langsteger W, Költringer P, Dimai HP, Passl R, Eber O. Immunoscintigraphy of inflammatory processes with a technetium-99m-labeled monoclonal antigranulocyte-antibody (Mab BW 250/183). *J Nucl Med* 31:417-423 (1990).
6. Oyen WJG, Netten PM, Lemmens AM, Claessens RMJ, Lutterman JA, van der Vliet JA, Goris RJA, van der Meer JWM, Corstens FHM. Evaluation of infectious diabetic foot complications with Indium-111-labeled human nonspecific immunoglobulin G. *J Nucl Med* 33: 1330-1336 (1992).
7. Peters AM. Editorial: Imaging inflammation: current role of labeld autologous leukocytes. *J Nucl Med* 33: 65-67 (1992).
8. Schwarz A, Steinsträßer A. A novel approach to 99m-Tc-labeled monoclonal antibody. *J Nucl Med* 28: 721 (Abstract) (1987).
9. Seybold K, Locher JT, Coosemans C, Andreas RY, Schubiger AP, Bläuenstein P. Immunoscintigraphic localization of inflammatory lesions: clinical experience. *Eur J Nucl Med* 13: 587-593 (1988).
10. Thakur ML, Lavender JP, Arnot RN, Silvester DJ, Segal AW. Indium-111-labeld autologous leukocytes in man. *J Nucl Med* 18: 1014-1021 (1977).
11. Weidlich G, Kroiss A, Auinger CH, Schernthaner G. Immunoscintigraphy for detection of foot infections in diabetic patients. *Diabetologia* 33: A24 (Abstract) (1990).

IMAGING INFLAMMATORY BOWEL DISEASE

J. Martin-Comin and M. Roca

S. Medicina Nuclear
Hospital de Bellvitge
Barcelona, Spain

The name of Inflammatory bowel disease refers to two well known diseases: ulcerative colitis (UC) and Crohn's disease (CD). Both are clinically similar though different in location and histology. The main feature of both is that after the initial diagnosis, new acute attacks may appear at any time, breaking symptom free periods.

Their incidence is variable from one country to another (table 1)[1] and their treatment is mainly medical though more than 50% of patients with CD undergo some surgery within 5 years after its diagnosis.

Table 1.

Incidence of IBD (new cases/100.000 h/year)

	Ulcerative Colitis	Crohn's disease
Denmark	8.1	1.8
France	2.9	4.2
Israel	5.8	1.3
Italy	1.9	0.8
Netherlands	6.8	3.9
Spain	0.8	0.7
Sweden	6.4	4.8
United Kingdom	11.3	2.7
U.S.A	7.2	4.0

Radiology, endoscopy and histology were the usual diagnostic methods and several clinical activity indexes have been described to evaluate the severity of the disease. Nevertheless they are sometimes contraindicated and not useful during the acute attacks of the disease. On the other hand, clinical indexes are difficult to obtain and they are not used in all centers.

Radiology, either barium enema or bowel transit, is less used than it was. It requires

Radiolabeled Blood Elements, Edited by J. Martin-Comin
Plenum Press, New York, 1994

patient preparation, takes long time, and it may produce serious complications, namely toxic megacolon. Actually it should not be performed in the first phase of the acute attack.

Endoscopy, is the most used procedure to obtain tissue samples to establish the diagnosis. However, though useful to establish the diagnosis, it is not useful to establish the extension of the disease because very often it is not possible to examine all the colon and the small bowel is dificult to examine.

Many Nuclear Medicine methods have been applied in the study of IBD, 67Ga scanning, 99mTc-DTPA scintigraphy, bowel permeability...but leucocyte labeled scintigraphy is the one that has really changed the management of the disease.

In 1981 Segal et al[2] and Saverymmuttu et al[3] described the use of 111In-labeled leucocyte scintigraphy in the management of IBD. The new method was really succesfull and today, 11 years later, labeled leucocyte scintigraphy has been incorporated into the IBD management protocols of most centers.

Unfortunately labeling leucocytes with 111In is a time consuming procedure, requires blood manipulation and is associated to relatively high radiation exposure. Therefore other labeling procedures and agents were introduced in the search of a better IBD scintigraphy tracer. Namely HMPAO, phagocyte labeling, monoclonal antibodies, human polyclonal immunoglobulin and nanocolloids[4 - 10].

This paper will review the usefulness of these agents in the clinical management of IBD. Their main characteristic are resumed in table 2.

Table 2

Scintigraphic relative uptake of different IBD seeking agents.

	L-In	L-HMPAO	MoAb	HIG
Liver	+++	++	+	+++
Spleen	+++	++	++	++
Kidney	-	+++	++	++
Urinary tract	-	+++	+	++
Bowel	-	++	+	+/-
Bone marrow	-	+	+++	+

L-In: 111In-leukocytes; L-HMPAO: 99mTc-HMPAO-Leucocytes
MoAb: Antigranulocyte monoclonal antibody BW 250/183
HIG: Human polyclonal immunoglobulin. +++: high, ++: moderate; +: low; -: absent.

In a patient where IBD is suspected the questions to answer are :
1. Diagnostic. Is it an IBD ?
if the answer is yes:
2. Extension. How much bowel is affected ?
3. The severity.

1. Diagnostic

Labeled leucocytes, whether with 111In or with 99mTc, and monoclonal antibodies have proved to be highly accurate in diagnosing IBD (table 3). HIG scintigraphy has been found accurate by some authors[8] while other[11, 12] found it useless. Nanocolloids seems not to be accurate enough for this purpose[9]. 111In-labeling scintigraphy is possibly the most used method. In fact once its diagnosis accuracy in comparison with endoscopy/radiology was demonstrated, it has been used as a reference method for the new procedures.

Scintigraphy is usually performed on a dual basis: early scan and late scan. The main scintigraphic features of IBD are: Labeled leucocyte deposits follow the intestinal pattern, while abscesses or tumours are more localized. IBD disease is usually well defined in the early scan while abscesses are frequently not seen in this early scan. Tomoscintigraphy in our experience may help in the localization of the disease and Kroiss et al[13] showed an increase from 71 to 90 % in sensitivity from planar to SPECT.

These false positive results have been described[14]: Yersinia infections, seudomembranous colitis, ischemic and bacterial colitis, abdominal tumours, gastrointestinal bleeding, radiation colitis, leucocyte swallowing and leucocyte uptake in the colostomy bag. In our opinion most of them may be identified in the patient anamnesis/physical examination. The true false positives are colitis of other ethiology, (especially infectious colitis).

It is important to know that patient treatment may modify significantly the accuracy of the technique. Becker et al[15] refer a decrease in sensitivity to 56 % with 2 weeks treatment. In our experience we have seen normal scans in patients with only 4-5 days of treatment.

Compared to other diagnostic modalities (endoscopy and radiology) scintigraphy is rapid, allows whole bowel examination and may be performed in the critically ill patient.

111In-chelates offer the most stable labeling, the time to diagnosis is about 6 hours (but to confirm it, it is sometimes necessary to wait up to the 18 hours image), and there is neither kidney nor bowel excretion. 99mTc-HMPAO labeling is less stable, time to diagnosis may be as short as 2-3 hours and the late scan is less necessary; its main drawback is that there is high kidney and bowel activity, especially in images obtained after 3 hours p.i (caudo-cranial or post-voiding views can be used to avoid missinterpretations). Monoclonal antibodies (BW 250/183) and HIG does not require blood manipulation, time to diagnosis is 24 h for the former and 3-4 h for the latter; both show kidney and bowel activity in late images.

Leucocyte scintigraphy is especially useful in identifying CD when terminal ileum is the only diseased segment. This area is difficult to approach by endoscopy, so scintigraphy which can examine the whole bowel (small and large) simultaneously, may be helpful. Isolated uptake in the ileo-caecal area is highly suggestive of CD. Cramma-Bohbouth et al[16] reported in 1990 that the accuracy of 111In-labeled leucocytes to diagnose small bowel disease was 85 % and increased to 91 % in the large bowel.

Table 3

Sensitivity, specificity and accuracy of different methods in the diagnosis of IBD.

	111In	99mTc-HMPAO	MoAb	HIG
Sensitivity	81-98	71-100	69-90	80
Specificity	75-100	81-100	87-93	87
Accuracy	72-99	75-100	76-91	83

2.- Extension:

Once the diagnosis is established the second question is how large the extension of bowel involved is. The answer is important for the treatment as well as for the follow up.

In the previous reports[17-23] good correlation between radiology, endoscopy and scintigraphic extension has been described using 111In labeling. Nevertheless, some authors[20] showed that correlation was better between endoscopy and scintigraphy (75 %) than between the latter and radiology (58%), reflecting that scintigraphy located disease better than radiology.

Correlation was also excellent between scintigraphy and surgical findings[18, 22]. Especially interesting is the work of Moisan et al[24] who showed that scintigraphy of the surgically resected bowel were identical to the pre-surgery scintigraphy.

Those results led to a less use of radiology, especially during the acute attack, and thereafter new procedures were compared with 111In-leucocyte scintigraphy.

Good agreement has been shown between 99mTc- HMPAO and 111In results[25, 26]. The HMPAO exam has the advantage that result are available less than 1 h post-reinjection. In fact, in our experience a 30 min image is used to analyze the presence of disease; if it is normal, IBD is very improbable. If leucocyte uptake is seen, the shape and location of activity is evaluated. Subsequently later images are obtained to evaluate complications or other possible diagnoses

Similar results have been shown with MoAb. Our group[6] showed an overall agreement of 89.3 % between 111In-oxine and 99mTc-BW 250/183 in the early scan. Agreement increased to 93.3 % in the late scan. However, if only diseased segment were evaluated agreement increase from 52.9 % to 80.4 %. In our opinion, this makes late scan mandatory when this MoAb is used.

Human polyclonal immunoglobulin does not seem to be as accurate as previous agents. Hebbardt et al[8] showed recently that they were useful for IBD diagnosis (sensitivity 80 %), but disease location was much less accurate with HIG than with other procedures (33 % agreement).

When using 99mTc-labeled agents, unespecific bowel activity may be seen, especially in late scans. Thus to evaluate rectal disease, caudo-cranial or post-voiding views must be obtained.

3. Disease severity

Since the first experiences with labeled leucocyte scintigraphy in IBD management, researchers have looked for a simple, useful, readily available index of disease activity. The most accurate is faecal excretion quantification. In normal patients or patients with quiescent disease it is less than 2 % in 48 h while it increases to up to 30 % in active disease, correlating with clinical activity index.

However, faecal collection and measurement is uncomfortable for the patients as well as for the clinical staff. Several scintigraphic indexes have been described[19, 21, 27], most of them have shown a significant correlation with clinical activity indexes. But those scintigraphic index have not been validated using the different agents with different distribution.

The spleen washout index used by the Rennes group[28], based on the fall in spleen activity from early to late scan, is perhaps the easiest to use with all the agents and in all patients (but spleenectomized).

Recently the Hammersmith group[29] described the whole body retention of 111In. They show good correlation with faecal excretion ($r=0.95$). Correlation was lower but still significant with CDAI ($r= 0.54$). However in our opinion it is not suitable for routine use as it may be influenced by injected patients present in the department.

In summary: 99mTc-leucocyte labeling is the most suitable agent for IBD evaluation. Early scans (less than 1 hour post-injection) must be used to evaluate both diagnosis and extension. Post-voiding or caudo-cranial views should be used to localize rectal involvement.

Monoclonal antibodies used today are a valuable option in centres without cell labelling facilities, but further research is needed in this field. They may also be useful in infectious patients (AIDS, hepatitis,..) to avoid blood manipulation.

111In-leucocyte labeling should be looked at as a reference method and used when other methods are not diagnostic.

REFERENCES

1. Solá R. A. Garcia-Pugés; J. Monés; C. Badosa; J. Badosa; F. Casellas; J. Pujol and V. Varea. Enfermedad Inflamatoria intestinal en Cataluña. *Rev. Esp. Enf. Digest.* 81: 7-14 (1992).
2. Segal A.W., Ensell J; Munro J.M. y colb. 111In tagged leukocytes in the diagnosis of inflammatory bowel disease. *The Lancet* 2: 230-237 (1981).
3. Saverymmutu S.H.; Peters A.M.; Lavender J.P. y colb. 111In-labelled autologous leukocytes in inflammatory bowel disease. *Gastroenterology* 80: 1273 (1981).
4. Peters A.M.; Danpure H.J.; Osman S. y colb. Clinical experience with 99mTc-HMPAO for labelling leukocytes and imaging inflammation. *The Lancet* 2: 946-949 (1986).
5. Martin-Comin J.; Moragas M.; Daumal J. y colb. Inflammatory bowel disease examination with 99mTc-HMPAO leukocytes. En Radiolabelled cellular blood elements. Progress in Clinical and biochemical research vol. 355. Ed. Sinzinger H y Thakur M. Wiley-Liss, New York 1990, pp. 165-172
6. Segarra I.; Roca M.; Baliellas C. y col. Granulocyte-specific monoclonal antibody 99mTc-BW 250/183 and 111In-oxine labelled leucocyte scintigraphy in inflammatory bowel disease. *Eur. J. Nucl. Med.* 18: 715-19 (1991).
7. Buscombe J.R; Lui D.; Ensing G.; de Jong R. and Ell P.J. 99mTc-HIG first clinical results of a new agent for localization of infection and inflammation. *Eur. J. Nucl. Med.* 16: 649-55 (1990).
8. Hebbard G.S.; Salehi N; Gibson PR; Lichtenstein N and Andrews JT. 99mTc-labeled IgG scanning does not predict the distribution of intestinal inflammation in patients with inflammatory bowel disease. *Nucl. Med. Commun.* 13: 336-41 (1992).
9. Wheeler J.G. N.F. Slack; A. Dunacan M. Palmer and O. Harvey. 99mTc-nanocolloid imaging in inflammatory bowel disease. *Nucl. med. Commun.* 11: 127-33 (1990).
10. Pullman W.E. Sullivan P.J. Barrat P.J. y colb. Assesment of inflammatory bowel disease by 99mTc phagocyte scanning. *Gastroenterology* 95: 989-996 (1988).
11. Spinelli F. Milella M; Sara R; Banfi F; Possa M and Vigorelli R. The value of 99mTc-labeled human immunoglobulin scan in the evaluation Crohn's disease. *Nuclearmedicine Suplem.* 27: 274-6 (1991).
12. Banzo J. Personal communication.
13. Kroiss A.; Weiss W; Auinger Ch y col. Immunoscintigraphy with I-123 and 99mTc labeled granulocytes antibody in patient with inflammatory bowel diseases. *Nuclearmedicine Sup.* 26: 394-396 (1989).
14. Estorch M and Martin-Comin J. Exploraciones isotópicas en el aparato digestivo. In "Estudios isotópicos en medicina. Ed. I. carrio et al. Springer-Verlag Iberica. Barcelona 1992. pp,127-144.
15. Becker W.; Fischbach W.; Weppler M. y colb. Radiolabelled granulocytes in inflammatory bowel disease: diagnostic posibilities and clinical indications. *Nucl. Med. Comm.* 9: 693-701 (1988).
16. Crama-Bohbouth G.E.; Pena AS; Arndt JW; Tjon R.T. et al. Value of 111In-tropolonate autologous granulocyte scintigraphy in the assesment of inflammatory bowel disease. *Scand. J. Gastroenterol.* 178: 93-98 (1990).
17. Daumal J.; Martin-Comin J.; Gasull M.A. y col. La gammagrafía con leucocitos-111In en el brote agudo de la enfermedad inflamatoria intestinal. Valoración de la localización, extensión y grado de actividad. *Med. Clin. (Barc)* 93: 325-330 (1989).
18. Saverymmuttu S.H.; Peters A.M.; Hodgson H.J. y colb. 111In autologous leukocyte scanning: comparison with radiology for imaging the colon in inflammatory bowel disease. *Br. Med. J.* 285: 255-257 (1982).
19. Ybern A.; Martin-Comin J.; Giné J.J. y colb. 111In-oxine labelled autologous leucocytes in inflammatory bowel disease: New scintigraphic activity indexEur. *J. Nucl. Med.* 11: 341-344 (1986).
20. Navab F.; Boyd C.M.; Diner W.C. y colb. Early and delayed 111In leukocyte imaging in Crohn's disease. *Gastroenterolgy* 93: 829-834 (1987).
21. Stein D.T.; Gray G.M.; Gregory P.B. y colb. Location and activity of ulcerative and Crohn's colitis by 111In leukocyte scan. *Gastroenterology* 84: 388-393 (1984).
22. Buxton-Thomas M.S.; Dickinson R.J.; Maltby P. y colb. Evaluation of indium scintigraphy in patients with active inflammatory bowel disease. *Gut* 25: 1372-1375 (1984).
23. Henry J.Y.; Moisan A; Le Cloirec J. y colb. 111In-autologous granulocytes in the diagnosis of abscess and in the assesment of inflammatory bowel disease. *Int. J. Nucl. Med. Biol.* 13: 185-190 (1986).
24. Moisan A.; Loreal O.; Bretagne J.F. y col. 111In-granulocyte scanning of resected intestinal specimens in inflammatory bowel disease. *Nuclear Medicine Suplem.* 25: 368-371 (1988).

25. Costa DC; Lui D and Ell PJ. Radiolabeled WBC in localisation of inflammatory bowel disease and detection of infection- comparison between 99mTc-HMPAO and 111In-oxine. *Nuclearmedicine suplem.* 25: 364-7 (1989).

26. Moisan A. Lecloirec J; Bretagne JF; Loreal O; Raoul JL and Henry JY. Imaging of IBD and scintigraphic assesment of resected colon: comparison of 111In-oxine and 99mTc-HMPAO leucocyte labeling. *Progress in Clinical and Biochemical Research.* Vol. 355: 159-64 (1990).

27. Saverymmuttu S.H.; Peters A.M.; Lavender J.P. y colb. Quantitative fecal 111In-labelled leukocyte excretion in the assesment of disease in Crohn's disease. *Gastroenterology* 85: 1333-1339 (1983).

28. Loreal O.; Moisan A.; Bretagne JF; Lecloirec J.; Raoul J.L.; Gastard J and Henry J.Y.Scintigraphic assesment of 111In-labeled granulocyte splenic pooling: a new approach to inflammatory bowel disease. *J. Nucl. Med.* 31: 1470-73 (1990).

29. Kaski M.C. A.M. Peters; D. Knight et al. 111In whole body retention: A method for quantification of disease activity in inflammatory bowel disease. *J. Nucl. Med.* 33: 756-62 (1992).

FAST DIAGNOSIS OF ABDOMINAL INFECTIONS AND INFLAMMATORY BOWEL DISEASE WITH 99mTc-HMPAO LEUKOCYTE SCAN

F. Spinelli, M. Milella, R. Sara, L. Ruffini, and R. Vigorelli

Department of Nuclear Medicine
Ospedale Niguarda-Ca'Granda
Milano, Italy

In a Editorial entitled "In search of the hot appendix - A clinician's view of inflammation imaging", published on the Journal of Nuclear Medicine in March 1990, Rubin[1] stated that "there is a compelling clinical need for an imaging approach that would allow the accurate assessment of a patient with acute abdominal sepsis, as exemplified by acute appendicitis", but that the 99mTc-HMPAO leukocytes scan cannot be employed for the rapid diagnosis of the acutely ill patient, because of too many false positive.

This statement was based on the results of a paper by Mountford et al[2], published on the same number of the Journal of Nuclear Medicine, in which the Authors yielded a relatively low specificity with 99mTc-HMPAO leukocytes due to the not specific activity in the bowel.

But, in their study, images were not recorded earlier than 4 hr after injection.

In a letter to the Editor[3] we referred our, at that time, limited experience, pointing out that early 99mTc-HMPAO leukocyte scan has the sensitivity required for diagnosing abdominal sepsis within the first few hours after injection, also quoting the first results of Vorne et al.[4]. The Finnish group published another paper in 1991[5], confirming the possibility of a fast diagnosis of abdominal infections with 99mTc-HMPAO leukocytes. On the contrary, Gibson et al[6] concluded that "a high rate of false positive scans occurs when 99mTc is used due to not specific intestinal accumulation".

Finally, in an Editorial[7] "Imaging Inflammation: current role of labeled autologous leukocytes", Peters stated that "acute sepsis for which an urgent answer is usually required or inflammatory bowel disease can be satisfactorily studied with 99mTc-HMPAO".

An accurate diagnostic method for the rapid assessment of acute abdominal infections and inflammation is a compelling clinical need. U S and C T are non specific and often insensitive for diagnosing an acute abdominal sepsis and inflammatory bowel disease (IBD). Compared to 111 In-oxine, the 99mTc-HMPAO has the advantage of convenience, selective labelling, improved image resolution, lower radiation dose, rapid focal uptake. However, because of nonspecific accumulation in the bowel, the suitability of the method is questioned.

PATIENTS AND METHODS

We present a retrospective study based on 157 consecutive patients scanned with 99mTc-HMPAO leukocytes. 37 were examined with suspicion of abdominal infection, including acute appendicitis, febrile postoperative and polytraumatic patients. 78 had Crohn's disease and 42 ulcerative colitis.

Of course, a rapid diagnosis is necessary in acute abdominal infection and not in IBD. However, it is convenient for a nuclear medicine service to use only one method and to end the examination in few hours.

Mixed leukocytes were isolated and labeled as described previously[8]. The activity injected was 185-222 MBq. Planar images were performed within 1 hr and at roughly 3 hr after the injection of labeled leukocytes. The diagnosis was confirmed by endoscopy and/or barium enema in IBD and by surgery or clinically in suspicious abdominal sepsis (SAS).

RESULTS

In the SAS group, of the 37 patients examined 8 were positive, 28 negative and 1 false positive.

In all cases the diagnosis was based on the 1 hr image. The pathological accumulation generally increased with time, but in no case the 3 hr image changed the diagnosis (Fig. 1). In the 78 patients with the diagnosis of Crohn's disease 61 were positive and 17 negative at 1 hr. A non-specific activity in the right lower abdomen (RLA) was found at 3 hr in 8 cases (10.2%). Three of the seven fistulae were not detected at any time.

42 patients were examined for ulcerative colitis; 31 were positive and 11 negative at 1 hr. In 3 patients (7.1%) a non-specific activity was detected at 3 hr in the RLA.

As in the SAS group, in the patients examined for Crohn's disease and ulcerative colitis the 3 hr scan did not change the ultimate diagnosis, although in most cases the pathological accumulation was more evident (Fig. 2 and 3).

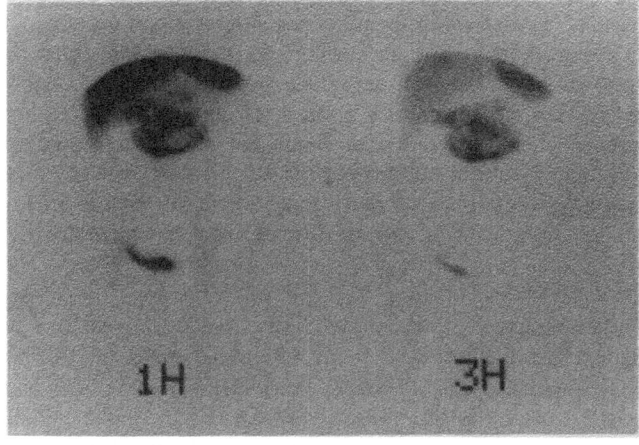

Figure 1. Patient with fever after colectomy for colon cancer. High uptake in the area of surgical intervention at 1 hr scan. At 3 hr scan the background is lower but the inflammation area is unchanged.

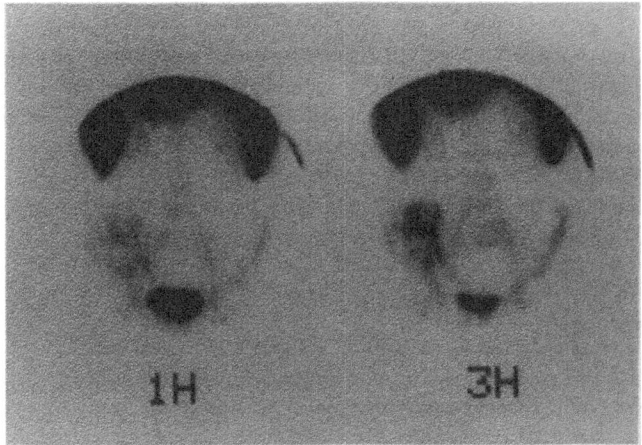

Figure 2. Crohn's disease located in the terminal ileum and in the ileocecal valve. The abnormal uptake is clearly evident in the 1 hr scan. At 3 hr the accumulation is more intense in the inflammatory sites but non specific activity is not seen.

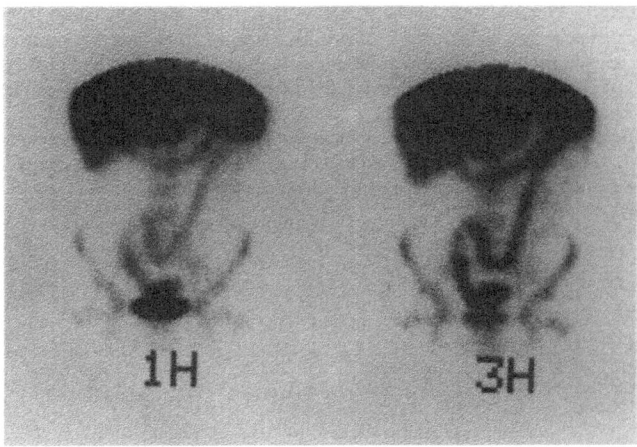

Figure 3. Ulcerative colitis involving the trasverse and descending colon, the sigma and rectum. The extension of the disease is rightly diagnosed in the 1 hr scan.

CONCLUSIONS

In acute abdominal sepsis early images (within 1 hr) yield high sensitivity and specificity. No further images are required.

In inflammatory bowel disease images at 1 hr are diagnostic and never show non-specific bowel activity, which is seen after 2 hr in a very small percentage of cases. We have found only 8.5% of non-specific bowel activity at 3 hr, always located in the RLA.

We do not believe that this faint non-specific accumulation, limited to a well defined abdominal site, could modify the accuracy of the test.

Since the pathological accumulation often increase with time, we could try to find a compromise between sensitivity and specificity, tentatively fixing at 1,5 hr the best time to image IBD.

Following these precautions, the concerns about the accuracy of 99mTc-HMPAO leukocytes in diagnosing abdominal infections should definitely end.

REFERENCES

1. Rubin RH. In search of the hot appendix. A clinicial's view of inflammation imaging (Editorial). *J. Nucl. Med.*; 32, 2029-2034 (1991).
2. Mountford PJ, Kettle AG, O'Doherty MJ, Cokley AJ. Comparison of technetium-99m-HM-PAO leukocytes with Indium-111-Oxine leukocytes for localizing intraabdominal sepsis. *J. Nucl. Med.; 31, 311-315* (1990).
3. Spinelli F, Milella M, Sara R. The usefulness of the 1-hr-technetium-99m-HMPAO leukocyte scan in the early diagnosis of acute abdominal sepsis (Letter). *J. Nucl. Med.; 31, 1734* (1990).
4. Vorne M, Soini I, Lantto T, Paakkinen S. Technetium-99m-HMPAO labeled leukocytes in detection of inflammatory lesions: comparison with gallium-67-citrate. *J. Nucl. Med.*; 30, 1332-1336 (1989).
5. Lantto EH, Tuomo J, Lantto T, Vorne M. Fast diagnosis of abdominal infections and inflammations with technetium-99m-HMPAO labeled leukocytes. *J. Nucl. Med.*; 32, 2029-2034 (1991).
6. Gibson P, Lichtenstein M, Salehi N, Hebbard G, Andrew J. Value of positive technetium-99m leukocyte scan in predicting intestinal inflammation. *Gut*; 32, 1502-1507 (1991).
7. Peters AM. Imaging inflammation: current role of labeled autologous leukocytes (Editorial). *J. Nucl. Med.*; 33, 65-67 (1992).
8. Spinelli F, Milella M, Sara R, Banfi F, Vigorelli R, Possa M, Bianchi Porro G, Ardizzone S, Gallitelli L. The 99mTc-HMPAO leukocyte scan: an alternative to radiology and endoscopy in evaluating the extent and the activity of inflammatory bowel disease. *J. Nucl. Biol. Med.*; 35, 82-87 (1991).

111In LABELED LYMPHOCYTE SCINTIGRAPHY IN PATIENTS WITH MALIGNANT LYMPHOMA

K. Uno, J. Kuyama, M. Saitoh, Y. Uchida, S. Minoshima, J.Okada, J. Itami and N. Arimizu

Department of Radiology
Chiba University School of Medicine
Chiba, Japan

INTRODUCTION

With the advent of the technique of 111In chelate cell labeling, the migratory properties of lymphocytes in patients with various lymphoid malignancies have been studied. Dr. Lavander[1] reported the kinetics of labeled lymphocytes in normal subjects and patients with Hodgkin's disease and observed radioactivities in cervical, external iliac, and inguinal lymph nodes in all subjects, then Dr. Wagstaff[2] studied the migration of lymphocytes in normal subjects and chronic lymphocytic leukemia. Dr. Cheng[3] also studied in nasopharyngeal carcinoma. Dr. Grimfors[4] reported this imaging technique as a staging method in Hodgkin's disease. We have used this imaging in Non-Hodgkin's lymphoma from 1989 and reported at the SNM in 1991[5]. Purpose of this study was undertaken to evaluate the usefulness of 111In labeled lymphocyte scintigraphy (InLLS) for imaging tumors as a staging method of malignant lymphoma (mainly Non-Hodgkin's lymphoma) and several other types of malignancies.

PATIENTS AND METHODS

111In tropolone labeled lymphocyte scintigraphy was done for 31 pretreatment lymphatic malignancies. All of them were pre-treated, and all had contracted malignancies for the first.

We evaluated 22 men and 9 women with a median age of 52 (range 28-76). The histologic diagnosis was obtained by lymph node biopsy in all of the patients, and the results were as follows: 27 with non-Hodgkin' lymphoma, 3 with Hodgkin's disease and 1 with Adult T-cell leukemia. The following staging procedures were also performed: CT (Head & Neck, chest, and abdomen) US (liver, spleen, and other abdominal organs), lymphangiography, bone marrow biopsy (bilateral iliac crest), CSF collection, and Gallium-67 scintigraphy. The clinical stagings were determined according to the Ann Arbor recommendations.

Radiolabeled Blood Elements, Edited by J. Martin-Comin
Plenum Press, New York, 1994

As a control group, InLLS was performed on 6 patients with inflammatory diseases, and 11 with malignant solid tumors. The Gamma camera was equipped with medium energy collimator and the dual energy peaks of 111Indium was selected as the energy window. Imaging was generally performed 24 hours after injection (acquisition time is 300 sec), and estimation of the comparision with Gallium scintigraphy was done along with this imaging.

To get a large amount of lymphocyte material, we used a Haemonetics cell separator. Canulas were inserted into cubital veins. The obtained buffy coat was layered onto Ficoll-Paque and centrifuged at 720G for 15 minutes.

In each patient, about 1.3×10^9 lymphocytes were acquired and labeled with 80 μCi of In-tropolone and then incubated for 20 minutes at room temperature. To remove free 111Indium, the lymphocytes were washed twice with saline at 270 G for 10 minutes. These procedures were carried out under strict sterile conditions, and were completed within 3 hours after obtaining buffy coats. The labeling efficiency was 53.4 % and total dose of Indium was 514 μCi/person.

Lymphocyte viability: In this procedure, the injected cell suspensions contained 91.7 % lymphocytes. 1×10^6 cells were incubated in 1 ml medium "RPMI1640" at 37°C in a humified atmosphere containing 5 % CO_2, and viability was determined in the firts 7 patients using a trypan blue exclusion test each day for 5 consecutive days.

Concurrently a T-cell activation test with mitogen PHA and Con A was executed. The day after labelling, we added mitogen PHA to one set of 1×10^6 cells and Con A to another identical set. The cell sets were prepared at 37° C, 5 % CO_2 in RPMI1640 medium. Furthermore, we added H-3 labeled thymidine to both sets on the third day, and uptake took place until the fifth day and destructed lymphocytes by trichole acetic acid. The count of H-3 uptake was done after 15 days. Consequently, the labeled lymphocytes revealed nearly a 73 % thymidine uptake compared to 100% uptake for the non-labeled control group, which contained either PHA or Con A individually (Fig.1).

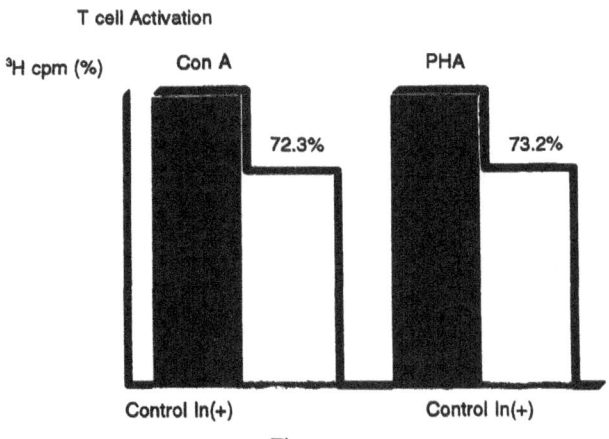

Figure 1.

We checked the lymphocytic viability in vivo study. InLLS showed no accumulation on the sites of skin metastases in one breast cancer patient at 24 hours after intravenous injection of InLLS.

Immediately after obtaining the image, OK432, a kind of BRM drugs, was injected subcutaneously in the left chest wall. A 24 hours image did not show the labeled lymphocyte accumulation (Fig.2).

After i.v. injection of InLLS
24 h   48 h

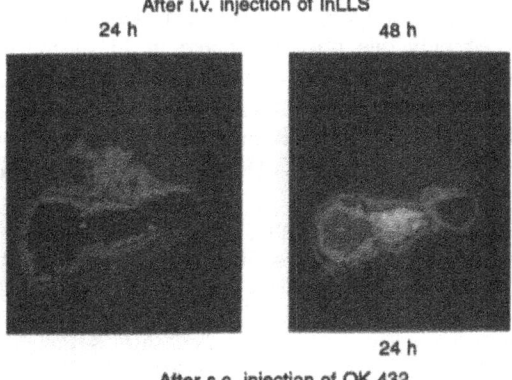

24 h
After s.c. injection of OK 432

Figure 2

Intense uptakes were indicated at the inflammatory site caused by OK432 at 48 and 72 hours after OK432 injection (Fig.3). This test indicated that lymphocytes preserve their migratory ability from 24 to 96 hours after Indium labeling.

After i.v. injection of InLLS
72 h   96 h

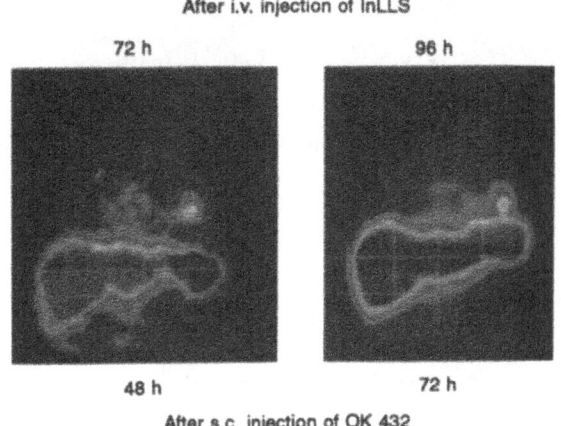

48 h   72 h
After s.c. injection of OK 432

Figure 3

RESULTS

Ga scintigraphy showed a sensitivity of 81 % (25/31), but of the 25 positive patients, 5 cases indicated some false negative sites. On the other hand, in the InLLS test group, all of the pathological sites were indicated with no false negatives sites. As for the detection of pathological sites, InLLS exhibited no specific anatomical affinity, and both lymph nodes and extranodal sites were displayed with InLLS as well (Sensitivity; 90 %).

In referrence to Hodgkin's disease, in comparison with NHL, InLLS showed more intense accumulation of labeled lymphocytes earlier in the lesion.

InLLS showed more intense accumulation from a very early timing in all cases of lymphatic inflamatory disease compared to NHL. On the other hand, in solid malignant tumors, InLLS indicated only one positive uptake in 11 of the cases. False positive accumulations were visible with InLLS in both the salivary glands and the inguinal lymph nodes. For nasopharyngeal cancer, InLLS shows no accumulation in the tumors.

A patient had left supraclavicular and axillar lymph node swelling. The left axillar lymph node was not demonstrated with Ga scintigraphy, but the effectiveness of InLLS was verified (Fig.4).

In 4 of the 31 patients with lymphatic malignancies, false positive accumulations were seen in the salivary glands and inguinal lymph nodes with InLLS. One must consider this fact when estimating these sites.

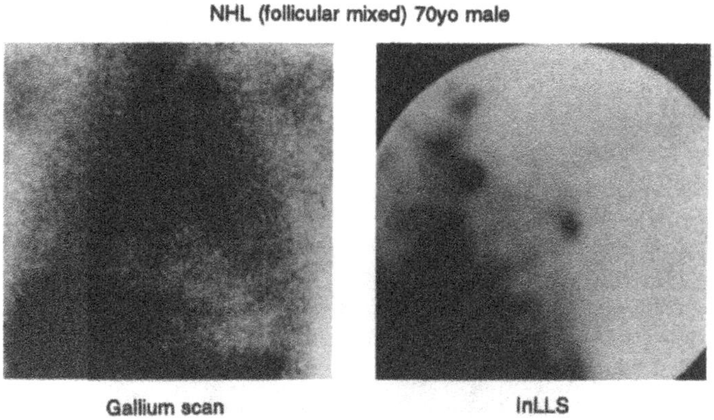

NHL (follicular mixed) 70yo male

Gallium scan   InLLS

Figure 4

DISCUSSION

With the introduction of 111In oxine as an alternative label, significant progress has been made in the evaluation of tumors. For 111In oxine, a dose of 40 μCi/10^8 cells is generally accepted as the upper limit above which radiation damage is likely to occur[2], and we used a labeled dose considering this condition. A trypan blue exclusion test, H-3 labeled thymidine uptake test and an inflammatory in vivo study induced by OK432 injection subcutaneously proved that the labeled lymphocytes were viable after labeling and preserved their migratory ability.

Although in patients with NHL there was marked sequestration of lymphocytes in the diseased lymph nodes and spleen, the relationship between the malignant grade of NHL and the detection of lymphoma involved lesions is not clear at present. From our data on the migration of lymphocytes in inflammatory diseases and Hodgkin's disease, InLLS showed intense accumulation from a very early timing compared to NHL. In some of the NHL patients, lymphocytic accumulation was still increasing 24 hours after injection, so the optimal timing of imaging needs to be examined still further. From these facts, InLLS appears to be a suitable radiolabeling isotope for NHL. For nasopharyngeal cancer[3], InLLS showed no accumulation in the solid tumors in our study. We have to investigate more patients with solid tumors in order to understand the mechanism of lymphocytes migration.

CONCLUSION

Even though the mechanism of InLLS accumulation in the tumor sites of malignant lymphoma patients is unknown, InLLS was useful as a staging method in NHL as well as Hodgkin's disease, and showed higher sensitivity (only with 24 hour images) than Ga.

REFERENCES

1. Lavender JP, Goldman JM, Arnot RN, Thakur ML. Kinetics of Indium-111 labelled lymphocytes in normal subjects and patients with Hodgkin's disease. *British Medical Journal*; 2:797-799 (1977).
2. Wagstaff J, Gibson C, Thatcher N, Crowther D. The migratory properties of Indium-111 oxine labelled lymphocytes in patients with chronic lymphocytic leukaemia. *British Journal of Haematology*; 49: 283-291 (1981).
3. Cheng PNM, Shiu WCT, Leung JOY, Ho SKW, Wong KKS, Metreweli C. A study of Lymphocyte Kinetics in nasopharyngeal carcinoma with Indium-111 oxine-labelled lymphocytes. *Clin. exp. Inmunol.*; 74: 398-403 (1988).
4. Grimfors G, Schnell PO, Holm G, Johansson B, Mellstedt H, Pihlstedt P, Bjorkholm M. Tumor imaging of Indium-111 oxine-labelled autologous lymphocytes as a staging method in Hodgkin's disease. *Eur J Haematol:* 42: 276-283 (1989).
5. Kuyama J, Maruno H, Minoshima S, Uchida Y, Okada J, Itami J, Imazeki K, Uno K, Saitoh M, Arimizu N. Indium-111 labeled lymphocyte scintigraphy in non-Hodgkin lymphoma. 32:917 (1991).

IN VIVO DETECTION OF LYMPHOCYTIC INFILTRATION: PRESENT STATUS AND NEW PROSPECTS

A. Signore

Nu. M.E.D. Group
Servizio Speciale Medicina Nucleare
Clinica Medica 2
Università "La Sapienza"
Roma, Italy

INTRODUCTION

After an initial enthusiasm, ten to fifteen years ago, in the development of new techniques for imaging in vivo lymphocyte traffic and pathological lymphocytic infiltrations in tissues, research in this field is now facing a slow progress.

The widely applyed technique of autologous labelled lymphocytes has been nearly completely abandoned because of the high radiosensitivity of these cells[1]. Furthermore, nanocolloids and polyclonal immunoglobulins have not yet proved to be very reliable in detecting sites of chronic inflammations.

Thus, research moved quickly and successfully to the field of acute inflammatory process but still it remains a major challenge for nuclear medicine researchers to develop a good radiopharmaceutical for targeting human lymphocytes in vivo.

Succeeding in this field will have important implications for the clinicians in terms of diagnostic and therapeutic decisions for diseases characterized by a chronic inflammation.

Amongst them, organ specific autoimmune diseases play a relevant role.

The possibility to early diagnose an autoimmune thyroiditis or Addison's disease, but also Crohn's disease or Ulcerative colitis, Rheumatoid arthritis or even Type 1 (insulin-dependent) diabetes mellitus, will allow early treatment and possible prevention of the disease itself. Moreover, from the clinical point of view, the possibility to monitor, in vivo, changes of mononuclear cell infiltration in target tissues is important for the therapy follow-up and for the early diagnosis of recurrence of disease.

These considerations strongly encourage the development of new radiopharmaceuticals.

In this manuscript, after briefly reviewing the radiopharmaceuticals that have been proposed to date in this field, I will discuss the present status and the future prospects in search of a new radiopharmaceutical suitable for in vivo detection of chronic inflammations.

Radiolabeled Blood Elements, Edited by J. Martin-Comin
Plenum Press, New York, 1994

PRESENT STATUS

Chronic inflammations are characterized from the histological point of view by a slow progressive accumulation of mononuclear white blood cells in the target tissue, with little increase of capillary permeability and exudate formation. Cells present in such inflammations are mainly T and B lymphocytes, monocytes and macrophages. Eosinophils and giant cells can also be found during folliculus and granuloma formation. Most important, these cells are thought to derive from locally proliferating cells; thus migration of committed cells from blood vessels to target tissues is only marginal.

The nuclear medicine techniques which have been proposed so far for in vivo detection of chronic inflammations are reported in table 1.

Table 1

Proposed techniques for imaging chronic inflammations

111In-oxine/tropolone autologous PBL's	2,3
99mTc-HMPAO autologous lymphocytes	4
99mTc-HSA Nanocolloids (30nm)	5
Polyclonal human Immunoglobulins (Ig or Fc)	6,7
Monoclonal antibodies CD3, CD4, CD5, CD25	8,9,10

Taking in consideration the physiopathological mechanism of chronic inflammation formation, it is possible to figure out why most of this techniques have given controversial results and why their sensitivity and specificity vary from disease to disease. Despite all these techniques have been tested in a number of different clinical conditions, the field of application has never been very wide for any of them. Moreover, they all have an important number of side effects and/or limitations. Table 2 summarizes the pros and cons of these techniques.

Table 2

Pros and Cons of different nuclear medicine techniques for imaging chronic inflammations

Technique	Pros	Cons
Autologous-PBL	No side effects	Tedious labelling Cell damage Low sensitivity
Nanocolloids	Not expensive No side effects Favourable dosimetry	Non specific Low sensitivity
HIG or Fc	Easy to use Good sensitivity	Non specific High GI uptake
Mo Ab	High specificity Good sensitivity	HAMA Expensive Not in follow-up

Based on our experience with labelled autologous lymphocytes[11] and on results published by other groups we started investigating a new approach for the in vivo detection of lymphocytic infiltrations.

Since most infiltrating lymphocytes express high numbers of interleukin-2 receptors (IL2R) on their surface[12, 13] we tested whether radiolabelled interleukin-2 (IL2) could target in vivo activated lymphocytes homing in sites of chronic inflammations.

After testing this technique in vitro[14] and in animal models such as the autoimmune BB/W rat[15] and the diabetes prone NOD mouse we applied this technique in humans for in vivo diagnosis of chronic lymphocytic infiltrations in different pathological conditions.

Results in diabetes prone mice showed that 123I-IL2 accumulates in the pancreas from 10 to 40 minutes after i.v. injection and remains in the organ until more than 90 minutes. Due to the fast blood clearance of the labelled protein the target/background ratio was very high as compared to other published techniques.

Figure 1 shows the comparison of 123I-IL2 and 123I-α Lactalbumin (a control protein with same molecular weight of IL2) in pre-diabetic NOD mice.

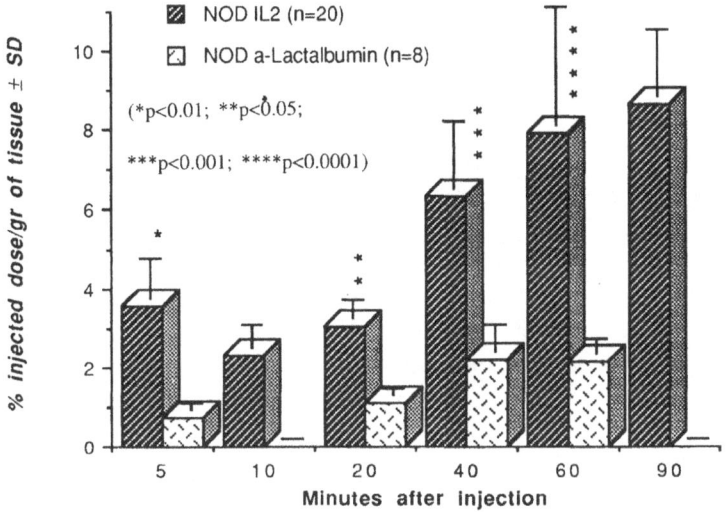

Figure 1. Pancretic accumulation of 123I-IL2 or 123I-αLA in diabetes prone NOD mice.

We also found a statistically significant correlation between the pancreatic radioactivity and the number of activated T-lymphocytes infiltrating the organ[16].

The same technique has been applied in humans and we concentrated on thyroid autoimmunity, Coeliac disease and Type 1 diabetes. In particular, autoimmune thyroid diseases have been studied with either 111In-oxine PBL's or 123I-IL2, whereas Coeliac disease and Type 1 diabetes have been investigated with either 123I-IL2 or 99mTc-HIG.

A total of 34 patients have been studied so far but data are still too preliminary to draw any significant conclusion.

As far as thyroid autoimmunity is concerned we were able to demonstrate the presence of activated lymphocytes also in Graves' disease, where 111In-oxine PBL's fail due to relatively low number of lymphocytes in the organ.

In Type 1 diabetes 123I-IL2 scan seems a superior imaging agent due to the relatively low uptake by gastrointestinal tract. This is even more important for Coeliac disease where 123I-IL2 scan allowed us to define the anatomical location and extent of the inflammatory lesions.

We are now progressing in labelling IL2 with 99mTc with retained receptor binding capacity thus allowing the injection of higher quantities of radioactivity at reasonable costs with improvement in image quality and sensitivity.

FUTURE PROSPECTS

The goal for NM in the next decade will be to design new radiopharmaceuticals (peptides or proteins) for different situations. Thus, we should be able to perform histological diagnosis of diseases and also a staging of the inflammatory process since this may have great relevance for therapeutic decisions.

Recent data indicates that chronic types of inflammation can be divided in two different sub-types based on the phenotype of infiltrating lymphocytes and on the cytokine production pattern in the microenvironment. This is relevant from the clinical point of view since the two types, named Th1 and Th2 derived, have a different evolution, a different prognosis and may require a different therapeutic approach.

As a consequence of the different cytokine production, different cytokine receptors are expressed by infiltrating cells in the two pathways. These can be the targets for selective imaging in search for a pathophysiology information (Figure 2).

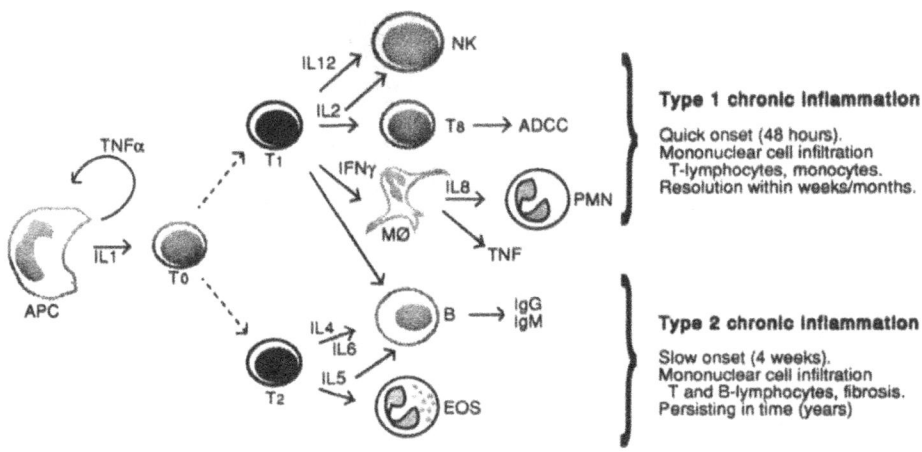

Figure 2. Types of chronic inflammation

A stage related diagnosis can also be attempted since therapeutic intervention may vary also according to the time of onset of the process.

In conclusion, the future prospects for in vivo imaging of lymphocytic infiltrations may include the use of different labelled peptides/proteins tailored to answer to different questions.

Cytokines or cytokine fragments, soluble receptors for cytokines, adhesion molecule ligands, Very Late Activation antigen binding peptides, octreotide and other hormones (VIP, GIP) can all be good candidates for achieving this ambitious goal.

REFERENCES

1. R.J.M. Ten Berge, A.T. Natarajan, M.R. Hardeman, E.A. Van Royen, and P. Schellekens. Labelling with Indium-111 has detrimental effects on human lymphocytes: concise communication. *J. Nucl. Med.*; 24:615 (1983).

2. B. Fisher, B.S. Packard, E.J. Reed, J.A. Carrasquillo, C.S. Carter, S.L. Topalian, J.C. Yang, P. Yolles, S.A. Larson and S.A. Rosenberg. Tumor localization of adoptively transferred Indium-111 labelled tumor infiltrating lymphocytes in patients with metastatic melanoma. *J. Clin. Oncol.*; 7:250 (1989).

3. J.P. Lavender, J.M. Goldman, R.N. Arnot and M.L. Thakur. Kinetics of Indium-111 labelled lymphocytes in normal subjects and patients with Hodgkin's disease. *Br. Med. J*; 2:797 (1977).

4. K.G. Shmidt, B.S. Poulsen, J.W. Rasmussen, J. Johansen and M. Ronne. Tc-99m-HMPAO as a lymphocyte label. In: Radiolabelled cellular blood elements. Ed. H. Sinzinger and M. L. Thakur. Wiley-Liss Inc. New York. 209 (1990).

5. M. De Schrijver, K. Streule, R. Senekowitsch and R. Fridrich. Scintigraphy of inflammation with nanometer-sized colloidal tracers. *Nucl. Med. Comm.*; 8:895 (1987).

6. D. Block, M.V. Ogtrop, J.W. Arndt, J.A.J. Camps, R.I.J. Feitsma, M. Goedemans and E.K.J. Pauwels. Detection of inflammatory lesions with radiolabelled immunoglobulins. *Eur. J. Nucl. Med.*; 16:303 (1990).

7. A.J. Fishman, R.A. Rubin, J.A. White, E. Locke, R.A. Wilkinson, M. Nedelman, R.J. Callahan, B. An Khan and H.W. Strauss. Localization of Fc and Fab fragments of nonspecific polyclonal IgG at focal sites of inflammation. *J. Nucl. Med.*; 31:1199 (1990).

8. R.M. Macklis, W.D. Kaplan, J.L. Ferrara, B.M. Kinsey, A.I. Kassis and S.J. Burakoff. Biodistrubution studies of anti-Thy 1.2 IgM immunoconjugates: implications for radioimmunotherapy. *Int. J. Radiat Oncol Biol Phys*; 15:383 (1988).

9. P. Thedrez, J. Paineau, Y. Jacques, J.F. Chatal, A. Pelegrin, C. Bouchard and J.P. Soulillou. Biodistribution of an anti-interleukin 2 receptor monoclonal antibody in rat recipients of a heart allograft, and its use as a rejection marker in gamma scintigraphy. *Transplantation*; 48:367 (1989).

10. I. Loutfi, P.M. Chisholm, D. Bevan and J.P. Lavender. In vivo imaging of rat lymphocytes with an indium 111-labelled anti-T cell monoclonal antibody: a comparison with indium 111-labelled lymphocytes. *Eur. J. Nucl. Med.*; 16:69 (1990).

11. P. Pozzilli, C. Pozzilli, P. Pantano, M. Negri, D. Andreani and A.G. Cudworth. Tracking of indium-111 oxine labelled lymphocytes in autoimmune tryroid disease. *Clin. Endocrinol*; 19:111 (1983).

12. W.S. Selby, G. Janossy, M. Bosil and D.P. Jewell. Intestinal lymphocyte subpopulations in inflammatory bowel disease: an analysis by immunohistological and cell isolation techniques. *Gut*; 25:32 (1984).

13. T.A. Waldmann, C.K. Goldman, R.J. Robb, J.M. Depper, W.J. Leonard, S.O. Sharrow, K.F. Bongiovanni, S.J. Korsmeyer and W.C. Greene. Expression of interleukin 2 receptors on activated human B cells. *J. Exp. Med.*; 160:1450 (1984).

14. A. Signore, P.C.L. Beverley, A. Parman, M. Negri and P. Pozzilli. Labelling of interleukin-2 (IL2) with 123-iodine with retention of its capacity to bind to activated lymphocytes. *Exp. Clin. Endocrinol*; 89:301 (1987).

15. A. Signore, A. Parman, P. Pozzilli, D. Andreani and P.C.L. Beverley. Detection of activated lymphocytes in endocrine pancreas of BB/W rats by injection of 123-interleukin-2: an early sign of type 1 diabetes. *Lancet*; 2:537 (1987).

16. A. Signore, M. Chianelli, A. Toscano, G. Ronga, L. Monetini, C.C. Nimmon, K.E. Britton, P. Pozzilli and M. Negri. A radiopharmaceutical for imaging areas of lymphocytic infiltration: 123I-Interleukin-2. Labelling procedure and animal studies. *Nucl. Med. Commun.*; 13:713 (1992).

CLINICAL EXPERIENCES WITH 111In LABELED HUMAN POLYCLONAL IgG

F.H.M. Corstens[1], W.J.G. Oyen[1], J.W.M. van der Meer[2] and
R.A.M.J. Claessens[1]

[1]Department of Nuclear Medicine
[2]Department of General Internal Medicine
University Hospital Nijmegen
Nijmegen, The Netherlands

INTRODUCTION

All currently available scintigraphic techniques to localize infection have serious limitations. 99mTechnetium(Tc) methylenediphosphonate lacks specificity. Physiological excretion of 67 gallium(Ga) in the gut hampers image interpretation of suspected abdominal infection. 67 Ga also accumulates in areas of bone remodelling and the physical characteristics of the radionuclide are not particularly good. Preparation of 111indium labelled autologous leucocytes (111In-WBC) is time consuming, complicated, costly and - in this HIV era - potentially dangerous for patients and staff. Moreover, in patients with decreased peripheral leucocyte counts the latter technique is practically impossible.

A few years ago, 111In labeled human non-specific immunoglobulin G (111In-IgG) was proposed as a radiopharmaceutical to delineate infectious and inflammatory foci[1,2]. In the University Hospital Nijmegen, The Netherlands, several groups of patients suspected of having infectious and inflammatory disease were studied using 111In-IgG as a scintigraphic imaging agent[3-8]. Particularly, patients with bone and joint infections including suspected infections around prostheses and diabetic foot complications, patients with abdominal inflammation/infection and patients with granulocytopenia were studied. Furthermore, in a prospective study the performance of 111In-WBC imaging was compared with 111In-IgG scintigraphy[9].

PREPARATION AND IMAGING PROTOCOL

Human non-specific polyclonal immunoglobulin G (Sandoglobulin[R], Sandoz AG, Nürnberg, Germany) was conjugated to diethylenetriaminepenta-acetic bicyclic anhydride (bicyclic DTPA) according to Hnatowich et al.[10]. The DTPA-coupled IgG preparation was labelled with sterile pyrogen-free 111In as indiumchloride. In all preparations, greater than 90 percent of the radioactivity was bound to IgG. A protein dose of 1.0 mg of IgG labelled with 2 mCi of 111In was injected intravenously.

Anterior and posterior whole body images, spot views of suspected areas and single photon emission computed tomography (SPECT) images in selected patients were acquired with a large field of view camera equipped with a medium energy collimator. Both 111In gamma peaks of 172 and 247 keV were used. Images were recorded at approximately 3 - 9, 24 and 48 hours post injection. An 111In-IgG scan was read as positive, if focally increasing accumulation of activity could be noted with time.

CLINICAL STUDIES

Bone, Joint and Joint Prosthesis Infection

In 113 patients, suspected of 120 infectious foci in bone (52 chronic and 8 acute infections), joint (15 localizations), joint arthroplasty (39 prostheses) and in soft tissue of the locomotor system (8 localizations), the diagnostic accuracy of 111In-IgG scintigraphy was studied[4]. The prevalence of infection was 59%. Overall sensitivity was 97%, specificity was 85%. 111In-IgG scintigraphy correctly identified presence, localization and extent of infections in 69 of 71 proven foci; 41 of 48 negative studies were correct. 111In-IgG accumulated not only in infectious foci but also in sterile inflammatory lesions, such as hematomas, callus formation in recent fractures and in sterile arthritis.

The results from a group of patients with suspected infected joint arthroplasty were particularly interesting. In 40 patients with a total hip or total knee prosthesis, we found 93% sensitivity, 88% specificity for infection and 100% specificity for inflammation[4].

In a group of diabetic patients with suspected infectious complications of the foot, 111In-IgG scintigraphy was useful in evaluating the presence or absence of osteomyelitis at gangrenous or ulcerative lesions[6]. The conventional bone scan was most sensitive for detecting pedal osteomyelitis, but was highly nonspecific in this group of patients. In contrast, 111In-IgG scintigraphy detected 6 of 7 proven osteomyelitic foci, while osteomyelitis was correctly ruled out in 16 out of 19 suspected sites.

Abdominal Inflammation and Infection

Preliminary results in twelve patients with active inflammatory bowel disease showed that all localizations, proven with colonoscopy, contrast radiography or during surgery, could be identified either on planar or on SPECT images[11]. In Nijmegen, The Netherlands, experience with 111In-IgG scintigraphy in patients with abdominal infections such as abscesses, infections in polycystic kidneys and around vascular prostheses, is limited but highly promising, being in agreement with vaster experience in Boston, USA[2].

Granulocytopenic Patients

Fever poses a major diagnostic therapeutic problem in patients with severe granulocytopenia. In these patients clinical signs of infection are often scarce and in the majority of the patients no cause of the fever can be detected. It has been estimated that in approximately one third of febrile granulocytopenic patients there is no infection. In these patients the fever is of paraneoplastic origin, or caused by drugs.

When a focus of infection is found, the identification of the causative microorganism and the start of adequate therapy is accelerated.

Twenty patients with granulocyte counts below 2.0 x 10^9/l were studied[7]. Sixteen suffered from different types of leukemia, three had malignant lymfoma and one had aplastic anemia. Most patients were granulocytopenic due to remission induction chemotherapy or conditioning regimen prior to bone marrow transplantation. One patient had granulocytopenia of unknown origin. Thirteen proven pulmonary, abdominal, joint and soft tissue infections of both bacterial and fungal origin, were detected adequately. 111In-IgG uptake, not due to verified inflammation, was observed in the large bowel of two patients. A thoracic wall infiltrate, that showed only mild inflammatory activity, was not detected. Small toxoplasmosis lesions in heart, liver and kidneys were obscured by physiologic 111In-IgG activity in these organs. The results of 111In-IgG scintigraphy in granulocytopenic patients provided further evidence that the accumulation of the radiopharmaceutical appeared not to be granulocyte mediated. It was concluded that 111In-IgG scintigraphy contributes to early diagnosing of focal infections in granulocytopenic patients and that it facilitates the installation of adequate therapy.

Fever of Unknown Origin

In a retrospective analysis of 24 immunocompetent patients with fever of unknown origin defined according to criteria by Petersdorf[12], 111In-IgG scintigraphy proved to be useful in 10 of 16 patients, whereas in other patients with normal studies no infection could be proven[13]. Proven inflammatory processes were missed in only one patient with endocarditis and infection of a renal cyst. A large size multicenter study in all Dutch University Hospitals is currently ongoing.

Comparative Study

In a prospective study the performance of 111In-IgG was compared to that of 111In-WBC in 35 patients[9]. Since both radiopharmaceuticals were labeled with 111In, the investigations had to be separated in time to allow clearance of the radiopharmaceutical that was administered first. The maximal 111In dose that can be safely injected with leucocytes is limited to 30 MBq. This strict limitation of the 111In does not apply to the IgG radiopharmaceutical. Therefore, in the study 111In-WBC scintigraphy was performed first and 111In-IgG scintigraphy one week later. Mean WBC count was 8,9 x 10^9/l (range 3,6 - 19,0 x 10^9/l). Most of the patients had subacute infections. Overall sensitivity and specificity was 74% and 100% for 111In-IgG scintigraphy and 52% and 75% for 111In-WBC scintigraphy respectively. Both techniques showed disappointing results in patients with disseminated Yersinia infection and in some patients with tuberculosis. Overall, 111In-IgG scintigraphy performed slightly but significantly better than 111In-leucocyte scanning. The first technique was particularly better in infections of the locomotor system, various soft tissue infections and in patients with subacute infections.

CONCLUSIONS

Many studies so far have shown good results of 111In-IgG for the imaging of infectious and inflammatory foci. The radiopharmaceutical has a constant high quality. It is convenient because it can be injected directly, thus overcoming the need of labelling blood cells with possible contamination of personnel with infected blood and erroneous administration of blood cells among patients, especially in those situations where a central radiopharmacy provides labelling services for several institutions. Unfortunately, at least several patients became HIV-positive and developed AIDS after in-vitro cell labelling for subsequent scintigraphic imaging[14, 15]. The IgG preparation used in the studies discussed above, is of human origin. Compared to using murine monoclonal antibodies directed against antigens on granulocytes, it overcomes the problem of human antimouse antibody response. Therefore precautions for follow-up scans are unnecessary.

111In-IgG scintigraphy showed a high accuracy for the detection of both acute and chronic low-grade infection. However, discrimination between sterile inflammation and infection is cumbersome. Among other limitations the high physiological background activity in liver and heart must be noted, thus obscuring infectious foci. Using 111In-IgG it is possible to localize infectious foci in patients with granulocytopenia. Besides bacterial also fungal infections show increased 111In-IgG uptake.

With regard to possible licensing of 111In-IgG it must be noted that in every country at least one human polyclonal immunoglobulin (unlabelled) has been approved for the treatment of immunodeficient conditions and for the prevention of hepatitis. In these instances gram doses of IgG are being administered, virtually without side effects, while for diagnostic radiopharmaceutical use only 1 mg has to be administered. In this respect it is not surprising that in over 1200 studies no single side effect after administration of radiolabeled human polyclonal IgG has been observed.

The mechanism of 111In-DTPA-IgG uptake and retention in foci of infection and inflammation has not been fully elucidated as yet. In preclinical studies on the biodistribution of various radiolabelled proteins, it was demonstrated that not only the protein, but also the radiolabel plays a major role in the dynamic distribution and focal uptake and retention of these agents[16]. In studies comparing 123I, 14C and 111In labelled IgG, the first two radionuclides, after initial accumulation, leaked out of the abscess parallel to the blood clearance, while 111In was retained in the focus, probably by release from the IgG[17]. These findings contribute to the understanding of preclinical and also clinical observations that show that the biological behaviour of 111In- and 99mTc-IgG are different.

REFERENCES

1. Fischman AJ, Rubin RH, Khaw BA, Callahan RJ, Wilkinson R, Keech F, Nedelman M, Dragotakes S, Kramer PB, LaMuraglia GM, Lind S, Strauss HW. Detection of acute inflammation with 111-Indium labeled non-specific polyclonal IgG. *Semin Nucl Med*; 18: 335-344 (1988).
2. Rubin RH, Fischman AJ, Callahan RJ, Khaw BA, Keech F, Ahmad M, Wilkinson R, Strauss HW. In-111 labeled nonspecific immunoglobulin scanning in the detection of focal infection. *N Eng J Med*; 321: 935-940 (1989).
3. Oyen WJG, Claessens RAMJ, van Horn JR, van der Meer JWM, Corstens FHM. Scintigraphic detection of bone and joint infections with indium-111 labeled nonspecific polyclonal human immunoglobulin G. *J Nucl Med*; 31: 403-412 (1990).
4. Oyen WJG, Van Horn JR, Claessens RAMJ, Slooff TJJH, Van der Meer JWM, Corstens FHM. Diagnosis of bone, joint and prothesis infections with indium-111 labeled nonspecific human immunoglobulin G scintigraphy. *Radiology*; 182: 195-199 (1992).
5. Oyen WJG, Van Horn JR, Claessens RAMJ, Slooff TJJH, Van der Meer JWM, Corstens FHM. Diagnosing prosthetic joint infections. *J Nucl Med*; 32:2195-2196 (1991).
6. Oyen WJG, Netten PM, Lemmens JAM, Claessens RAMJ, Lutterman JA, Van der Vliet JA, Goris RJA, Van der Meer JWM, Corstens FHM. Evaluation of infectious diabetic foot complications with indium-111 labeled human nonspecific immunoglobulin G. *J Nucl Med*; 33:1330-1336 (1992)

7. Oyen WJG, Claessens RAMJ, Raemaekers JMM, De Pauw BE, Van der Meer JWM, Corstens FHM. Diagnosing infection in febrile granulocytopenic patients with indium-111 labeled human IgG. *J Clin Oncol*; 10:61-68 (1992).

8. Oyen WJG, Claessens RAMJ, Van der Meer JWM, Rubin RH, Strauss HW, Corstens FHM. Indium-111 labeled human nonspecific immunoglobulin G: a new radiopharmaceutical for imaging infectious and inflammatory foci. *Clin Inf Dis*; 14:1110-1119 (1992).

9. Oyen WJG, Claessens RAMJ, van der Meer JWM, Corstens FHM. Detection of subacute infectious foci with indium-111 labeled autologous leukocytes and with indium-111 labeled human nonspecific immunoglobulin G: a prospective comparative study. *J Nucl Med*; 32:1854-1860 (1991).

10. Hnatowich DJ, Childs RL, Lanteigne D, Najafi A. The preparation of DTPA-coupled antibodies radiolabeled with metallic radionuclides: an improved method. *J Immunol Meth*; 65:147-157 (1983).

11. Oyen WJG, Naber AHJ, Claessens RAMJ, van der Meer JWM, Corstens FHM. Evaluation of inflammatory bowel disease activity with indium-111 labeled human nonspecific immunoglobulin G. *J Nucl med*; 33:919 (1992).

12. Petersdorf RG and Beeson PB. Fever of unexplained origin: report of 100 cases. *Medicine*; 40:1-30 (1961).

13. De Kleijn EMHA, Oyen WJG, Claessens RAMJ, Corstens FHM, Van der Meer JWM. Scintigraphy with indium-111 labeled polyclonal human immunoglobulin G (in-111-IgG) in patients with fever of unknown origin (FUO). *Nucl Med Commun*; 13:626 (1992).

14. Lange JMA, Boucher CAB, Hollak CEM, Wiltink EHH, Reiss P, Van Royen EA, Roos M, Danner SA, Goudsmit J. Failure of zidovudine prophylaxis after accidental exposure to HIV-1. *N Eng J Med*; 322:1375-1377 (1990).

15. Rojas-Burko J. Health officials reactions to infection mishaps. *J Nucl Med*; 33:13-27N (1992).

16. Oyen WJG, Claessens RAMJ, van der Meer JWM, Corstens FHM. Biodistribution and kinetics of radiolabeled proteins in rats with focal infection. *J Nucl Med*; 33:338-394 (1992).

17. Claessens RAMJ, Oyen WJG, Koenders EB, Tibben JG, Massuger LFAG, Corstens FHM. Potentials and pitfalls of indium labeled and iodinated proteins for scintigraphy of infectious disease and malignancy. *Eur J Nucl Med*; 19:700 (1992).

COMPARISON OF TECHNETIUM-99m-LABELLED HUMAN POLYCLONAL IMMUNOGLOBULIN SCINTIGRAPHY WITH CONVENTIONAL BONE SCINTIGRAPHY IN PATIENTS WITH RHEUMATOID ARTHRITIS AND OSTEOARTHRITIS

M.H.W. de Bois[1], J.W. Arndt[2], E.A. van der Velde[3], E.K.J. Pauwels[2] and F.C. Breedveld[1]

[1]Departments of Rheumatology
[2]Diagnostic Radiology and Nuclear Medicine
[3]Medical Statistics
University Hospital
Leiden, The Netherlands

ABSTRACT

The ability of technetium 99m labelled polyclonal human immunoglobulin G (99mTc-IgG) scintigraphy and conventional bone scintigraphy with technetium 99m labelled hydroxymethylene diphosphonate (99mTc-HDP) to detect and to differentiate between the different degrees of arthritis activity was studied in 24 patients with rheumatoid arthritis (RA) and 10 patients with osteoarthritis (OA). The patients with RA were divided into 4 groups based upon clinical and radiological observations: 1: non-erosive, in remission (n=5); 2: non-erosive, active (n=5); 3: erosive, in remission (n=7); 4: erosive, active (n=7). The patients were scored for joint pain, swelling and uptake of the radiopharmaceutical on a 4-point scale. The mean joint scores of 99mTc-IgG scintigraphy in RA patients with active disease was significantly ($p < 0.001$) higher than of patients with inactive disease. The mean joint scores were also higher in patients with erosions compared to patients without erosions but the difference was less significant ($p < 0.05$). For 99mTc-HDP scintigraphy no significant differences were found between the mean scores of these patient groups. When 99mTc-IgG scintigraphy is regarded as a test to detect arthritis as defined by joint swelling, this test has a sensitivity that ranged between 64 and 100% for the different joints. Comparison of scintigraphic results between patients with RA and OA revealed that the mean joint score of 99mTc-IgG scintigraphy was significantly ($p < 0.001$) higher in the patients with RA than in patients with OA whereas for 99mTc-HDP scintigraphy this difference was not significant.

This study shows that 99mTc-IgG scintigraphy, in contrast to, 99mTc-HDP scintigraphy is a sensitive and specific method to detect synovitis and differentiates between the different degrees of disease activity in RA.

INTRODUCTION

Rheumatologists continue to seek improvement in accurate assessment of disease activity in rheumatoid arthritis (RA). There is no golden standard to quantify arthritis activity. The availability of an objective parameter to evaluate disease activity in RA would be of great value in patient management and in the examination of therapeutical effects. 99mTc-IgG scintigraphy has been suggested as a reliable objective method to detect arthritis activity in RA.

AIM OF THE STUDY

This study was performed to ascertain the following:

- How does 99mTc-IgG scintigraphy compare to 99mTc-HDP scintigraphy in the detection of arthritis activity ?
- Can 99mTc-IgG scintigraphy detect different degrees of arthritis activity ?

For this purpose, 24 patients with RA selected for various levels of disease activity or joint destruction and 10 patients with osteoarthritis (OA) were investigated with both 99mTc-IgG- and 99mTc-HDP scintigraphy.

PATIENT AND METHODS

Twenty-four patients (7 males, 17 females) with RA, and 10 patients (2 males, 8 females) with clinical and radiological features of primary OA, were studied. The mean age of the patients with RA was 55 years (range 20-80 years) and they had a mean disease duration of 7 years (range 0-21 years). The patients with RA were divided into 4 groups based upon clinical and radiological observations: 1: non-erosive, in remission (n=5); 2: non-erosive, active (n=5); 3: erosive, in remission (n=7); 4: erosive, active (n=7). The mean age of the patients with OA was 67 years (range 56-80 years) and they had a mean disease duration of 6 years (range 1-21 years). Imaging was performed 4 hours after 99mTc-IgG injection and 2 hours after 99mTc-HDP injection. The period between the 2 scintigraphic investigations was between 2 and 7 days. Anterior and posterior total body views and anterior spotviews of the joints were obtained. The following joints were investigated; shoulder, elbow, wrist, 5 separate metacarpophalangeal (MCP) and proximal interphalangeal (PIP) joints, 4 distal interphalangeal (DIP) joints, hip, knee, ankle and forefoot. All joints were scored for pain, swelling and radiopharmaceutical uptake on a 4 point scale. CRP, ESR levels and X rays of the hands, wrists and feet were obtained.

RESULTS

The group of patients with active RA had, in contrast to patients with RA in remission significantly higher scores for joint pain, swelling, CRP and ESR. The mean joint scores of 99mTc-IgG scintigraphy in RA patients with active disease (8.14) was significantly ($p < 0.001$) higher than of patients with in remission disease (2.58), whereas such differences were not significant for 99mTc-HDP scintigraphy (active RA 9.96; RA in remission 6.67). The group of RA patients with erosions had a significantly higher mean joint score with 99mTc-IgG scintigraphy when compared to the group of patients with RA without erosions (erosive RA 6.51; non-erosive 3.75; $p < 0.05$). No significant differences in the mean joint scores of 99mTc-HDP scintigraphy were detected between patient groups with or without erosions (erosive RA 9.83; non-erosive RA 6.30). The mean scores of all joints for 99mTc-IgG scintigraphy were significantly ($p < 0.001$) higher in the RA patients (mean value 5.36) than in OA patients (mean value 1.01). Whereas in the case of 99mTc-HDP scintigraphy the difference between scintigraphic scores of the 2 patient groups was not significant (mean value RA 8.36; mean value OA 6.63). The sensitivity of 99mTc-IgG scintigraphy used as a test to detect joint swelling in 24 RA patients ranged between 64% for the ankles and 100% for the wrists. The specificity was lower, varying from 41% for the wrists to 83% for the DIP joints. In the case of 99mTc-HDP scintigraphy the specificity was lower, varying from 16% for the wrist to 71% for the DIP joints.

CONCLUSION

The results of this study have shown that 99mTc-IgG scintigraphy, when compared to 99mTc-HDP scintigraphy, is a more specific method to detect synovitis and is more sensitive in the detection of different degrees of arthritis activity in RA. These conclusions are based upon the observations that the 99mTc-IgG scintigraphic scores were significantly ($p < 0,001$) higher in patients with RA than in patients with OA, whereas 99mTc-HDP scintigraphy this difference was not significant. The 99mTc-IgG scintigraphic scores were also significantly higher ($p < 0.001$) in the RA patients with active disease than in the patient group with inactive disease; such differences were not significant for 99mTc-HDP scintigraphy.

ANTIGRANULOCYTE ANTIBODY BONE MARROW SCANS IN CANCER PATIENTS WITH METASTATIC BONE SUPERSCAN APPEARANCE

G. Torres, Ll. Berná, I. Carrió, M. Estorch, J.R. Germá and C. Alonso

S. Medicina Nuclear
Hospital de Sant Pau
Barcelona

INTRODUCTION

Superscan is defined as a special appearance of bone scan, characterized by homogeneous and symmetrical increased uptake of bone radiopharmaceuticals in the skeleton. That appearance has been described as "too good" or beautiful scan and it include some features as faint or absent renal images, presence of some nonhomogeneity of tracer uptake throughout the skeleton, and faint representation of skull and long bones.

In clinical practice however, homogeneous symmetrical increased uptake of bone tracer may be difficult to identify. Therefore, it may be sometimes difficult to distinguish a superscan appearance from a normal bone scan.

The aim of this work is to determine if assessment of bone marrow is helpful in the diagnosis of bone invasion in patients with suspected superscan.

PATIENTS

We studied 10 consecutive patients selected from a series of 1200 cancer patients referred to our department for conventional bone scanning: 7 females, aged from 32 to 61 years, presenting with breast cancer (stage I, 1 patient; stage II, 4 patients; stage III, 1 patient; stage IV, 1 patient) who were studied from 13 to 74 months after diagnosis of the primary tumour; 3 males, aged from 61 to 82 years, presenting with prostate cancer stage D2, who were studied from 1 to 3 months after diagnosis of the primary tumour.

METHODS

Conventional bone scans, bone marrow scans with antigranulocyte monoclonal antibody, bone X-ray surveys and conventional laboratory tests were performed in all patients. Bone marrow biopsy could be obtained in 3 patients with breast cancer and in one patient presenting with prostate cancer.

Radiolabeled Blood Elements, Edited by J. Martin-Comin
Plenum Press, New York, 1994

Whole-body bone scans consisting of multiple views were performed after the intravenous injection of 740 MBq of 99mTc-DPD using a conventional large field of view camera with a high resolution, low-energy collimator. Images were interpreted by consensus among three experienced observers who assessed: increased uptake of bone tracer relative to soft tissue or "too good" general appearance, faint or absent renal image, presence of some nonhomogeneity of tracer uptake, and skull/long bones relative tracer uptake. Whole-body bone marrow scans were performed within the same week. Multiple views were acquired 6 hours after the intravenous injection of 740 MBq of 99mTc-antigranulocyte monoclonal antibody BW 250/183 using the same instrumentation. An average of 600 kilo-counts per view was obtained. Images were interpreted by consensus among the same three observers. Defects in the central bones were interpreted as corresponding to tumour replacement. Bone marrow expansion was defined as the presence of tracer uptake distal to the first one-third of the femoral an humeral shafts and was graded as: grade 1, activity present in the second third of the shaft, and grade 2, activity present in the last third of the shaft.

RESULTS

Bone Scans: all patients presented bone scans interpreted as superscan appearance suggesting diffuse bone involvement. Eight bone scans were evaluated as "too good" due to a high uptake of tracer in the skeleton, with increased contrast between bone and soft tissue. Renal images were evaluated as abnormal in all scans; kidneys were faintly seen in 6 cases and not seen in 4 cases. In 8 scans, presence of some nonhomogeneities of tracer uptake throughout the skeleton were observed. Skull and long bones were faintly seen in 5 scans.

Bone Marrow Scans: all patients presented bone marrow scans showing marked absence of tracer uptake in the central skeleton indicating tumour replacement. All bone marrow scans showed bone marrow expansion, grade 1 in 7 scans and grade 2 in 3 scans.

Laboratory Tests: Eight patients had increased serum alkaline phosphatase and two patients presenting with prostate carcinoma had marked increased serum prostatic acid phosphatase. All patients presented decreased haemoglobin levels, less than 12 grams per decilitre; and 7 patients had haemoglobin less than 9 grams per decilitre. Five patients had marked leucopenia with less than 3.500 leucocytes per millilitre, and 6 patients had severe thrombocytopenia with less than 100.000 platelets per millilitre. Bone marrow biopsy demonstrated metastatic bone marrow infiltration in all patients in whom it was performed (Table 1).

X-Ray Surveys: In 9 patients bone X-ray examinations were reported as definitive of bone metastatic involvement with diffuse blastic lesions. One patient presented only with one doubtful lesion in the pelvis.

DISCUSSION

In clinical practice, to distinguish a normal scan from a superscan in a cancer patient may represent a diagnostic dilemma, since superscan appearance may sometimes resemble a normal scan.

Bone marrow is the primary soil of metastatic bone disease. Seeding of tumour cells in the bone marrow is followed by invasion of bone tissue matrix and finally by invasion of the cortical bone. Antigranulocyte antibody bone marrow scans provide excellent bone marrow visualization and have been shown to be useful in the diagnosis of metastatic bone disease. Decrease in uptake or focal defects in bone marrow scans are interpreted as metastatic bone marrow invasion. In this way, when diffuse metastatic involvement of the cortical bone renders an almost normal appearance of bone scan, it could be easier to visualize absent bone marrow due to tumour replacement in a bone marrow scan.

In our study, all patients presented marked absence of central bone marrow as a result of tumour replacement, suggesting that patients with superscan appearance on their bone scans have extensive bone involvement despite subtle changes on conventional bone scans.

In conclusion, antigranulocyte bone marrow scans show extensive bone marrow invasion in cancer patients with suspected bone superscan. This reinforces the concept of these patients having extensive bone invasion despite mild global abnormalities in the bone scan. Confirmation of extensive bone invasion in patients with suspected bone superscan may contribute to a proper staging of these patients.

Table 1. Blood tests and bone marrow biopsy results

Patient	sAlP	sPAcP	Hb	Leucocyte	Platelet	BMB
1	432		6,1	2.900	70.000	Nd
2	218		6,4	3.200	147.000	+
3	262		6,5	2.100	65.000	+
4	461		8,5	6.300	56.000	Nd
5	860		10,3	6.690	58.000	Nd
6	338		10,9	2.290	283.000	Nd
7	291		8,0	3.270	113.000	+
8	754	190	11,2	4.700	225.000	Nd
9	282	2,3	8,6	4.400	78.000	Nd
10	1987	38,4	7,6	6.500	69.000	+

sAlP: serum alkaline phosphatase (normal: 81-263 U/l)
sPAcP: serum prostatic acid phosphatase (normal: < 2 U/l)
Hb: haemoglobin
BMB: bone marrow biopsy
Nd: not done

IMAGING OF RA INFLAMED JOINTS WITH 99mTc-LABELED SPECIFIC MURINE ANTI-CD4- AND NONSPECIFIC HUMAN IMMUNOGLOBULIN

R.W. Kinne[1], W. Becker[2], J. Schwab[3], G. Horneff[3], A. Schwarz[4], J.R. Kalden[3], G.R. Burmester[3], F. Emmrich[1], and F. Wolf[2]

[1]Max-Planck-Society, Clinical Research Unit for Rheumatology/ Immunology
[2]Department of Nuclear Medicine
[3]Institute of Clinical Immunology and Rheumatology, Department of Medicine III
University of Erlangen-Nuremberg, Erlangen
[4]Radiochemical Laboratory of the Behring Werke (Hoechst AG)
Frankfurt, Germany

ABSTRACT

The presence of CD4-molecules on T-helper cells and macrophages, both abundantly present in human rheumatoid arthritis (RA) inflammatory infiltrates, provides the rationale for the use of radiolabeled anti-CD4 monoclonal antibodies (mAbs) to image RA arthritic joints (Becker et al. 1990). The imaging properties of a 99mTechnetium (99mTc)-labeled murine anti-human CD4 mAb (MAX.16H5; 200-300 μg, 370-550 MBq) were compared to those of polyclonal human immunoglobulin (HIG; Technescan[R], MDH-67, Mallinckrodt Diagnostica; 1 mg, 370 MBq) after intravenous injection into 8 patients with severe, active RA; in one RA patient the anti-human CD4 mAb was compared to an isotype-matched murine control mAb (BW 431/26; anti-human carcino-embryonic-antigen; Behringwerke; 2 mg; 810 MBq), and to HIG on separate occasions. Whole body and joint scans in anterior and posterior views were obtained 1, 4 and 24 h after injection.

As early as 4 h after injection, the anti-human CD4 mAb showed a higher target-to-background ratio in arthritic knee and elbow joints in comparison to either polyclonal HIG or, in one case, the murine isotype matched control mAb. Specific detection of inflammatory infiltrates rich in CD4$^+$ cells may allow a superior quality in the imaging of RA inflamed joints.

INTRODUCTION

In the inflamed synovium of RA joints there is a high number of both T-helper cells and macrophages, which express CD4 target molecules (Janossy et al. 1981). A mAb directed against the CD4 molecule therefore appears to be a promising candidate for specific imaging of RA joints.

A radiolabeled (99mTc) anti-human CD4 mAb (MAX.16H5; Emmrich et al. 1986) has been shown to clearly depict arthritic joints (Becker et al. 1990). This suggests that the anti-CD4 mAb acts through specific recognition of its target molecule, although a nonspecific accumulation solely due to its immunoglobulin (Ig) moiety cannot be excluded. To clarify this point, the accumulation of a 99mTc-labeled specific anti-CD4 mAb in arthritic joints was compared to that of nonspecific murine and human control Ig.

MATERIALS AND METHODS

Patients

Eight patients with severe, active RA according to the 1987 criteria of the American Rheumatism Association (ARA) (Arnett et al. 1988) were studied. Clinical and laboratory findings of the patients at the times of the studies are listed in Table 1. The study protocol was reviewed and approved by the Ethics Committee of the University of Erlangen-Nuremberg. Written consent was obtained from all patients after they had been fully informed about possible risks of the antibody injection.

Antibodies

Nonspecific polyclonal HIG (Technescan^R HIG; MDH-67) was prepared by and purchased from Mallinckrodt Diagnostica (Holland).

The anti CD4 mAb MAX.16H5 (IgG$_1$ isotype) was prepared according to the guidelines of the German Society for Immunology, the Paul Martini Endowment and the regimens of the European Community Committee for Proprietary Medical Products (Emmrich 1987).

The anti-CEA mAb BW 431/26 (IgG$_1$ isotype; Behringwerke, Frankfurt, Germany) reacts with the carcino-embryonic-antigen on the majority of colon carcinomas (Bosslet et al.1985).

Radiolabeling and i.v. Injection

One mg of HIG was incubated for 20 min with 370 MBq 99mTc-pertechnetate before i.v. injection, achieving a labeling yield of > 95 %.

The anti-human CD4-(200-300 μg), as well as the anti-human carcino-embryonic-antigen mAb (2 mg), were radiolabeled according to the mercaptoethanol method of Schwarz and Steinstraesser (1987).

Image Acquisition

Static gamma-camera images of whole body, knees, ankles, elbows, and hands were acquired in anterior and posterior views 1, 4, and 24 h after injection using a gamma-camera (Rota-Camera) interfaced to a computer system (Micro-Delta; both Siemens, Germany). Integrated radioactivity distribution on a 128 x 128 matrix was measured using a high resolution, low energy collimator.

Table 1. Clinical characteristics of RA patients (n=8) on the dates of i.v. injection of 99mTc-labeled HIG, the anti-CEA or the anti-CD4 monoclonal antibody.

Pat.	Age (yrs) sex	Disease duration (yrs)	Previous Treatment	Date	Ig injected	Ritchie articular index	Number of swollen joints	Morning stiffness (h)	RF	ESR	CRP
F.H.	50/M	8	Gold, IFNγ, MTX DP, Cyc, Lym anti-CD4, Ster	6.07.89	anti-CD4	122	29	4	+	55/87	48
				15.01.91	HIG	130	21	24	+	25/76	12
				25.07.91	HIG	n.d.	n.d.	n.d.	+	35/50	0
M.S.	59/F	11	Gold, IFNγ, MTX anti-CD4, Ster	22.03.90	HIG	n.d.	n.d.	4	+	n.d.	48
				4.04.90	anti-CD4	108	34	5	+	82/119	0
				31.07.91	HIG	n.d.	n.d.	n.d.	+	110/∞	48
R.W	51/F	10	Gold, Chlo, MTX DP, anti-CD4 Ster, Aza	4.04.90	anti-CD4	98	25	0.75	+	120/124	24
				18.10.90	anti-CD4	65	18	2	+	127/140	48
				8.11.91	HIG	n.d.	n.d.	n.d.	+	42/70	6
K.H.	62/F	20	Gold, MTX, Sala anti-CD4, Ster	31.10.89	anti-CD4	103	25	4.5	+	50/90	48
				13.03.90	HIG	89	14	3	+	28/63	48
R.F.	74/F	14	Gold, Chlo, MTX Sala, anti-CD4 Ster, Cyc	30.10.90	HIG	59	13	10	+	63/100	48
				15.04.91	anti-CEA	60	10	8	+	60/106	48
				24.04.91	anti-CD4	45	6	2	+	82/127	96
N.K.	22/F	12	Gold, Chlo, MTX Sala, anti-CD4 Ster, Aza	29.11.89	anti-CD4	93	20	2	+	47/72	48
S.M.	76/F	20	Gold, Chlo, Ster	8.03.90	HIG	n.d.	n.d.	n.d.	+	112/∞	96
H.R.	51/F	17	Gold, IFNγ, MTX DP, anti-CD4 Ster, Aza	22.10.90	HIG	77	14	0.5	-	10/13	0

RF = rheumatoid factor, ESR = erythrocyte sedimentation rate, CRP = C-reactive protein, IFNγ = Interferon gamma, Chlo = chloroquine, MTX = methotrexate, DP = D-penicillamine, Sala = salazosulfapyridine, Cyc = cyclophosphamide, Lym = lymphapheresis, Ster = glucocorticoids, Aza = azathioprin, n.d. = not determined

Evaluation of Whole Body and Joint Scans

Whole body scans of RA patients and normal volunteers were evaluated using the region of interest (ROI) technique. By placing regions over organs and joints in anterior and posterior views, the radioactivity accumulated 1, 4, and 24 h following injection of the different Igs was determined. The geometric mean of the counts in both views was calculated and divided by the geometric mean of the whole body region. Values were expressed as the percentage of the whole body counts accumulated in the ROI.

Statistics

The non-parametric Mann-Whitney (U) test was applied to analyze differences between the counts accumulated in different regions of interest in whole body scans. Significant differences were accepted at $p \leq 0.05$.

RESULTS

Whole Body Distribution

The anti-CD4 mAb accumulated to a significantly higher degree than HIG in the liver of RA patients 24 h after i.v. injection (Fig. 1). Higher accumulation of the anti-CD4 mAb than HIG was also observed in the spleen, although the difference only approached significance. In contrast, blood pool levels of the radiolabeled Igs, as inferred by placing a ROI over the heart, were significantly lower for the anti-CD4 mAb than for HIG 24 h following injection (Fig. 1).

In all arthritic joints the accumulation of the anti-CD4 mAb, expressed as % of whole body counts, was not significantly different from that of the control Ig (Fig. 1).

Target/Background (T/B) Ratio in Joints

In knee joint scans of RA patients a high T/B ratio between inflamed knee joint and adjacent vessels, higher than with HIG, was observed 4 h after injection of the anti-CD4 mAb (Fig. 2).

Using semiquantitative visual scoring, the T/B ratio of the anti-CD4 mAb was significantly higher in arthritic knees and elbows than after injecting nonspecific polyclonal HIG (data not shown).

A favourable T/B ratio for the anti-CD4 mAb was observed also in comparison to an isotype-matched murine anti-CEA mAb, as demonstrated in one patient (R.F.), who received all 3 different Igs (Fig. 3).

DISCUSSION

The present study shows on one hand that no differences in the total amount of radioactivity accumulated in RA arthritic joints can be detected after injection of either a radiolabeled specific anti-CD4 mAb or nonspecific HIG (Fig. 1). An increased endothelial permeability in inflamed joints, leading to high concentrations of proteins with large molecular weight in synovial tissue and synovial fluid (Kushner et al. 1971) may obscure differential accumulation; the 2 Igs employed in this study may therefore be taken up into the inflamed joint irrespectively of their immunological specificity.

On the other hand a ROI placed over the whole joint detects the radioactivity not only in the joint itself, but also in adjacent blood vessels and muscles. The levels of circulating radioactivity of the anti-CD4 mAb and HIG were significantly different (Fig. 1, 2). Therefore, differences in the tissue-bound fraction of radioactivity in the joint may not became apparent if one only compares total levels of radioactivity within the joint ROI.

When this factor is taken into account, e.g. by evaluating the ratios between levels of radioactivity in the synovial membrane region and those in either blood vessels or

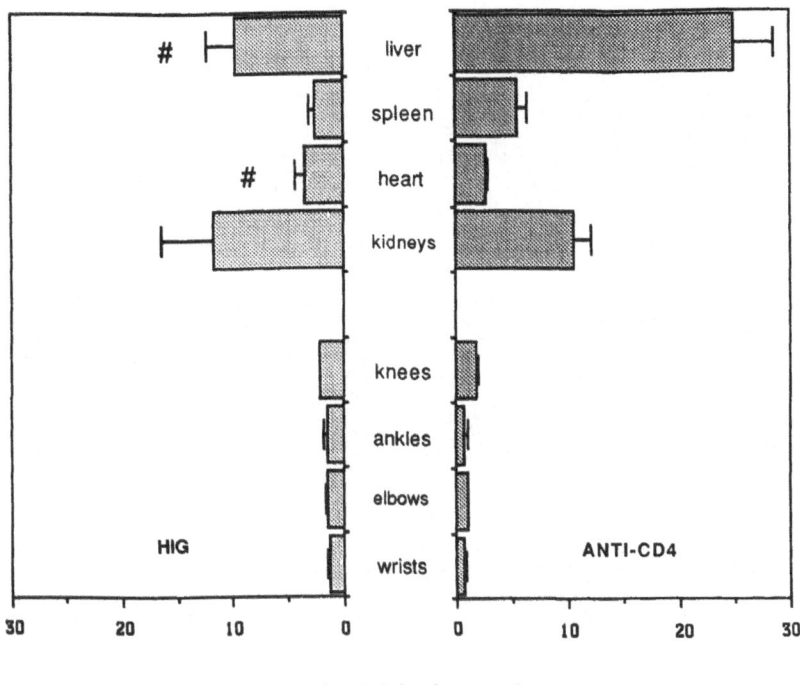

Figure 1. Evaluation of whole body scans 24 h after injection of radiolabeled HIG or the labeled anti-CD4 mAb using ROI placed over different organs and joints. # = p ≤ 0.05 Mann-Whitney (U) test.

muscle, the anti-CD4 mAb shows a significantly higher T/B ratio in arthritic knees and elbows compared to control HIG (Fig. 2). This finding is further confirmed by a study performed in one RA patient, in which the imaging properties of the anti-CD4 mAb were superior not only to those of HIG but also to those of an isotype-matched mouse mAb with irrelevant specificity (Fig. 3).

The disease activity in individual joints was mostly comparable when the scans with different Igs were performed (data not shown); therefore, the superior imaging properties of the anti-CD4 mAb as a tracer seem to be based on a more specific detection of inflammatory infiltrates rich in CD4-positive cells.

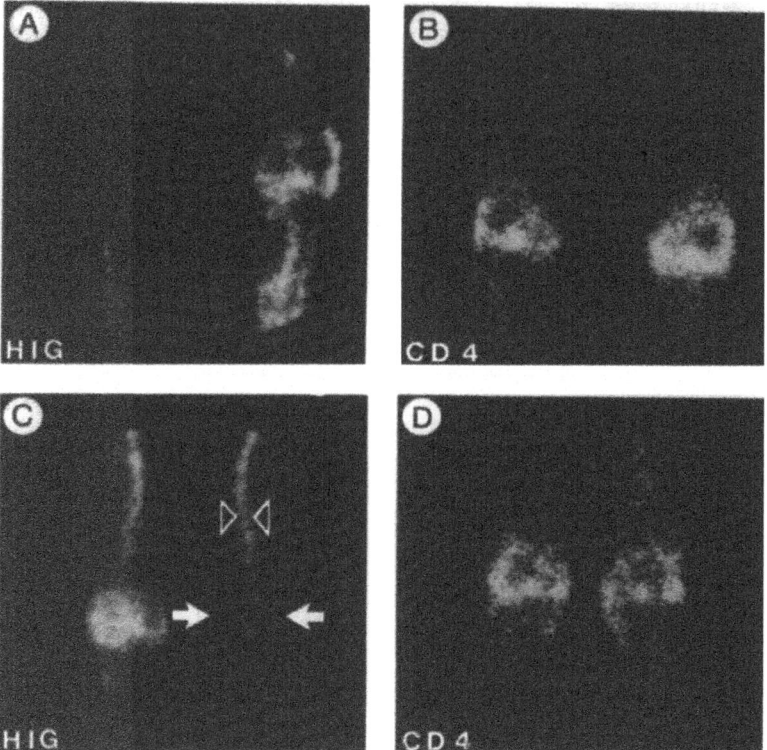

Figure 2. Scans of knee joints from 2 RA patients who received both radiolabeled HIG (A,C) and the labeled anti-CD4 mAb (B,D). A and B, C and D represent subsequent scans with HIG or the anti-CD4 mAb in the same patient, in each case 4 h after injection of the Ig. The time elapsed between the two studies was 12.5 (A-B) and 16 (C-D) months. Colors from black to white represent levels of radioactivity ranging from low (black) to high (white), respectively.

In the case of labeled HIG (A,C) large blood vessels (arrowheads) are clearly visible; the inflamed joints are outlined but the levels of radioactivity in the inflamed joint (arrows) are not higher than in the adjacent vessels. In contrast, the level of radioactivity in the knee joints in the case of the anti-CD4 mAb (B,D) is clearly higher than in the adjacent vessels and the vessels cannot be clearly delineated.

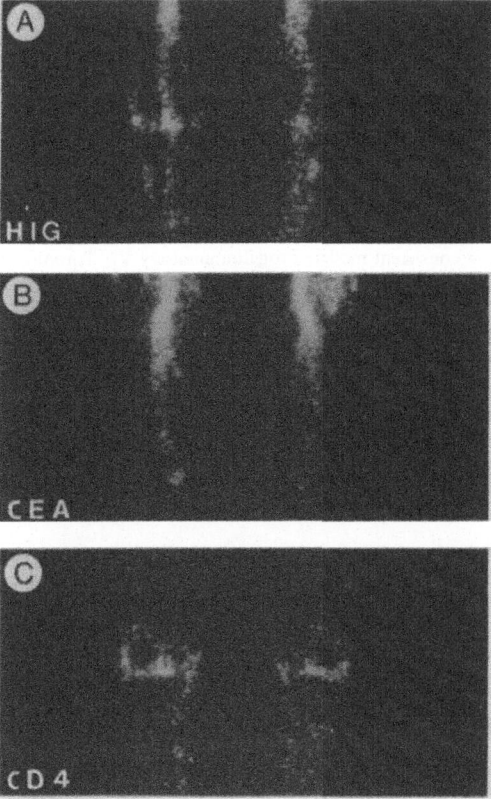

Figure 3. Scans of knee joints from 1 RA patient who received 3 different Igs, in each case 4 h after their injection. The time elapsed between the studies was 5.5 months (A-B) and 9 days (B-C). Colors from black to white represent levels of radioactivity ranging from low (black) to high (white), respectively.

In the case of labeled HIG (A) large blood vessels are clearly visible; the inflamed joints are delineated but the levels of radioactivity in the inflamed joint are not higher than in the adjacent vessels. In the case of the control anti-CEA mAb (B) the joint region shows clearly lower radioactivity levels than adjacent vessels; in fact, the inflamed joint is not outlined. In contrast, the level of radioactivity in the knee joints after injection of the anti-CD4 mAb (C) is clearly higher than in the adjacent vessels, which in this case cannot be distinguished from the tissue background.

ACKNOWLEDGEMENTS

U. Vorderwuelbecke is acknowledged for expert technical assistance and Dr. E. Palombo-Kinne for helpful suggestions. The Clinical Research Unit for Rheumatology of the Max-Planck-Society is funded by the German Ministry for Research and Technology (BMFT).

REFERENCES

Arnett FC, Edworthy SM, Bloch DA, McShane DJ, Fries JF, Cooper NS, Healey LA, Kaplan SR, Liang MH, Luthra HS, Medsger TA Jr, Mitchell DM, Neustadt DH, Pinals RS, Schaller JG, Sharp JT, Wilder RL, Hunder GG, 1988. The American Rheumatism Association 1987 revised criteria for the classification of rheumatoid arthritis. *Arthritis Rheum* 31: 315-324.

Becker W, Emmrich F, Horneff G, Burmester GR, Seiler F, Schwarz A, Kalden JR, Wolf F, 1990. Imaging rheumatoid arthritis specifically with technetium 99m CD4-specific (T-helper lymphocytes) antibodies. *Eur J Nucl Med* 17: 156-159.

Bosslet K, Lüben G, Schwarz A, Hundt E, Harthus HP, Seiler FR, Muhrer C, Klöppel G, Kayser K, Sedlacek HH, 1985. Immunohistochemical localization and molecular characteristics of three monoclonal antibody-defined epitopes detectable on carcinoembryonic antigen (CEA). *Int J Cancer* 36: 75-84.

Emmrich F, 1987. Empfehlungen für die Herstellung und Prüfung in vivo applizierbarer monoklonaler Antikörper. *Dtsch Med Wochenschr* 112: 194-198.

Emmrich F, Eichmann K, Weltzien HU, 1986. The generation of the repertoire of T cell specificities and functions: towards a consistent model. Prog Immunology VI, Toronto, pp 406-417.

Janossy G, Duke O, Poulter LW, Panayi G, Bofill M, Goldstein G, 1981. Rheumatoid arthritis: A disease of T-lymphocyte/macrophage immunoregulation. *Lancet* 839-842.

Kushner I, Somerville JA, 1971. Permeability of human synovial membrane to plasma proteins. *Arthritis Rheum* 14: 560-570.

Schwarz A, Steinstraesser A, 1987. A novel approach to Tc-99-labeled monoclonal antibodies. *J Nucl Med* 28: 721.

99mTC-HMPAO RADIOLABELLED LEUCOCYTES IN INFLAMMATORY BOWEL DISEASE: SPECT VS PLANAR SCINTIGRAPHY

N. Prandini[1], L. Feggi[1], D. Cantarini[2], F. Macario[2], S. Gamberini[2], R. Scagliarini[2], R. Reverberi[3] and L. Lodi[3]

[1]Nuclear Medicine Department
[2]Gastroenterology Unit
[3]Blood Transfusion Service
S.Anna Hospital
Ferrara, Italy

INTRODUCTION

The scintigraphy with radiolabelled WBC plays an important role in the diagnosis and management of the patients with inflammatory bowel disease (IBD) because of the limitations of both endoscopy and radiography. Barium radiography is important in the diagnosis of IBD and of strictures of bowel but can to fail in the diagnosis of disease activity or in the detection of such complications as abscesses[1]. Endoscopy has a very high sensitivity in the diagnosis of large bowel inflammation but sometimes it can miss the localizations in both the small bowel and the right colon because of an incomplete examination in active disease[2, 3]. The sensitivity of scintigraphy in the diagnosis of the disease and in the assessment of the disease activity in IBD is higher than radiography and like endoscopy plus biopsy, and it is an indispensable means in the diagnosis of abdominal sepsis[4, 5, 6, 7]. Moreover, is a simple, rapid and noninvasive procedure because it does not require enema or intubation for the evaluation of the patients[3].

In most of the experiences the results of scintigraphy are reported as global sensitivity and specificity of either or both planar and SPECT scans and we did not find any paper concerning the comparison of SPECT versus planar imagings[4, 5, 6, 7, 8]. Therefore, we compared the two techniques to assess if SPECT can significantly improve the sensitivity of leucocyte scintigraphy in IBD.

MATERIAL AND METHODS

We retrospectively compared the results of 65 scintigraphies imaged in 61 patients with both planar and SPECT scans. All the patients (30 females and 31 males), aged 9-74 years (mean 37), also underwent to at least 2 examinations (endoscopy plus biopsy and radiography or ultrasonography) and a clinical long-term follow-up of more than 6 months. Fifty-five patients had pathologically proven diagnosis (4 patients underwent a bowel resection after scintigraphy) and 6 patients had clinical diagnosis and long term-follow up.

The WBC, separated from a 42 ml blood sample, were resuspended in 1 ml of platelets poor plasma and labelled at room temperature with 2 ml of 99mTc-HMPAO and an activity of 30 mCi. The mean labelling efficiency of 99mTc-HMPAO was 93% with a little amount of secondary bound (4.74%), hydrolyzed (1.57%) and free technetium (0.54%). The mean labelling efficiency of WBC was 67% with a mean activity injected of 20 mCi (young patients received a proportionally smaller activity than adults). Scintigraphies were performed with a single head camera (409 Elscint) equipped with a LFOV, parallel holes, high resolution collimator. Planar scans were acquired at 30 minutes, 2 and 20 hours with a matrix of 256x256 pixels and more than 1 million counts. SPECT were imaged with a matrix of 64x64 pixels, with a 360 degrees rotation (steps of 6 degrees, 20 sec each). The images were processed by reconstruction, (Hanning back projection filter with coefficients of 0, 1, 1) and by correction of attenuation (0.125/cm factor). Transaxial, coronal and sagittal views with slice of 2 pixels (1.25 cm) were shown in the final report.

Retrospectively all the images were separated according to their kind (planar or SPECT) and were independently read by two expert nuclear medicine physicians. The small and large bowel was divided in 6 segments (small, ascending, transversum, descending, sigmoid and rectum) and all segments were assessed as positive or negative. All results were put together and all the disagreements discussed.

RESULTS

Our histological findings were 42 Crohn disease, 13 ulcerative colitis and 10 unspecific colitis.

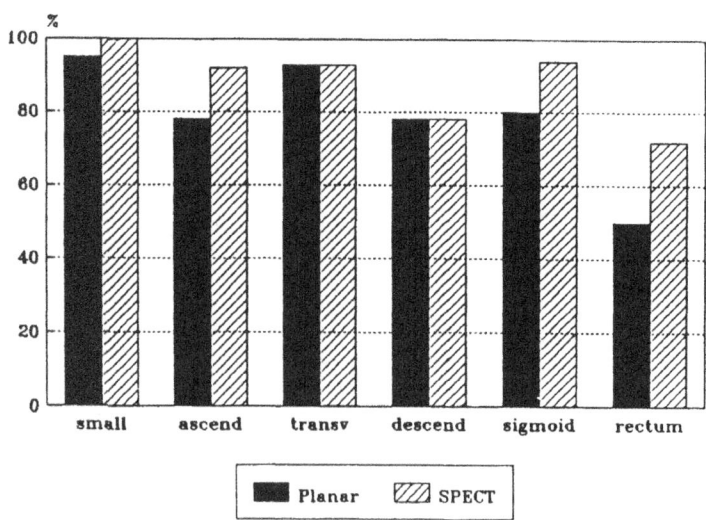

Figure 1. Sensitivity of both planar and SPECT WBC scintigraphies in inflammatory bowel disease concerning all bowel segments.

In order to consider the extension of disease in the segments of small and large bowel the best results of both techniques were found in the localizations in small bowel with a sensitivity of 94.3% for planar and 100% for SPECT (fig 1). The sensitivity was in all localizations better for SPECT than planar but decreases for both techniques in distal bowel with a sensitivity in sigmoid of 79.4% and 91.4%, respectively, for planar and SPECT, and in rectum of 50% and 70.6%, respectively, for planar and SPECT (fig. 2).

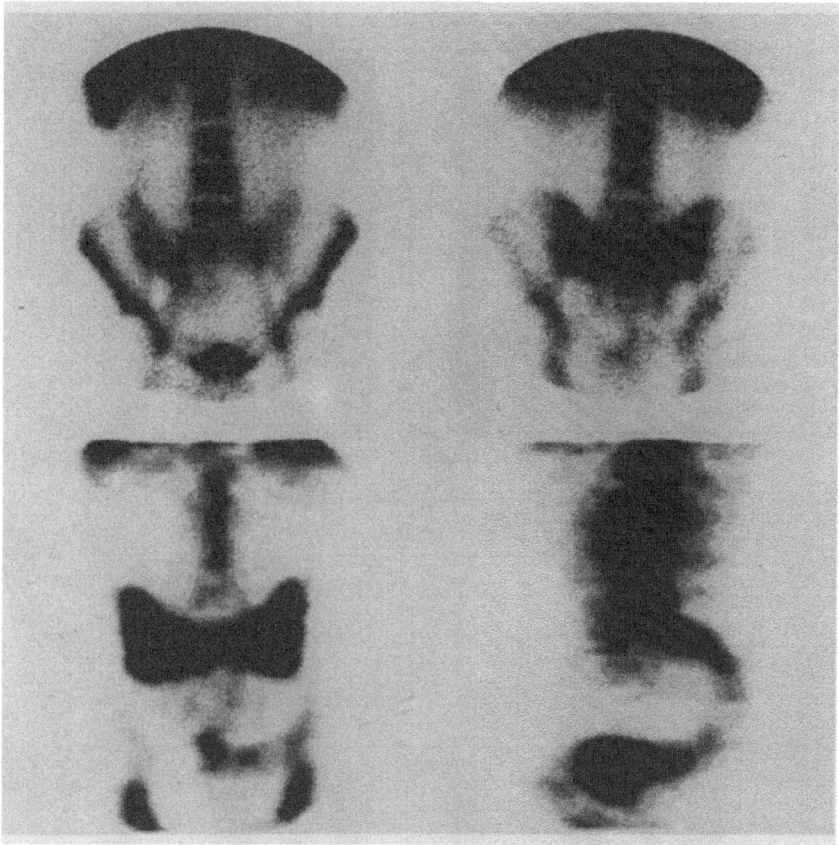

Figure 2. WBC scintigraphy in ulcerative colitis, planar (top) and SPECT scan (bottom): uptake of WBC in small bowell and little areas of uptake in rectum showed only on SPECT scan.

The specificity of both techniques was similar and very high in all segments (fig. 3). SPECT obtained the same or better results than planar in all segments but in sigmoid, in which 2 cases false positive in SPECT were correctly assessed by planar at late imagings.

Figure 4 shows the diagnostic accuracy of both techniques for all segments: SPECT has better results than planar.

The overall sensitivity, specificity and diagnostic accuracy of both techniques are 78.5%, 94.5%, 87.8%, respectively for planar, and 82.8%, 94.9%, 89.7%, respectively for SPECT. The Wilcoxon test for unpaired data shows a significant difference (P = 0.049) between the two series of results.

The overall results of both techniques for the presence of disease were 54 TP, 10 TN and 1 FP with a sensitivity of 100%, a specificity of 90% and a diagnostic accuracy of 98.5%.

In our experience endoscopy plus biopsy yelded a sensitivity of 80.1% considering each segment individually and radiography a sensitivity of 55%. The worst results were obtained by ultrasonography with a sensitivity of 43%.

Specificity of LS in IBD

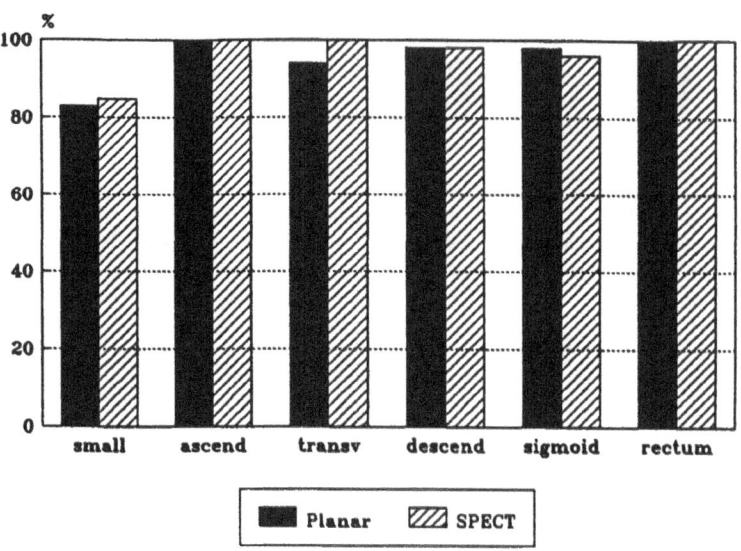

Figure 3. Specificity of both planar and SPECT techniques in the same segments.

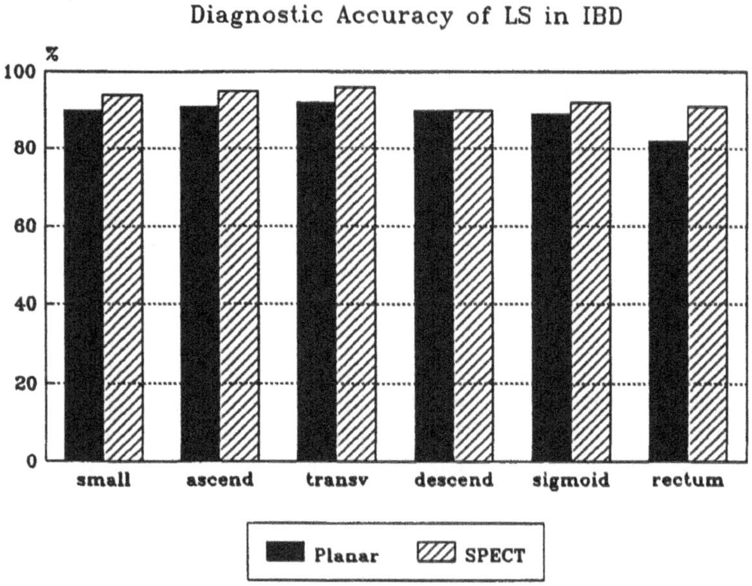

Diagnostic Accuracy of LS in IBD

Figure 4. Diagnostic accuracy of both techniques.

DISCUSSION AND CONCLUSION

Our data confirm that WBC scintigraphy has the best diagnostic accuracy in the management of IBD in spite of a not very high sensitivity to diagnose all the segments involved correctly. The diagnostic accuracy decreases in the segments close to liver and spleen because of their high activity. In the little pelvis the results of the scintigraphies worsen and they were lower than those of endoscopy. In fact, in these cases endoscopy was treated as a gold standard. Moreover, most localizations in distal bowel were of ulcerative colitis in which the uptake of WBC is lower than in Crohn's disease. Nevertheless, the employ of endoscopy is reduced in the follow up to avoid complications or to intolerance of the patients to intubation; in these cases scintigraphy plays the first role assessing the activity of the disease[3].

SPECT provides significantly better results than planar scans in the study of the distal large bowel, especially in the localizations with low activity or close to bladder. However, we only performed the SPECT scan 2 hours p.i. of labelled WBC but in this way the specificity decreases. Three phase scintigraphy with planar scan and a SPECT scan performed at the moment of the maximum specificity of uptake (2 hours p.i.) can better distinguish the segments involved and improve both sensitivity and specificity of WBC scan in IBD[10].

In conclusion, our data confirm that scintigraphy is very useful in the global diagnosis of disease although sensitivity is not uniformly high for all segments. SPECT provides significantly better results than planar in all bowel segments and improves the sensitivity of WBC scintigraphy in distal large bowel.

BIBLIOGRAPHY

1. M.L.Janower: in Radiology, Taveras Editor, Lippincott Company; 32: 1-15 (1990).
2. L.E.Smith: *Dis. Colon Rectum*; 19: 407-12 (1976).
3. S.H.Saverymuttu: *Br Med J*; 285: 255-7 (1982).
4. R.D.Rothstein: *JNM*; 32: 5, 856-9 (1991).
5. S.Saverymuttu: *Gastroenterology*; 85: 1333-9 (1983).
6. J.Scholmerich: *Gastroenterology*; 95: 1287-93 (1988).
7. A.Furno: *Eur J Nucl Med*; 19: 8, 232-5 (1992).
8. R.Laitinen: *Clin Nucl Med*; 15; 597-602 (1990).
9. B.H.Guze: *Clin Nucl Med*; 15: 8-10 (1990).
10. W.Becker: *J Nucl Med*; 27: 1109-15 (1986).

FIRST YEAR EVOLUTIONARY PATTERNS OF 99mTc-HMPAO-LEUKOCYTE UPTAKE IN UNEVENTFUL PROSTHETIC KNEE JOINT REPLACEMENT

J.M. González, M. Ysamat, J. Verdú, N. Jou[1], J. Castell, A. García and M. Fraile

Serveis de Medicina Nuclear i Rehabilitació[1]
Hospital Universitari Vall d'Hebron
Barcelona

Tecnetium-WBC imaging seems a promising technique for the evaluation of suspected bone and joint sepsis. Leukocyte scanning may be used to rule out infection in painful Total Knee Arthroplasty (TKA). However, a complete knowledge of the postoperative patterns of leukocyte uptake is lacking. Therefore, our aim was to establish the the time-course of WBC deposition during the first year after TKA surgery in patients without complications.

POPULATION

We studied 20 patients (16 women), with a mean age of 63 years (range 52 to 73). One year after surgery, all patients had had an uneventful clinical course, with no signs or symptoms of complication, such as infection or aseptic loosening. Patients were followed at one, six, and twelve months postoperatively. At each time point, prosthetic knees were clinically evaluated, and blood chemistry including WBC count and ESR was obtained, together with plain X-ray examination and WBC scanning. The clinical parameters were always within normal limits. Altogether, 26 TKA were evaluated, including the following controls: 21 at one month, 11 at 6 months, and 16 at 12 months.

METHOD

Cell Labeling

Sampling was done by collecting 44 ml of blood in 6 ml of ACD-A solution. Leukocyte labeling with about 444 MBq of 99mTc-HMPAO was achieved after facilitated red blood cell sedimentation using 8 ml of 6% hydroxyethylstarch in 0.9% sodium chloride. The leukocyte pellet was resuspended and incubated with cell poor plasma. Labeling efficiency was 58.3 ± 7% (mean ± SD) in 37 consecutive procedures.

Imaging and Analysis

Ten minute anterior planar views of both knees were obtained 4 to 6 hours after reinjection. Qualitative assessment was achieved through inspective analysis by three independent observers, the diferences being solved by agreement. Uptake was graded using a four point scale as follows: 0 - no uptake, similar to background activity, 1 - activity in TKA slightly more than background, 2 - more than grade 1 and less than marrow uptake, 3 - equal to or more than marrow uptake. 8 sites were considered per arthroplasty: 5 femoral (1 intercondyleal, 2 condyleal, 2 supracondyleal) and 3 tibial (1 at the metallic tip, 2 at the tibial plateau) (Figure 1).

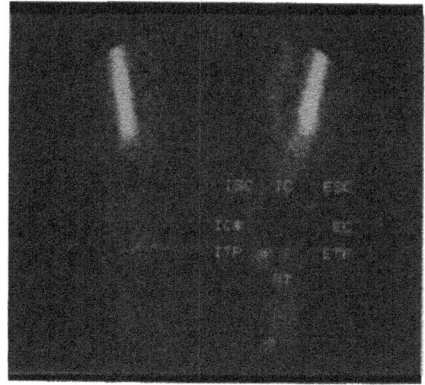

Figure 1. For the qualitative assessment, 8 different periprosthetic sites were considered as follows (clockwise): IC - intercondyleal, ESC -external supracondyleal, EC - external condyleal, ETP - external tibial plateau, MT - metallic tip, ITP - internal tibial plateau, IC* - internal condyleal, ISC - internal supracondyleal. The scoring system consisted of a four-point scale from 0 - no uptake, to 3 - equal to or more than marrow uptake.

Also, quantitative assessment was approached by the activity ratio of periprosthetic tissues (both femoral and tibial halves) to a nonvascular background region within the thigh, using irregular ROIs (Figure 2).

RESULTS

Figure 3 is a plot of uptake scores for the eight periprosthetic sites considered, one, six, and twelve months after surgery, respectively. It can be seen that WBC uptake significantly decreases over time (Chi-square analysis, $p < 0.001$), especially between one and six months. The tissues around the metallic tip seem to be more leukocyte-avid than the rest, although the differences among sites were not statistically significant at any time.

Figure 4 is a plot of the quantitative assessment for both the femoral and the tibial halves of TKAs at one, six, and twelve months, using the bone-to-background ratio. It can also be seen that leukocyte uptake around the prosthesis decays over twelve months, the differences being highly significant between time points (paired t-test, p < 0.001). No differences were seen between the femoral and the tibial halves of TKAs. The 95 percentile value for the uptake ratio at six months amounts 1.96, and this can be used as the cut-off to separate abnormal uptake.

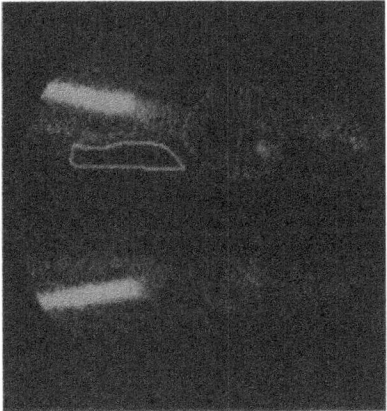

Figure 2. For the quantitative assessment, the ratio of bone-to-background activity was derived using irregular ROIs.

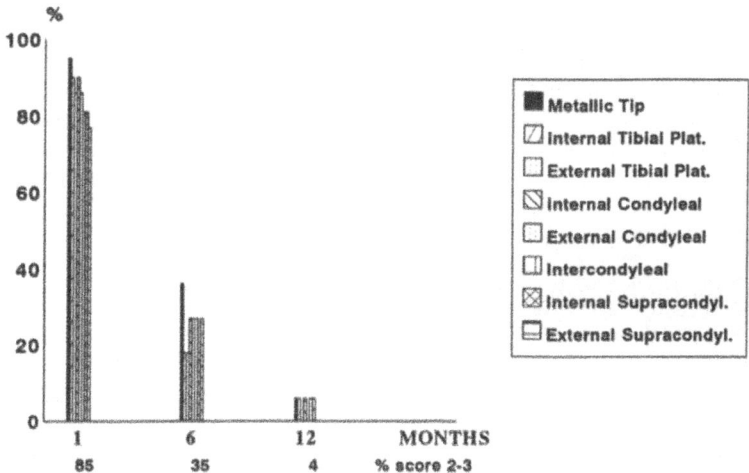

Figure 3. Each of the 8 bars is a graph of the percentage of regions with an uptake score equal to or higher than 2 at the three time point under consideration. Uptake of WBC in tissues around TKAs clearly decays over time, especially between one and six months postoperatively.

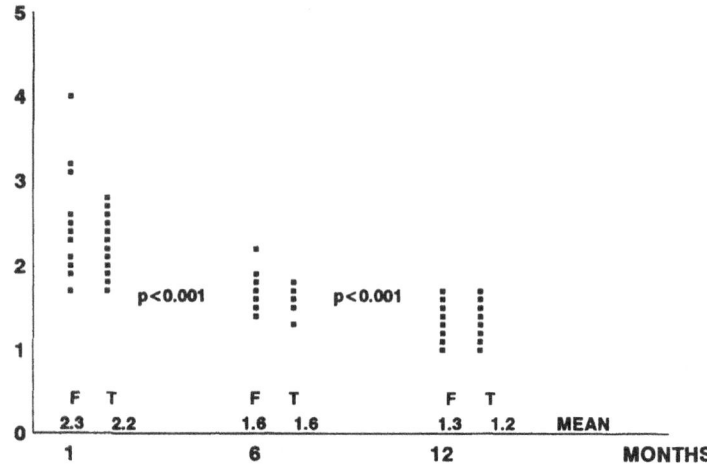

Figure 4. Each point in the graph represents the activity ratio between periprostetic bone and a non-vascular background region, both for the femoral (F), and the tibial (T) halves of TKAs. Also, the mean values for the correspondig activity ratios are displayed.

COMMENTS

Leukocyte imaging has proved superior to combined technetium-gallium scanning in the diagnosis of bone infection[1]. Although infection is uncommon after TKA, it is an ominous complication, usually leading to prosthetic replacement[2]. Bone pain after surgery is the main presenting complaint of infection, although it may also be due to aseptic loosening, which in fact is a more frequent complication than sepsis itself. Differentiation between both is clinically relevant. Therefore, the use of leukocyte scanning has been suggested in the evaluation of patients with painful TKAs[3]. Some inflammatory changes are, nevertheless to be expected postoperatively, and one can anticipate a certain degree of abnormal WBC deposition.

To our knowledge, the time-course of leukocyte uptake in tissues surrounding the prosthetic implant has not been previously addressed. Based both on visual inspection and on quantitative assessment, our study shows that TKAs take-up WBC very avidly one month after surgery, which renders the technique quite unuseful during the early postoperative period. Later on, leukocyte deposition decreases, with a slowing rate of decrease over twelve months. This applies to all sites around the prosthesis, although a non-significant trend can be seen for the tissues close to the tibial metallic tip to be more WBC-avid than the rest at one and six months.

Assessment of TKAs at six months may prove especially difficult, as there is still a marked uptake of WBC in patients with an uneventful clinical course. In this setting, the use of cut-off value for the bone-to-backgorund ratio of about 2 seems to separate abnormal uptake, thus giving an indication that infection could be present.

In summary, WBC scanning may contribute in the evaluation of patients with painful TKAs. However, early postoperative changes are associated with abnormal leukocyte uptake in "normals" (during the first six months). After that period of time, and up to one year postoperatively, quantitation of the bone-to-background activity ratio may be used to rule out infection.

REFERENCES

1. Merkel KD, Brown ML, Dewanjee MK, Fitzgerald RH: Comparison of Indium-labeled-leukocyte imaging with sequential Technetium-Gallium scanning in the diagnosis of low-grade musculoskeletal sepsis. *J Bone Joint Surg*; 67: 465-476 (1985).
2. Rand JA, Fitzgerald RH: Diagnosis and management of infected total knee arthroplasty. *Orthopedic Clinics of North America*; 20:201-210 (1989).
3. Rand JA, Brown ML: The value of 111-Indium leukocyte scanning in the evaluation of painful or infected total knee arthroplasty. *Clinical Orthopedics and Related Research*; 259: 179-182 (1990).

DETECTION AND QUANTITATIVE ANALYSIS OF JOINT INFLAMMATION WITH 99mTc-POLYCLONAL HUMAN IMMUNOGLOBULIN G

F. Pons[1], F. Moyá[2], R. Herranz[1], M. Solá[1], JA. del Olmo[2], FJ. Setoain[1], J. Muñoz-Gómez[2] and J. Setoain[1]

[1]Service of Nuclear Medicine
[2]Service of Rheumatology
Hospital Clínic. University of Barcelona
Barcelona (Spain)

Radiolabelled non-specific polyclonal human immunoglobulin G (HIG) has been recognized as a reliable modality for localization of infection and inflammation. The assessment of active joint inflammation is of great interest in some rheumatologic diseases, however it is prone to subjective variables as a gold standard is not available.

The aim of this study was to evaluate the suitability of 99mTc-HIG scintigraphy as an objective method for detecting active joint inflammation and to assess the degree of activity in noninvolved and inflamed joints.

MATERIALS AND METHODS

Twenty eight patients (8 males and 20 females) were studied. Fourteen (mean $\pm$ SD: 55 $\pm$ 11 years) presented with rheumatoid arthritis (RA) and were suffering from clinically active synovitis in several joints. The remaining 14 (mean $\pm$ SD: 64 $\pm$ 10 years), with osteoarthritis, were taken as a control group.

HIG (1 mg) was labelled with pertechnetate Tc99m and the patients were injected intravenously with 740 MBq. Scintigraphy was performed at 4 and 24 hours and anterior spot views of the shoulders, elbows, hands, hips, knees, ankles and feet were obtained. Forty-two joints of each patient could be used for evaluation. The metacarpophalangeal, proximal and distal interphalangeal joints of hands were evaluated separately. The metatarsophalangeal and interphalangeal joints of the feet were considered as one region (forefeet).

All joints (total of 1176) were assessed clinically for pain and swelling on a 4-point scale by the same investigator. The scans were analysed subjectively by two independent observers who were unaware of the patients's clinical data. All the above mentioned joints were scored in both scans on a 4-point scale depending on the degree of uptake. We also performed a quantitative analysis of scans and joint to background (J/B) ratios of uptake were obtained by dividing the average counts per pixel in each joint by the average counts per pixel in a region of interest located around soft tissue of the thigh.

RESULTS

The labelling efficiency was $98.5 \pm 0.6\%$.

Visual analysis of scans: In RA patients, 204 joints presented signs of pain and/or swelling. 99mTc-HIG scintigraphy showed an increased uptake in 177 (87%) of them at 4 hours (Fig. 1) and 167 (82%) at 24 hours. Most of the joints without positive uptake corresponded to joints with mild pain and without swelling. Scores of joint uptake correlated with clinical scores of pain and swelling in both scans ($r = 0.7$, $p < 0.01$).

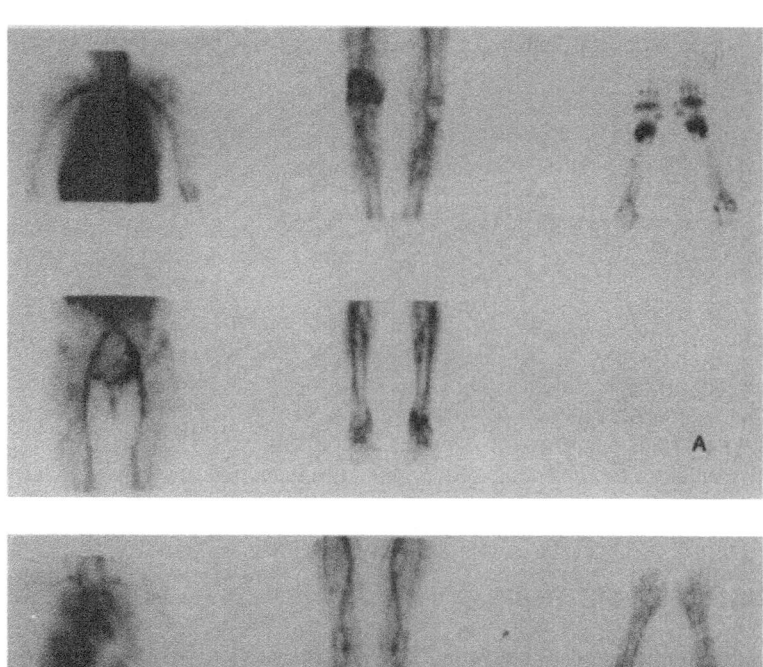

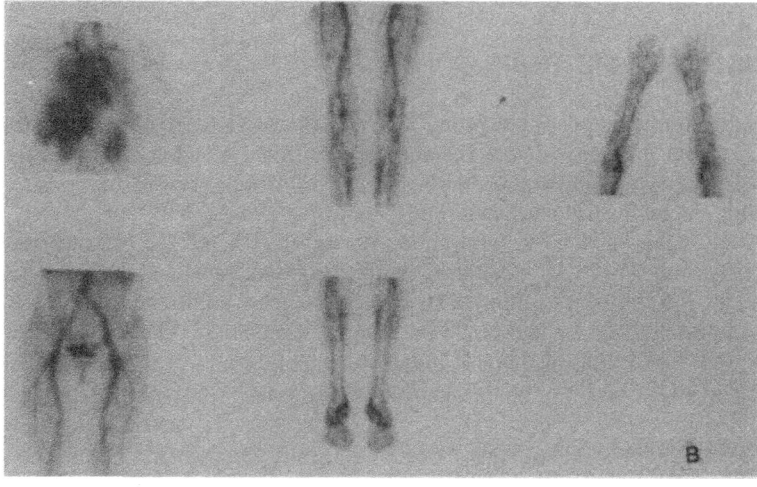

Figure 1. 1A. Images obtained at 4 hours in different patients suffering from clinically active synovitis. Abnormal uptake of the radiopharmaceutical is seen in several joints. **1B.** Scintigraphy performed at 4 hours in a patient from the control group that shows physiological distribution of the radiopharmaceutical.

Quantitative analysis of scans: In both groups of patients, J/B ratios were significantly higher in scans performed at 4 hours compared with those at 24 hours (p < 0.0001). When we analysed these ratios in the control group, we found significant differences between the diverse joints as it can be seen in Fig. 2.

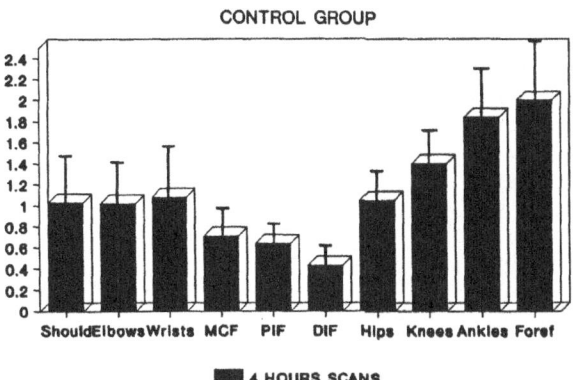

Figure 2. Joint to background ratios of uptake in scans performed at 4 hours (values are expressed as the means and one standard deviation for each group of joints).

Quantitative analysis of scans demonstrated that joints with absent pain or swelling in RA patients had significantly higher J/B ratios than the osteoarthritis group, and lower J/B ratios than joints clinically involved.

CONCLUSIONS

The results of this study show that 99mTc-HIG scintigraphy can localize synovitis in clinically involved joints. A greater number of affected joints was seen in scans performed at 4 hours in spite of its high blood-pool activity. 99mTc-HIG clears rapidly from both the background and target, so that this relatively rapid washout at sites of inflammation and the physical half-life of 99mTc probably makes scans performed at 24 hours less suitable. The differences found in J/B ratios of uptake between the diverse joints in the control group makes it difficult for quantitative analysis to establish ratios for the different degrees of synovitis. However, it could be helpful in some particular joints for the management of these patients. We believe that 99mTc-HIG scintigraphy can be useful in rheumatologic patients in whom it is difficult to assess the presence of pain and swelling by clinical examination. It might provide an objective method of detecting more accurately synovitis and measuring the activity of the disease.

REFERENCES

Berná LL, Torres G, Diez C, Estorch M, Martínez-Duncker D, Carrió I. Technetium-99m human polyclonal immunoglobulin G studies and conventional bone scans to detect active joint inflammation in chronic rheumatoid arthritis. *Eur J Nucl Med*; 19: 173-176 (1992).

Bois MHW de, Arndt JW, Velde EA van der et al. 99mTc Human Immunoglobulin Scintigraphy. A reliable method to detect joint activity in rheumatoid arthritis. *J Rheumatol*; 19: 1371-1376 (1992).

Buscombe JR, Lui D, Ensing G, de Jong R, Ell PJ. Tc-99m- human immunoglobulin (HIG)-first results of a new agent for the localization of infection and inflammation. *Eur J Nucl Med*; 16: 649-655 (1990).

Fischman AJ, Rubin RH, Khaw BA, et al. Detection of acute inflammation with 111In-labeled nonspecific polyclonal IgG. *Semin Nucl Med*; 18: 335-344 (1988).

Liberatore M, Clemente M, Lurilli AP et al. Scintigraphic evaluation of disease activity in rheumatoid arthritis: a comparison of technetium-99m human non-specific immunoglobulins, leucocytes and albumin nanocolloids. *Eur J Nucl Med*; 19: 853-857 (1992).

Lubbe PAHM van der, Arndt JW, Calame W, Ferreira TC, Pauwels EKJ, Breedveld FC. Measurement of synovial inflammation in rheumatoid arthritis with technetium 99m labelled human polyclonal immunoglobulin G. *Eur J Nucl Med*; 18: 119-123 (1991).

Oyen WJG, Claessens RAMJ, Horn JR van, Meer JWM van der, Corstens FHM. Scintigraphic detection of bone and joint infections with indium-111-labeled nonspecific polyclonal human immunoglobulin G. *J Nucl Med*; 31: 403-412 (1990).

INCREASED LUNG ACTIVITY OF 111In LABELLED POLYCLONAL IgG IN PATIENTS WITH AIDS AND ACTIVE CHEST INFECTION

J.R. Buscombe, W.J.G. Oyen, R.F. Miller, A. Grant, R.A.M.J. Cleassens, J.M.W. Van der Meer, D. Lui, F.H.M. Corstens and P.J. Ell

UCLSM, London, U.K. and University Hospital, Nijmegen
The Netherlands

Patients infected with the human immunodeficiency virus (HIV) are at risk of life threatening infection. Consequently the most common cause of morbidity and death in HIV infected patients within the United Kingdom remains pulmonary infection often with *Pneumocystis carinii* pneumonia[1]. Functional imaging techniques using scintigraphic methods provide unique information which will demonstrate the presence of infection before there are changes on planar or computed tomography X-ray. Imaging with [67]Gallium citrate has become established as the method of choice in the initial investigation of HIV infected patients presenting with symptoms or signs of chest infection[2,3]. Unfortunately the agent is non-specific and may accumulate in sites of tumour or benign pathology such as rib fractures[4]. 111Indium labelled polyclonal human immunoglobulin (111In-HIG) has been shown to have a high sensitivity and specificity in localising infection in immunocompromised patients and those who are infected with HIV[5]. In some patients the study demonstrates intense accumulation of 111In-HIG in the presence of active infection (Fig 1) but often the changes are more subtle.

The aim of this study was to confirm that significantly greater uptake of 111In-HIG seen in patients with active chest infections can be confirmed quantitatively when compared with those patients in whom no chest infection is present.

METHODS

A retrospective analysis was performed on 55 111In-HIG studies performed on 51 HIV infected patients (50 patients were male, mean age 32, range 17-57). All patients presented with signs and/or symptoms of either an active chest infection or infective disease elsewhere. Typical presenting symptoms were fever, night sweats, malaise, loss of weight and cough. Physical examination normally confirmed fever but localising signs were often absent.

All patients were imaged 48 hours after administration of 37MBq of 111In-HIG. Anterior and posterior images (600kcounts each)of the chest were performed on a standard gamma camera fitted with a medium energy collimator. All images were read by two clinicians unaware of the patient's diagnosis or presenting symptoms or signs.

To quantify lung uptake regions of interest were draw over the upper, mid and lower zones of the right lung. Regions were placed so that the both the periphery and the hilum of the lung were excluded. By using the mean counts in both anterior and posterior projections of the lung a geometric mean of lung activity was obtained. This was divided by the geometric mean of activity in the left ventricle obtained using regions of interest drawn over the heart in anterior and posterior images.

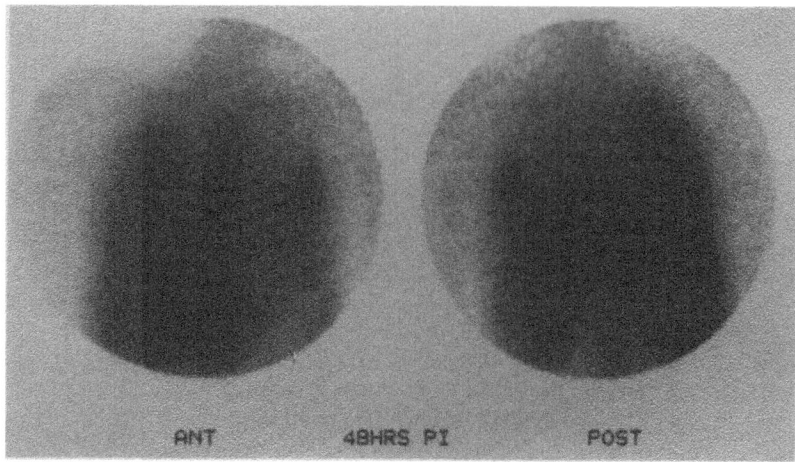

Fig 1. Patient with *Pneumocystis carinii* pneumonia and marked uptake of 111In-HIG in both lungs.

RESULTS

Qualitative reporting of the studies demonstrated that all patients subsequently confirmed to have active chest infection had positive accumulation of 111In-HIG in the chest (Table 1).

Table 1

Final diagnosis	Positive study	Negative study
P. Carinii	17	0
Other infections	21	0
Normal	1	16

In one patient with severe renal failure there was diffusely increased accumulation of 111In-HIG in both lungs but no infection was found in the lungs even at post mortem. There was significantly greater activity in the lungs (measured as lung/heart ratio of

111In-HIG activity) in patients infected with *Pneumocystis carinii* ($p < 0.05$) or other infective agents ($p < 0.05$) when compared with patients in there was no evidence for active chest infection. (Table 2).

Table 2

Final diagnosis	lung/heart ratio (mean)	lung/heart ratio (s.d.)
P. Carinii	0.66	0.05*
Other infections	0.59	0.09*
Normal	0.51	0.06

* $p < 0.05$ compared to normal group, student's t test.

In one patient studied on three occasions for recurrent fever the initial scan demonstrated positive accumulation of 111In-HIG in the chest, subsequently the patient was found to have cytomegalovirus pneumonitis. This was treated with the anti-viral Ganclocovir and there was a subsequent fall in the lung/heart activity (Fig 2).

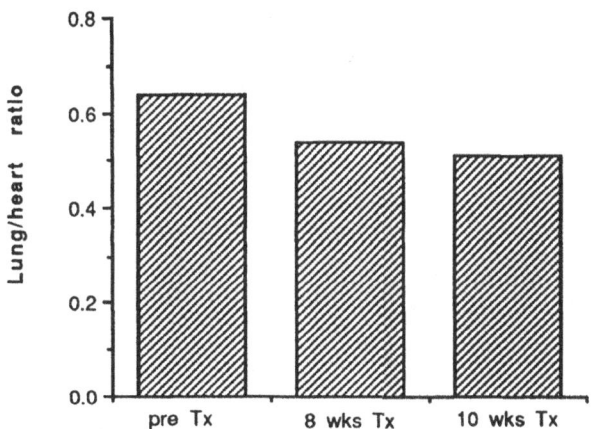

Fig 2. Sequential lung/heart ratio of 111In-HIG in a patient with cytomegalovirus pneumonitis treated with Gancyclovir.

CONCLUSION

Quantitative analysis of the lung/heart ratio of 111In-HIG activity confirms the qualitative finding that there is significant accumulation of this tracer in HIV antibody patients with active chest infection. The single patient with a falling lung/heart activity is response to specific antiviral therapy suggests that 111In-HIG may be used to monitor the effect of treatment.

REFERENCES

1. Peters B.S., Beck E.J. Coleman D.G., Wadsworth M.J.H., McGuiness O., Pinching A.J. (1991) Changing disease patterns in patients with AIDs in a referral centre in the United Kingdom: The changing face of AIDS. *Brit Med J.* 302; 203-206.

2. Bitran J, Beckerman C, Weinstein R, Bennet C, Ryo U, Pinsky S. Patterns of gallium-67 scintigraphy in patients with acquired immune deficiency syndrome and AIDS related complex. J Nucl Med. 28: 1103-1106 (1987).

3. Kramer EL, Sanger JJ, Garay SM, Greene JB, Tiu S, Banner H, McCauley DI. Gallium-67 scans of the chest of patients with acquired immunodeficiency J Nucl Med. 28: 1107-1114 (1987).

4. Buscombe JR, Miller RF, Lui D, Ell PJ. Combined Ga-67 citrate and Tc-99m human immunoglobulin imaging in human immunodeficiency virus-positive patients with fever of determined origin Nucl Med Comm.; 12: 583-592 (1991).

5. Oyen WJG, Claessens RAMJ, Peamekers JMM, Pauw BE Van der Meer JWM, Corstens FHM. Diagnosing infection in febrile granulocytopaenic patients with indium-111 labelled human immunoglobulin *J Clin Oncol*; 10:61-68 (1992).

111In-PLATELETS AND 99mTc-HUMAN POLYCLONAL IMMUNOGLOBULIN (HIG) SCINTIGRAPHY IN PATIENTS WITH CEREBROVASCULAR DISEASE

L. Prat[1], M. Roca[1], J. Rubio[2], X. Ferrer[2], Y. Ricart[1], L. Mairal[1], and J. Martin-Comin[1]

[1]Serveis de Medicina Nuclear
[2]Servei de Neurologia
Hospital Universitari de Bellvitge
Barcelona, Spain

INTRODUCTION

Atherosclerosis is the main cause of morbidity and mortality in the industrial countries.

Although its ethiopatogenesis is not exactly known, it is accepted that the atheromatous plaque progresses in cycles of activity and quiescence.

The process is initiated when the endothelium is injured and some of the cells die. Subsequently the necrotic area is covered by platelets and posteriorly new endothelial cells grow on this surface. These new endothelial cells have increased permeability to lipids and lipoproteins, and fatty material is deposited in the subendothelial space. This fatty material is very irritating and produce an inflammatory reaction. As a reaction macrophages migrate to the subendothelial space and phagocytize the fatty material and damaged endothelial cells. The macrophages full of lipids are called the foam cells and they express Fc receptors on the surface.

Standard imaging techniques (sonography, doppler, computed tomography,angiography and magnetic nuclear resonance) used in the diagnosis of atherosclerotic disease allows identification of changes in wall thickness, in the turbulence of blood flow or in lumen diameter. Unfortunately all these changes appear once the atheromatous plaque is evolutionated, and they are not useful in the early diagnosis of lesions.

In the search for a non invasive technique that allows the diagnostic of the atheromatous plaques in the early stages, different tracers have been used, the most significant being platelets[3, 4, 5] and low density lipoproteins[12, 15, 16]. In this study we have used two different tracers the 111In-platelets and the 99mTc-polyclonal immunoglobulin G (HIG), in patients with cerebro-vascular disease.

MATERIAL AND METHOD

Patients

Twenty-one patients (14 men, mean age 53.3 y, range 34-76 y.) having suffered a cerebro vascular accident were studied within a week of the accident.

All patients underwent scintigraphy, doppler sonography and arteriography of the neck arteries in non selected order. All exams were performed within 14 days of the accident.

Scintigraphy Studies

Fourteen patients were studied with In111-platelets, and seven patients with 99mTc-HIG.

1.- Platelet labeling:
Autologus platelets were labeled with In111-Oxine as previously described[22].
Administered dose was 300 uCi.

2.- Immunoglobulin labeling:
Human polyclonal immunoglobulin G was labeled with 15-20 mCi Tc99m. To a vial containing 1 mg HIG, 4.2 mg of Disodium tartrate and 8 ug of stannous chloride, 15-20 mCi of pertechnetate were added and after 20 minutes of incubation the preparation was ready for injection.
Administered dose was 15-20 mCi.

In the fourteen patients studied with In111-platelets a scintigraphy of the neck was obtained at 24 and 48 hours post injection. The images were obtained with a large field of view scintillation camera fitted with a medium energy parallel-hole collimator. Window was centered over the In-111 peak.

In the seven patients studied with Tc99mHIG scintigraphy images of the neck were obtained at 4 and 24 hours post injection. The images were obtained with a large field view scintillation camera fitted with a low energy parallel-hole collimator. Window was centred over the Tc99m peak.

Scans were analyzed by two independent observers, who did not know the results of the other examinations, and final agreement was obtained in all cases.

The visualization of activity in the right brachycephalic trunk was considered normal. The scan was considered positive (abnormal) if an asymmetric uptake between both carotid regions was seen.

3.-Other studies:
Doppler sonography and arteriography were performed in all patients (arteriography could not be obtained in one case).

Depending on the results of the Doppler sonography and the arteriography, carotid arteries were classified into four groups: Group 1: Normal (no stenosis or less than 15%), Group 2: Atheromatous lesions with stenosis between 15-50%, Group 3: Atheromatous lesions with stenosis greater than 50% and group 4: Atheromatous lesions with carotid occlusion.

RESULTS

Tables 1 and 2 show the results of the platelet scan and the HIG scan.

Table 1 PLATELETS-In111. (14 patients, 28 carotids).

	SCINT.(+)	SCINT. (-)
NO ATHEROMATOUS LESIONS	2	11
ATHEROMATOUS LESIONS STENOSIS < 50%	0	2
ATHEROMATOUS LESIONS STENOSIS > 50%	4	7
ATHEROMATOUS LESIONS OCCLUSION	1	1
TOTAL	7	21

In-111-platelet uptake was seen in only 5 out of the 15 carotid arteries with atheromatous lesions.

Eleven out of the 13 normal arteries had a normal scan, while unexpected platelet uptake was seen in 2 normal arteries by doppler sonography or angiography.

Table 2 HIG-Tc99m.(7 patients, 14 carotids).

	SCINT.(+)	SCINT. (-)
NO ATHEROMATOUS LESIONS	2	8
ATHEROMATOUS LESIONS STENOSIS < 50%	0	1
ATHEROMATOUS LESIONS STENOSIS > 50%	3	0
ATHEROMATOUS LESIONS OCCLUSION	0	0
TOTAL	5	9

The HIG scan was positive in 3 out of the 4 arteries with atheromatous lesions. There were two scans that were positive and have not atheromatous lesion. The first corresponded to a right carotid abnormality and showed kinking in the arteriography, the left artery was normal. In the second one the doppler was normal and the angiography could not be done.

DISCUSSION

Our data with In-111-platelets shows low accuracy (57%) in the detection of atheromatous lesions.

Those results are in agreement with previously reported experimental and clinical results. McAffe et al. showed, in dogs, that thrombus older than 24 h were not seen in the labeled platelets scan. Henninger et al[5] describe platelet accumulation only in the atheromatous plaque, if it is heterogenous and unstable. The plaques with a fibrotic component do not show platelet uptake, these fenomena can explain the low accuracy that we have seen in our data and the great variability of results that we can see in the literature. Powers et al 1982[2] found a sensitivity of 43%, Davis et col 1980[3] found a sensitivity of 75% and Goldman et col[4] report a sensitivity of 51% for the detection of atheromatous plaques.

Although most of the authors demonstrate activity in the evolved plaques, the usefulness of labeled platelets for detecting early lesions has not been established. Some authors have employed radiolabeled low density lipoprotein as a tracer for detecting metabolically active plaques. The experience in animals published by Lees et al in 1985[6] using 99mTc-LDL and the one made by Virgolini et col 1991[10] using 125-I-LDL show intense activity in the damaged artery.

Radiolabeled LDL has also been employed in hipercholesterolemics patients and patients with atherosclerotic disease, Lees et col 1985[12], Sinzinger et col 1986[13], Ryan et col 1988[14], Ginsberg et col 1990[15] and Virgolini et col 1991[16]. All of them conclude that there is activity in the atheromatous plaques and that the activity accumulation depends in part on the number of foam cells. Although these studies are promising, autologous LDL are tedious, expensive and difficult to isolate. So, other components of atheromatous plaque have been investigated as potential scintigraphic tracers.

Because of the important role of foam cells in the formation of plaques and because these cells expressed Fc receptors on the surface, Fischman et al thought that Immunoglobulin G might be a good tracer[17]. They demonstrated the utility of HIG and Fc fragment in detecting experimental atherosclerosis.

On the other hand the study made by Carrio et al[23] in rabbits, with injured arteries showed HIG activity in arteries with injury but without atheromatous plaque. They conclude that the activity seen in the arteries with atheromatous plaque might be produced by the inflammatory process secondary to the lesion, independent of the Fc receptor mechanism of the foam cells that are in the atheromatous plaque.

Our results with HIG showed a better accuracy (78%), compared to the radiolabeled-platelets, in the detection of atheromatous lesions. In spite of that, we do not know if the activity is due to the foam cells in the atheromatous plaque or to the local inflammatory process secondary to the atheromatous disease.

Because of the small number of patients that we have studied with HIG, statistics are not valuable. Larger studies are needed.

CONCLUSIONS

1. 111In-labeled platelets scintigraphy does not seem to be useful in evaluating the activity of atheromatous lesions in carotid arteries.

2. Though only 7 patients have been studied, 99mTc-HIG scintigraphy seems more useful. Image quality was better and it allows the identification of 75% of atheromatous lesions.

3. However further studies are necessary to elucidate whether it expresses inflammation or atheromatous activity.

REFERENCES

1. ML.Thakur, LL.Walsh, HL.Malech, A.Gottschalk. Indium111-labeled human platelets: Improved method,efficacy and evaluation. *J.Nucl.Med* 22: 381-385 (1981).
2. W.Powers, BA.Siegel, HH.Davis, CJ.Mathias, HB Clark, MJ.Welch. Indium-111 platelet scintigraphy in cerebrovascular disease. *Neurology* 32: 938-943 (1982).
3. HH.Davis, BA Siegel, LA:Sherman, WA Heaton, TP.Naidich, JH Joist, MJ.Welch. Scintigraphy detection of carotid atherosclerosis with Indium-111-labelled autologous platelets. *Circulation* 61: 982-988 (1980).
4. M.Goldman, JO.Leung, A.Aukland, RJ.Haeker, Z.Drolc, CN.McCollum. 111-Indium platelet imaging. Doppler spectral analysis and angiography compared in patients with transient cerebral ischemia. *Stroke* 14: 752-756 (1983).
5. H.Henningsen. Platelet scintigraphy of the carotid artery: comparison with the histology of thrombendarterectomy specimens.In: K.Poeck, Ringelstein (eds).New trends in diagnosis and management of stroke.Springer-Verlag, Heidelberg New York.
6. R.Lees, H.Garabedian, A.M.Lees, D.J.Schumacher, A.Miller, J.Isaacsohn, W.Strauss. Technetium-99m Low density lipoproteins: Preparation and biodistribution. *J.Nucl.Med.* 26: 1056-1062 (1985).
7. Vallabhajosula, M.Paidi, JJ.Badimon, N.Le, J.Goldsmith, V.Fuster, H.Ginsberg. Radiotracers for low density lipoprotein biodistribution studies in vivo: Technetium-99m low density lipoprotein versus radioiodinated low density lipoprotein preparations. *J.Nucl.Med* 29: 1237-1245 (1988).
8. J.Rosen, P.Butler, G.Meinken, T.Wang, R.Ramakrishnan, S.Srivastava, P.Alderson, H.Ginsberg. Indium-111 labeled LDL: A potencial agent for imaging Atherosclerotic disease and lipoprotein biodistribution. *J.Nucl.Med.* 31: 343-350 (1990).
9. S.Vallabhajosula, S.Goldsmith. 99mTc-Low density lipoprotein : Intracellularly trapped radiotracer for noninvasive imaging of low density lipoprotein metabolism in vivo. *Seminars in Nuclear Medicine*, vol XX,n 1, 68-79 (1990).
10. I.Virgolini, P.Angelberger, J.O'Grady, H. Sinzinger. Low density lipoprotein labelling characterizes experimentally induced atherosclerotic lesions in rabbits in vivo as to presence of foam cells and endothelial coverage. *Eur.J.Nucl.Med.* 18: 944-947 (1991).
11. R.Lees, A.Lees,W.Strauss. External imaging of human atherosclerosis. *J. Nucl. Med.* 24: 154 - 156 (1983).
12. R.Lees, A.Lees, H.Strauss, J.Isaacsohn, M.Barlai-Kovach, A.Fishman, K.McKusick, H.Garabedian. The distribution and metabolism of 99mTc labeled low density lipoprotein in human subjects. *J.Nucl.Med.* 26.n5.(1985).
13. H.Sinzinger, J.Kaliman, P.Angelberger, P.Fitscha, H.Bergmann,R.Höfer. Radiolabeled human LDL for the diagnosis of in vivo kinetics and the increased entry into the arterial wall in human. Nuklearmedizin. Ed. H.Schmidt, D.Emrich.F.K.Schattauer Verlag.Stuttgart-New York (1986).
14. J.Ryan, P.Harper, R.Hay, K.Williams, K.Lathrop, V.Stark R.Fleming. Human biodistribution of I-123 and Tc99m labeled LDL. *J.Nucl.Med* 29.N5 (1985).
15. H.Ginsberg,S.Goldsmith, S.Vallabhajosula. Noninvasive imaging of 99mTechnetium labeled low density lipoprotein uptake by tendom xantomas in hypercholesterolemic patients. *Arteriosclerosis* 10: 256-262 (1990).
16. I.Virgolini, F.Rauscha, G.Lupatelli, A.Ventura, J.O'Grady, H.Sinzinger. Autologous low-density-lipoprotein labelling allows characterization of human atherosclerotic lesions in vivo as to presence of foam cells and endothelial coverage. *Eur.J.Nucl.Med* 18: 948-951 (1991).
17. A.Fischman, R.Rubin, B.Khaw, P.Kramer, R.Wilkinson, M.Ahmad, M.Needelman, E.Locke, N.Nosull, W.Staruss. Radionuclide imaging of experimental atherosclerosis with nonspecific polyclonal immunoglobulin G. *J.Nucl.Med.* 30: 1095-1100 (1989).
18. B.Khaw, E.Calenoff, E.Chen, S.O'Donell, N.Nossiff, W.Strauss. Localization of experimental atherosclerotic lesion with monoclonal antibody Z2D3. *J.Nucl.Med.*32 N5 (1991).
19. A.Fischman, R.Rubin, J.White, E.Locke, R.Wilkinson, M Nedelman, R.Callahan, B.A.Khaw, W.Strauss. Localization of Fc and Fab fragments of nonspecific polyclonal IgG at focal sites of inflammation. *J.Nucl.Med*; 31: 1199-1205 (1990).
20. M.Juweid, W.Strauss, H.Yaoita, R.Rubin, A.Fischman. Accumulation of immunoglobulin G at focal sites of inflamation. *Eur.J.Nucl.Med* 19: 159-165 (1992).

21. A.Serafini, I.Garty, R.Vargas-Cubas, A.Friedman, D.Rauh, M.Neptune, L.Landress,G.Sfakianakis. Clinical evaluation of a Scintigraphic method for diagnosing inflamations/infections using Indium-111-labeled nonspecific human IgG. *J.Nucl.Med*; 32: 2227-2232 (1991).

22. J.Martin-Comin, M.Roca, JM.Griño, C.Paradell, A.Caralps. In111-oxine autologous labeled platelets in the diagnosis of kidney graft rejection. *Cli.Nucl.Med*. 8: 7-10 (1983).

23. I. Carrió, L. Berná, L. Prat, M. Roca, V. Riembau, G. Torres, D. Duncker and M. Storch. 111In-polyclonal IgG and 125I LDL uptake in experimental arterial wall injury. *J. Nucl. Med*. 33: 845 (1992). (abstract book).

DIAGNOSIS OF VASCULAR GRAFT INFECTION BY 99mTc-HMPAO-LABELED LEUKOCYTE SCAN

E. Prats, J. Banzo, M.D. Abós, F. García, M. Delgado, T. Escalera, T. García Miralles and R. Gastón

Nuclear Medicine Department
University Hospital, Zaragoza
Spain

Prosthetic vascular graft infection is one of the most serious and potencially catastrophic complications in vascular surgery. The symptons are usually nonspecific, and the diagnosis of sinthetic vascular graft infection is difficult by conventional radiographic methods.

The aim of this study was to determine the usefulness of 99mTc-HMPAO-labeled leukocyte scan in the diagnosis of prosthetic vascular graft infection.

METHODS AND MATERIALS

We have performed 62 scans in 51 patients with vascular graft. Vascular reconstructive surgery was due to abdominal aortic aneurysm in 11 patients, oclusive atherosclerotic disease in 39 patients, and in 1 patient was due to vascular injury.

We studied a total of 54 grafts. The most frecuent type was the aorto-bifemoral graft, present in 40 patients, axilo-bifemoral was present in 4 patients, ilio-femoral in 3, femoro-femoral in 2, axilo-femoral in 2, femoro-popliteal in 1, aorto-femoral in 1 and ilio-popliteal in 1.

Patients were evaluated from 7 days to 13 years after their graft placement. Thirty-seven scans were performed due to graft infection suspiction, and 25 were control patients.

Leukocytes were labeled with 99mTc-HMPAO according to Hammersmith Hospital method[1], and scintigraphic images were obtained at 30 minutes, 3 hours, and, ocasionally, 24 hours. A whole-body scan was performed at 3 hours.

We have considered to be evidence of graft infection all persistent increased uptake along the expected area of the graft.

Correlative CT studies were done in 11 cases, and 6 confirmed infected grafts were also evaluated with 99mTc-HIG. A perigraft fluid and/or gas collection was considered as evidence of graft infection on CT.

The diagnosis of infected graft was confirmed by culture in all cases.

Radiolabeled Blood Elements, Edited by J. Martin-Comin
Plenum Press, New York, 1994

RESULTS

Vascular graft infection was present in 18 patients. In the culture, staphylococcus aureus was found in 9 cases (50% of all the positive cultures), corinebacterium in 3, pseudomona aeruginosa in 2 and other pathogens were found in 4 cases (S. aureus + enterococcus durans in 1, enterobacter + corinebacterium in 1, enterobacter + actinobacter in 1 and E. coli + klebsiella pneumoniae in 1).

All the 18 graft infections were detected by 99mTc-HMPAO-labeled leukocyte scan, showing an early (30 m) uptake of labeled leukocytes. No false-positive scans were found. There were 44 negative scans in patients who subsequently showed to have noninfected grafts, so, no false-negative scans were found. The sensibility and specificity of the scan in the detection of prosthetic graft infection were100%.

We also detected extragraft migration of labeled leukocytes in 2 pelvic absceses, 2 infected fistulas, 3 ischemic colitis, 1 infected hematoma, 1 soft tissue infection and 1 non-infected hematoma. One superficial groin infection presented negative scan. Five pseudoaneurysm didn't show scintigraphic evidence of graft infection.

CT was also performed in 11 patients with graft infection suspicion. All the 6 vascular graft infection of this group were detected by 99mTc-HMPAO-labeled leukocyte scan, whereas CT was positive only in 4. A pelvic abscess was detected by both methods.

99mTc-HIG scan was performed in 6 confirmed infected grafts. Only 2 infected grafts were detected with 99mTc-HIG scan.

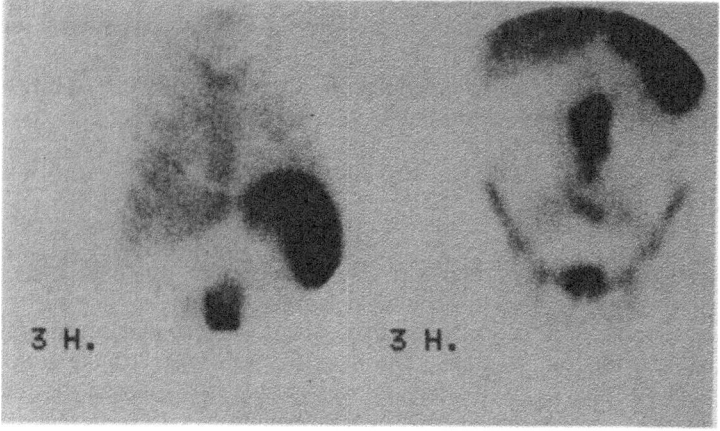

Figure 1. Infected aorto-bifemoral graft (E. coli + klebsiella pneumoniae): Intense uptake of 99mTc-HMPAO-labeled leukocytes along aortic and left ilio-femoral limbs of the graft.

DISCUSSION

The progress of reconstructive vascular surgery has led to an increased use of synthetic prosthetic materials. Although the incidence of infection after implantation is low (2%-6%) these numerically few patients present serious problems with respect to treatment of the infection. These problems are reflected by the high rates of amputation and mortality[2].

Early infections usually appear first in subcutaneous positions and become apparent by the discharge of pus. Late infections may present as graft-enteric erosion or fistula, or as ill-defined abdominal pain and fever.

The diagnosis of sinthetic vascular graft infection is difficult by conventional radiographic methods. Promising results using 111In-leukocyte scintigraphy have been reported[3-9]. In this paper we determine the usefulness of 99mTc-HMPAO-labeled leukocyte scan in the diagnosis of vascular graft infection. All the 18 graft infection present in our study were detected by 99mTc-HMPAO-labeled leukocyte scan. No false-positive or

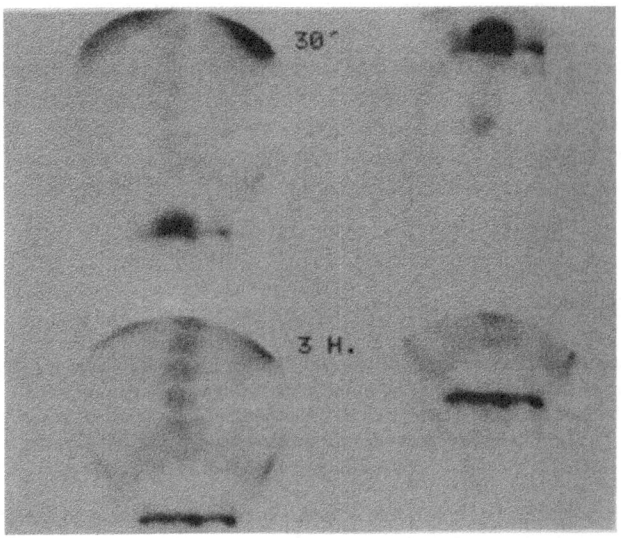

Figure 2. Infected femoro-femoral graft (E. aureus): Early and persistent uptake along the infected graft.

false-negative scans were found. So, the sensibility and specificity of the scintigraphy in the detection of vascular graft infection was100%. Similar results were reported by Vorne et al[10].

We also detected extragraft migration of labeled leukocytes in 2 pelvic absceses, 2 infected fistulas, 3 ischemic colitis, 1 infected hematoma, 1 soft tissue infection and 1 non-infected hematoma. In our 2 patients with hematoma the localization of the hematoma was far from the prosthetic area, and so, we could evaluate the graft without problems.

Five pseudoaneurysm didn't show scintigraphic evidence of graft infection. Usually, pseudoaneurysms have been considered a potential cause of false positive results in labeled leukocyte scintigraphy[11]. In the 99mTc-HMPAO-leukocyte scan pseudoaneurysms are always visualizated like a hot spot in the dynamic study, which is easily detected in very early (5 m) and early (30 m) images, whereas significant uptake of labeled leukocytes is never seen in delayed (3 h) scans. The most likely explanation for false positive results is the labeling of "contaminating" platelets and eritrocytes. In the HMPAO scan, the contamination of platelets and eritrocytes is lesser, and in our hospital, if we suspect pseudoaneurysm, we also perform a dynamic study and images at 5 minutes.

CT has been shown to be effective in detecting graft infections, but the CT features of graft infection, however, can be non-specific[12]. We performed CT in 11 patients with graft infection suspicion. A perigraft fluid and/or gas collection was considered as evidence of graft infection on CT ("specific findings"). All the 6 vascular graft infection of this group were detected by 99mTc-HMPAO-labeled leukocyte scan, whereas CT was positive only in 4. A pelvic abscess was detected by both methods.

Indium-111-labeled human polyclonal inmunoglobulin G (HIG) has been used in the diagnosis of vascular graft infection with promising results[13]. We performed 99mTc-HIG scan in 6 confirmed infected grafts. Only 2 were detected with 99mTc-HIG scan. In our experience, the most important problem in the evaluation of vascular grafts with 99mTc-HIG is the high vascular pool which difficults the interpretation of the images.

In conclusion: The 99mTc-HMPAO-labeled leukocyte scan is the most accurate and valuable diagnostic method for evaluation of suspected prosthetic vascular graft infection. All the positive scans showed an early uptake of labeled leukocytes. No false positive 99mTc-HMPAO-labeled leukocyte scans were obtained in the evaluation of the vascular graft. In our experience, 99mTc-HIG imaging is not useful in the detection of vascular graft infection.

REFERENCES

1. Peters AM, Dampure HJ, Osman S et al. Clinical experience with 99mTc-hexamethylpropylenamineoxine for labelling leukocytes and imaging inflammation. *Lancet*; 2: 946-949 (1986).
2. Lorentzen JE, Nielsen OM, Arendrup H et al. Vascular graft infection: An analysis of sixty-two graft infections in 2411 consecutively implanted synthetic vascular grafts. *Surgery*; 98:81-86 (1985).
3. Stevick CA, Fawcet HD. Aortoiliac graft infection: Detection by leukocyte scan. *Arch Surg*; 116: 939 (1981).
4. Wilson DG, Seabold JE, Lieberman LM. Detection of aortoarterial graft infections by leukocyte scintigraphy. *Clin Nucl Med*; 8: 421-423 (1983).
5. Williamson MR, Boyd ChM, Read RC et al. 111-In-labeled leukocytes in the detection of prosthetic vascular graft infection. *AJR* ; 147: 173-176 (1986).
6. Berridge DC, Earnshow JJ, Frier M et al. 111In-labeled leukocyte imaging in vascular graft infection. *Br J Surg*; 76: 41-44 (1989).
7. Becker W, Dusel W, Berger P et al. The 111In-granulocyte scan in prosthetic vascular graft infections: Imagin technique and results. *Eur J Nucl Med*; 13: 225-229 (1987).
8. Forstrom LA, Dewanjee MK, Chowdhry BS et al. Indium-111 labeled purified granulocytes in the diagnosis of synthetic vascular graft infection. *Clin Nucl Med*; 13: 859-862 (1988).
9. Mark AS, McCarthy SM, Moss AA et al. Detection of abdominal aortic graft infection: Comparasion of CT and In-labeled white blood cell scans. *AJR*; 144:315-318 (1985).
10. Vorne M, Laitinen J, Lehtonen J et al. 99mTc- leukocyte scintigraphy in the prosthetic vascular graft infections. *Nucl. Med*; 28: 95-99 (1989).
11. Gilbert BR, Cerqueira MD, Vea HW et al. Indium-111 labeled leukocyte uptake: False-positive results in noninfected pseudoaneurysms. *Radiology*; 158:761-763 (1986).
12. Johnson KK, Russ PD, Bair JH et al. Diagnosis of synthetic vascular graft infection: Comparasion of CT ang Gallium scan. *AJR*; 154: 405-409 (1990).
13. La Muragla GM, Fishman AJ, Straus HW et al. Utility of the indium-111 labeled human inmunoglobulin G scan for the detection of focal vascular graft infection. *J Vasc Surg*; 10:20-28 (1989).

LABELED PLATELETS IN IDIOPATHIC THROMBOCYTOPENIC PURPURA

A. Moisan, T. Lamy, A. Devillers, J. Le Cloirec, P.Y. Le Prise and
J.Y. Herry

CAC - CHU - Rennes, France

Idiopathic thrombocytopenia purpura (ITP) in adults is a relatively common hematologic problem. Splenectomy is seen as therapeutic means to increase the incidence of definitive remission in patients with chronic ITP. The predictive factors at short and long term success of splenectomy are still ill-defined and questioned[13].

The diagnosis of chronic ITP is one of exclusion. The classically accepted ITP criteria[11] are :
- isolated thrombocytopenia (platelets $< 50 \times 10^9/l$) with normal leukocyte and erythrocyte counts, bone marrow aspirate with no quantitative cytological abnormality and normal or elevated megakaryocyte count ;
- no clinical or echographic splenomegaly ;
- no evidence of hereditary abnormality ;
- no signs of any situation that could be associated with thrombocytopenia ; drugs, viruses (CMV, HBs, HIV, EBV) , systemic lupus erythematosis, leukemia, lymphoma or disseminated intravascular coagulation.

Antiplatelet antibody IgG (PAIgG) measurements are positive in 60 to 90 % of the cases. This is a non specific finding, present in many other types of immune and nonimmune thrombocytopenia.

Most of the patients are treated with prednisone at 0,25 to 2 mg/kg/day for at least 30 days. Primary failures (no increase in platelet count above $50 \times 10^9/l$) and relapses led to resumption of steroid therapy, danazol, vincristine or high dose immmunoglobulins (400 mg/kg/day for 5 days). Persistence of severe and drug resistant thrombocytopenia beyond 6 months after diagnosis led to propose splenectomy in nearly 50 % of cases[1]. This period is shortened for patients at risk, those with hypertension, over 65 years old or in the presence of threatening thrombocytopenia ($< 20 \times 10^9/l$). It's generally in these circumstances that platelet kinetics could take place. Over the last 30 years number of studies have tried to define predictive factors of the efficacy of splenectomy such as subject's young age[3, 4, 5, 10], the quality of initial response to steroid therapy[3, 14] and the results of labeled platelet kinetics[7, 15, 16, 17, 21, 24].

The main interests of kinetics studies are to confirm ITP diagnosis (95 % cases) with a lifespan < 4 days and specify the sequestration site. In less than 5 % of cases, lifespan is normal, so the diagnosis of ITP is challenged despite a normal bone marrow aspiration, a preleukemia syndrome or pure refractory thrombocytopenia can be suggested[18].

Radiolabeled Blood Elements, Edited by J. Martin-Comin
Plenum Press, New York, 1994

Platelets kinetics studies with chromium 51 (51Cr) can only be performed in autologous transfusion, when thrombocytopenia is moderate (platelets $> 50 \times 10^9/1$) leading most often to the exploration with donor platelets (risk of isoimmunization and viral transmission). With 51 Cr, however, labeling efficiency is low (< 15 %) and external counts are performed with a probe which preclude quantitative measurements of the uptake in spleen, liver and heart. As early as 1976, platelet kinetics were studied by labeling with a liposoluble marker, 111Indium (111In) oxinate[26] or tropolonate[2]. The advantages of 111In over 51Cr are well known : kinetics studies with autologous platelets even in presence of severe thrombocytopenia (platelets : $10 \times 10^9/1$), high labeling efficiency (50 to 90 %) and the ability to perform a biodistribution study with gammacamera. The ICSH[9] published new recommandations in 1988, based on the method of THAKUR et al[26].

According to the degree of thrombocytopenia, 50 to 100 ml of blood are collected and acidified by an ACD-A solution (20 %). The platelet rich plasma (PRP) is obtained by one or two slow centrifugations (150 G, 20 min). A rapid centrifugation at 900 G isolates the platelet pellet which is preserved in less than 1 ml of plasma poor in platelets (PPP). Three to 5 MBq of 111In oxinate or tropolonate are added drop wise to the platelet button. After incubation (5-10 min) the platelet solution is washed with 10 ml of PPP at pH 6,5. For 10×10^{10} platelets in solution, labeling efficiency raised 90 %.

Lifespan is determined from 5 to 10 blood samples taken from 15 min after injection until radioactivity disappeared. The contamination by other blood cells must be calculated (generally < 10 %). The recovery rate at equilibrium is normal varying from 50 to 70 %. In ITP, the lifespan calculated according a monoexponential, a multihit or a linear model is shortened 1 to 4 days. The shape of the survival curve is exponential in most cases. The mean platelet turnover is markdely lower than normal[8]. This parameter has to be analyzed according to the medical treatment underway at the time of the study especially prednisone, since this therapy may influence the rate of platelet production[6]. The predictive value for splenectomy efficacy, of platelet turnover' increase, reported by Siegel[24] is non evident.

Dynamic images and time activity curves over spleen, liver and heart in posterior view are performed with a large field of view gamma camera peaked for 173 and 247 kev and interfaced with a computer. At equilibrium mean 111In activity in the liver (10 to 15 %) and the spleen (25 to 30 %) correspond to that of normal subjects. PETERS et al[19] attempt to analyse factors concerning platelet destruction : radioactivity present in the spleen depends on 3 variables : splenic blood flow, intrasplenic transit time and platelet destruction. In ITP splenic platelet pooling appears to be normal.

The first hour and daily thereafter static images or whole body scanning can be realized to quantify late platelet destruction in organs. Different methods have been proposed to calculate the late 111In platelet sequestration. Localization studies performed using 51Cr labeled give counts rate from small non imaging probes variably positioned over the liver, spleen and heart. Ratios spleen/heart and liver/heart are calculated daily.

From static images of 111In labeled platelets, regions of interest (ROI) over spleen and liver give the uptake or the decrease of radioactivity in each organ after correction of decay of 111In. A quantification from ROI in anterior and posterior views has been proposed by VAN ROONEN[27]. The geometrical mean (GM) is an accurate and practical method for the in vivo quantification of 111In platelets in organs. Quantification from whole body images, using the GM method is interesting[25], but the time-consuming gammacamera is too important to be proposed in routine.

Multicentric studies of sequestration sites seemed to be somewhat contradictory. The spleen appears to be the preferential site of platelet destruction although in variable proportions (28 to 85 %)[15, 17, 21, 23]. Mixed or mainly hepatic uptake or diffuse uptake are consequently variable. The different methods used to label platelets (autologous or homologous, 51Cr or 111In) and to quantify platelet sequestration (probes, numeric images) could explain some discording results.

The table 1 summarizes the results of main series studying the correlation of sequestration sites with effectiveness of splenectomy, in short term and long term follow-up. Some reports indicate the value of platelet sequestration site : high percentage of total remission (85 to 90 %) after splenectomy, associated to a splenic uptake[5, 6, 7, 12, 16, 17, 21]. Other studies contradict these conclusions[8, 22, 23, 24], with relatively good results in cases of mixed or hepatic uptake.

Table 1 - Results of main series analysing the correlation of sequestration sites with effectiveness of splenectomy

Number of patients	Method (isologous platelets vs autologous platelets)	Splenectomized patients	Duration of assessment (months)	% Complete remission according to the sequestration site			Ref
				splenic	mixed	hepatic	
563	51Cr:iso	206	≥ 6	81	38	9	(16)
34	51Cr: iso	34	3-56	92	87		(23)
197	51Cr: iso: 164	111	≥ 12	80		45	(7)
190	111In: auto	64	6	98	40	0	(15)
181	51Cr: iso: 133 111In: auto 48	181	≥ 3	83		42	(5)
59	111In: auto	21	< 1	60	66	66	(24)
222	111In: auto	103	6	86	55	7	(17)
96	111In: auto: 78 iso: 18	36	?	CR 29/36, 6/7 failures without splenic sequestration			(21)
105	111In: auto	51	6-72	87	22	0	(12)

The total remission after splenectomy in large series averages 70 %. This result could be improved (> 85 %) when there is a splenic sequestration site confirmed by 111In autologous platelet kinetics. A splenic uptake appears as a good predictive factor of effectiveness of splenectomy, and platelet kinetics should be performed before surgery. The low success rate in the cases with mixed or hepatic sequestration seems to be a valuable predictive index to exclude splenectomy.

In conclusion, the lifespan study of 111In labeled platelets in patients with persistance of severe and drug resistant thrombocytopenia beyond 6 months after diagnosis of ITP or sooner for patients at risk, presents 2 mean interests. First the study confirms the diagnosis of ITP in most cases (95 %) and can show that some thrombocytopenias with usual clinical and biological criteria of ITP are not necessarily caused by excessive destruction (< 5 % cases). Secondly, it guides clinicians in deciding whether or not splenectomy should be performed, as the chances of success are greatly reduced, in our opinion, in cases of mixed or hepatic sequestration.

REFERENCES

1. Berchtold P, McMillan R. Therapy of chronic idiopathic thrombocytopenic purpura in adults. *Blood*; 74: 2309-2317 (1989).
2. Danpure HJ, Osman S, Peters AM. Labelling autologous platelets with 111In tropolonate for platelet kinetic studies : limitations imposed by thrombocytopenia. *Eur. J. Haematol.*; 45: 223-230 (1990)
3. Difino SM, Lachant NA, Kirshner JJ and al. Adult idiopathic thrombocytopenic purpura : clinical findings and response to therapy. *Am. J. Med*; 69: 430-442 (1980).
4. Fabris F, Zanatta N, Casonato A and al. Response to splenectomy in idiopathic thrombocytopenic purpura: prognostic value of the clinical and laboratory evaluation. *Acta Haemat.*; 81: 28-33 (1989).
5. Fenaux P, Caulier MT, Hirschauer MC and al. Reevaluation of the prognostic factors for splenectomy in chronic idiopathic thrombocytopenic purpura (ITP) : a report on 181 cases. *Eur. J. Haematol.*; 42: 259-264 (1989).
6. Gernsheimer T, Stratton J, Ballem PJ, Slichter SJ. Mechanisms of response to treatment in autoimmune thrombocytopenic purpura. *N. Engl. J. Med.*; 320: 974-980 (1989).
7. Gugliotta L, Isacchi G, Guarini A and al. Chronic idiopathic thrombocytopenic purpura (ITP) : site of platelet sequestration and results of splenectomy. A study of 197 patients. *Scandinavian Journal of Haematol.*; 26: 407-412 (1981).
8. Heyns A du P, Badenhorst PN, Lotter MG and al. Platelet turnover and kinetics in immune thrombocytopenic purpura : results with autologous 111In-labeled platelets and homologous 51Cr-labeled platelets differ. *Blood*; 67: 86-92 (1986).
9. International Commitee for standardization in Hematology panel on diagnostic applications of Radionuclides (ICSH). *J. Nucl. Med.*; 29: 564-566 (1988).
10. Julia A, Araguas C, Rossello J and al. Lack of useful clinical predictors of response to splenectomy in patients with chronic idiopathic thrombocytopenic purpura. *Br. J. Haematol.*; 76: 250-255 (1990).
11. Karpatkin S. Autoimmune thrombocytopenic purpura. *Blood*; 56: 329-343 (1980).
12. Lamy T, Moisan A, Dauriac C, Ghandour C, Morice P, Le Prise PY. Splenectomy in idiopathic thrombocytopenic purpura : ITS correlation with the sequestration of autologous indium-111-labeled platelets. *J. Nucl. Med.*, 34: 182-186 (1993).
13. McVerry BA. Management of idiopathic thrombocytopenic purpura in adults. *Br. J. Haematol.*; 59: 203-208 (1985).
14. Mintz S, Petersen SR, Cheson B and al. Splenectomy for immune. Thrombocytopenic Purpura. *Arch. Surg.*; 116: 645-650 (1981).
15. Moisan A, Le Prise PY, Le Cloirec J and al. 111-Indium labelled platelets in thrombocytopenic purpura survival and biodistribution studied with scintillation camera. A review of 485 patients. In Kessler Ch, Hardeman M.R., Henningsen H. and Petrovici J.N. (Eds), Clinical application of radiolabelled platelets, Kluwer Academic Publishers 1990; 248-257.
16. Najean Y, Ardaillou N. The sequestration site of platelets in idiopathic thrombocytopenic purpura : its correlation with the results of splenectomy. *Br. J. Haematol.*; 21: 153-164 (1971).
17. Najean Y, Dufour Y, Rain JD, Toubert ME. The site of platelet destruction in thrombocytopenic purpura as a predictive index of the efficacy of splenectomy. *Br. J. Haematol.*; 79: 271-276 (1991).
18. Najean Y, Lecompte T. Chronic pure thrombocytopenia in elderly patients. *Cancer*; 64: 2506-2510 (1989).
19. Peters AM, Saverymuttu SH, Wonke B and al. The interpretation of platelet kinetic studies for the identification of sites of abnormal platelet destruction. *Br. J. Haematol*; 57: 637-649 (1984).
20. Pizzuto J, Ambriz R. Therapeutic experience on 934 adults with idiopathic thrombocytopenic purpura: multicentric trial of the cooperative latin american group on hemostasis and thrombosis. *Blood*; 64: 1179-1183 (1984).
21. Reiffers J, Vuillemin L, Broustet A, Ducassou D. Kinetic study of Indium-111 labelled platelets in idiopathic thrombocytopenic purpura (in french). *Nouv. Press Med.*; 11: 2335-2338 (1982).
22. Richards JDM, Thompson DS. Assessment of thrombocytopenic patients for splenectomy. *J. Clin. Pathol.*; 32: 1248-1252 (1979).
23. Ries CA. Platelets kinectics in auto-immune thrombocytopenia : relation between splenic platelet sequestration and response to splenectomy. *Ann. Intern. Med.*; 86: 194-195 (1977)
24. Siegel RS, Rae JL, Barth S and al. Platelet survival and turnover :Important factors in predicting response to splenectomy in immune thrombocytopenic purpura. *Am. J. Hematol.*; 30: 206-212 (1989).
25. Stratton JR, Ballem PJ, Gernheimer T, Cerqueira M, Slichton SJ. Platelet destruction in autoimmune thrombocytopenic purpura : Kinetics and clearance of Indium 111-labeled autologous platelets. *JNM,*;30: 629-737 (1989).
26. Thakur ML, Welch MJ, Joist JH, Coleman RI. Indium-111-labeled platelets : studies on preparation and evaluation of in vitro and in vivo functions. *Thrombo Res.*; 9: 345-357 (1976).

27. Vanreenen O, Lotter MG, Heyns AP, Kock F, Herbst C. Kotle H, Pieters H, Minnaar PC, Badenhorst PN. Quantification of the destribution of 111In labelled platelets in organs. Eur. J. Nucl. Med.; 780-784 (1982).

CLINICAL ROLE OF RADIONUCLIDE BASED TECHNOLOGY FOR THROMBUS IMAGING IN 1992

M.D. Ezekowitz

Yale University School of Medicine
Cardiovascular Medicine Section 3 FMP
New Haven

INTRODUCTION

Radionuclide imaging of thrombosis became a reality when Thakur and McAfee in the mid 1970's, were successful in labelling platelets with 111indium. Since that time, competing technologies with the potential application of directly imaging thrombosis have evolved in parallel with radionuclide imaging. These technologies include; magnetic resonance imaging and ultrasound in its various forms. These non-invasive techniques have all competed with invasive contrast fluoroscopic techniques and in the case of venous thrombosis with another non-invasive technique impedance plethysmography. Since the symposium has dealt exclusively with radionuclide based techniques, I felt it important to take a step backwards and to describe the advantages and disadvantages of radionuclide imaging as compared to available technology in 1992.

CORONARY THROMBOSIS

In the area of cardiac investigation it is clear that the most rewarding application of these technologies would be the rapid identification of coronary thrombi. Numerous attempts have been made to image coronary thrombi with radionuclide based techniques. We were successful in a single case, using 111Indium labelled platelets. This patient had massive symmetric left ventricular hypertrophy as a consequence of unrecognized hypertension. Successfully imagingwas only possible because the extra cardiac coronary vessels could be separated from the cardiac blood pool. This, however, proved to be an exceptional situation and in spite of the use of tomographic imaging and a variety of MRI and Ultrasound subtraction techniques, the reliable identification of cooronary thrombosis using radionuclide based technologies has been elusive.

Radiolabeled Blood Elements, Edited by J. Martin-Comin
Plenum Press, New York, 1994

INTRACARDIAC MASSES

We showed in 1979 that using radiolabelled platelets it was possible to image, left ventricular thrombi. Simultaneously, several studies found that the rapidly evolving technology of two-dimensional echocardiography also provided a convenient and accurate method of identifying left ventricular clot. Echocardiography is not only useful in identifying the clot, but aslso identifying the predisposing condition, that of either regional or global reduction in left ventricular function. The disadvantage of radionuclide techniques is that the images have to be acquired 48-72 hours after the injection of labelled platelets and that the techniques rely on the hematological activity of the thrombus. John Stratton showed that active thrombi, as identified by platelet imaging, were more likely to embolize than thrombi that were seen by ultrasound and had negative images by platelet imaging. Thus, with the wide availability of ultrasound and its proven diagnostic accuracy, platelet imaging has been superseded by ultrasound for the clinical identification of clots in the ventricle.

An area of investigation needing active attention is that of imaging thrombosis in the left atrium. Transesophageal echocardiography is the only technique that is currently available for the identification of clots in the body or left atrial appendage. This technique is minimally invasive requiring esophageal intubation and imaging of the heart while the patient is sedated. Attempts at using radionuclide based technologies to identify clots in the left atrium have been unsuccessful. Magnetic resonance imaging can be used to identify thrombi in either the left ventricle or left atrium; however, it is an expensive technology requiring transportation of the patient to the imaging suite and is not widely used for this purpose.

DEEP VEIN THROMBOSIS

Three technologies compete against venography for the diagnosis of venous thrombosis. These are duplex ultrasound, impedance plethysmography and platelet imaging. Platelet imaging has been useful as a surveillance tool in high risk postoperative patients. Labelled platelets can be injected immediately after surgery and because of the half-life of the platelets and the radioisotope, 111Indium can be imaged for at least 5 to 7 days after injection. Ultrasound is useful for the diagnosis of acute venous thrombosis. Three criteria are used; lack of compressibility of the vein, the demonstration of a thrombus or the failure to identify an increase blood flow within the vein with compression of the calf. Using these three criteria the diagnosis is usually accurate wiht sensitivities and specificities in the nineties. Ultrasound is suitable for study of patients in the intensive care unit because it is portable. The major limitation of this technology is the technical quality of the study. Currently it is the test of choice for the diagnosis of venous thrombosis. Magnetic resonance imaging is highly accurate for the diagnosis of venous thrombosis, allowing accurate detection of thrombi from the ankle through to the right atrium. Images can be acquired in twenty minutes. The disadvantage of the technology is its costs, the availability of equipment and the fact that the patient has to be transported to the imaging suite. It is therefore, not widely used for this purpose.

SUMMARY

In summary the ideal radionuclide label has not been achieved. The ideal label should have a short and simple labelling procedure that can be used in most community hospitals. The label and its parent molecule should be non-toxic and the label should remain attached to the substrate and not elute. It should have a high affinity for its target and should be rapidly cleared from the circulation. This latter characteristic is the most difficult to achieve.

The promise for the future rests on the identification of coagulation factors other than those that have been currently used which may not circulate in the bloodstream but be adherent to the vessel wall. The use of peptides have theoretical advantage because of their rapid clearance time. However, it is important to recognize that the off-time of peptides is often so rapid that a continuous infusion of these agents needs to be achieved in order to maintain the peptide attached to its target. This would obviously provide a continuing background and therefore, in my view, is not the solution to solving the problem of optimizing the target to background ratio for high resolution imaging. It is possible that application of positron emission tomographic imaging might obviate this problem.

CLINICAL APPLICATIONS OF RADIOLABELED PLATELETS : KIDNEY AND PANCREAS TRANSPLANTATION

F. Lomeña and C. Piera

Nuclear Medicine
Hospital Clinic
University of Barcelona
Spain

INTRODUCTION

Since 1981 we have been using 111In-labeled platelets scintigraphy as evolutive control after renal and/or pancreas transplantation. From 1981 to 1986 we have used oxine to label platelets and in 1986 we changed the labeling agent introducing mercaptopyridine.

In our hospital the main indication for labeled platelets scan after renal and pancreas transplantation has been the early diagnosis of kidney and pancreas acute allograft rejection. Nowadays because of several factors which we will discuse later the labeled platelet scan is only used in pancreas transplantation and to discriminate the origin of fever in patients with irreversibly non-functioning renal graft.

EARLY DIAGNOSIS OF ACUTE RENAL GRAFT REJECTION

Early and accurate diagnosis of acute graft rejection (AR) is very important because it is neccessary to carry out a correct antirejection therapy before functional impairment has begun.

From 1981 to 1986 we have labeled the platelets with 111In-oxine using a method modified[1] from Thakur's[2] and the scans were obtained by the follow-up technique described by Sinzinger in Toronto in 1981. To evaluate the platelet uptake in the kiney allograft we calculated the platelet uptake index (PUI) as the relationship between activity in the region of interest over the graft and activity in a contralateral area.

The schedule of our follow-up technique is not complicated. A first labeling and reinjection of 111In-platelets (100 μCi) were performed 48-72 hours after transplantation. A daily scan during one week was obtained with a minimum of five scans. If the patients presented AR we continued the follow-up to valorate the evolution after therapy. In the patients without signs and simptoms of AR we continued the control with a new labeling and reinjection. A maximum of three labelings were used to complete the method.

Pathological platelet uptake was only seen in patients with AR[3]. The uptake appeared in most cases before renal functional impairment, simultaneously with other signs of AR as fever. We studied 170 patients under conventional immunossupresive therapy (azathioprine). The PUI was 1.0 ± 0.1 in the group with functioning graft and 1.1 ± 0.1 in cases of acute tubular necrosis. The PUI was higher for AR (2.0 ± 0.4) without difference between vascular and interstitial or cellular AR. After steroid antirejection therapy, the PUI became lower in cases of good evolutive response. This feature was typical for interstitial or non vascular AR. In cases of vascular AR with bad evolution after therapy the PUI did not decrease. Patients with chronic rejection had a PUI lower than in cases of AR (1.4 ± 0.3) and without significant difference in comparison with the non AR group.

In 40 patients treated with cyclosporine as immunossupresive therapy the PUIs were similar in non AR and AR groups. We did not find graft platelet uptake in cases of cyclosporine nephrotoxicity. The PUI in this group was 1.2 ± 0.1.

Since 1986 we have been using mercaptopyridine to label platelets following the method of Thakur[4]. Our labelling efficiency is 49.8 ± 18 ($n = 176$). The in vitro agregability of merc-labeled platelets is better than for oxine-labeled platelets[5]. The results for AR are similar than with oxine but the PUIs are significantly higher for merc (table 1).

Table 1

| | PUI | | |
	MERC	OXINE	
NO REJECTION	1.2 ± 0.2	1.1 ± 0.1 (n.s.)	($n = 29$)
ACUTE REJECTION	2.9 ± 1.8	1.8 ± 0.3 ($p < 0.001$)	($n = 37$)
CYCLOSPORINE NEPHROTOXICITY	1.1 ± 0.1	1.0 ± 0.1 (n.s.)	($n = 14$)

Labeled platelets scan has only two relative limitations using oxine or merc, abdominal hematomas[1,3] and thrombocytopenia[1,3]. Hematomas are frequent in the abdomen of patients in early postoperative transplantation and may cause false positive results. The use of a lateral view in the scan permits to differentiate the abdominal wall hematoma. Habitually the shape of hematomas is different from renal shape and it is easy to carry out a correct diagnosis. Thrombocytopenia can produce false negative results.

Our results are similar to others described by several authors and are different in interstitial AR and cyclosporine neprotoxicity[6,7]. Leithner et all reported pathological uptake in vascular AR but not in interstitial type and in cyclosporine toxicity he found PUI higher than in well-functioning grafts. These results probably are true for patients with AR treated with cyclosporine and prednisolone but in patients treated with azathioprine and prednisolone there is patological uptake in interstitial AR. The patological uptake in vascular AR is due to endothelial damage with intravascular thrombotic phenomena. Probably in intersticial AR there are loose thrombocyte aggregates into the lumen of vessels in combination with acute blast-cell infiltration[8]. These aggregates may be the cause of pathological uptake of labeled platelets and they disappear from the graft when the inflammation is overcome after steroid therapy.

The explanation for cyclosporine toxicity may be the doses used in immunossupresive therapy. When initially was introduced the doses of cyclosporine were considerably higher than are now and produced a microvascular arteriopathy with endothelial damage and endovascular thrombosis. Logically the PUI were higher than in well-functioning grafts. Now using lower doses of cyclosporine the toxicity is only a tubular impairment and it produces a PUI similar to those cases of acute tubular necrosis no different from well-functioning grafts.

During the period 1988-1992 the number of labeled platelets scan done for early AR diagnosis decreased dramatically. Several reasons there are implicated. The improvement in tissue typing and the changes in immunossupresive therapy have diminished the number and severity of AR. The availability to label platelets with 111In is not the same during all the week and the labeled platelets scan does not give functional information. Other non-isotopic techniques as doppler may allow an accurate and early diagnose of renal AR. Now we use the labeled platelets scan only when there are difficulties to establish a correct diagnosis of AR by other methods.

PANCREAS TRANSPLANTATION

We are using de same protocol for pancreas transplantation. A diffuse uptake in pancreas graft was seen in cases of AR. The scans became positive before changes in biochemical test. We did not have seen platelet uptake in normally functioning grafts. Venous thrombosis and hematomas have a focal aspect different to diffuse uptake of AR[9].

IMMUNOLOGICAL FEVER IN PATIENTS WITH IRREVERSIBLY NON-FUNCTIONING RENAL GRAFT

This is a new approach of labeled platelets in renal transplantation. Many patients on hemodialysis with irreversibly non-functioning renal allograft develop fever when immunossupresive therapy is at minimal doses or has been withdrawn. This prolonged fever may be due to persistence or reactivation of immunological phenomena of rejection. It also could be due to a systemic infectious disease or to have other etiology.

Many explorations and complementary techniques are necessary for an accurate diagnosis and to establish a correct therapy. If the fever has an immunological origin the definitive treatment could be the nephrectomy, when the fever does not appear with steroids.

PATIENTS AND CONTROLS

We have studied 40 patients (20 males) on hemodialysis (time on dialysis = 5.27 (1-23) months) due to irreversibly renal graft failure (AR=23, chronic rejection=16, de novo nephropaty=1). The patients age was 37.5 ± 12.1 years. They had fever during 3.4 (1-12) weeks. Only 13 patients were under minimal steroid doses and the other 27 were without immunosupression.

As controls we have studied 6 patients without fever and with irreversibly non-functioning renal graft. The renal graft failure was due to AR (4 patients) or chronic rejection (2 patients). The time on dialysis was 6.15 (3-10) months.

METHOD

We reinjected 3.7-7.4 MBq of 111In-mercaptopyridine-platelets and 24 and 48 hours scans were performed. We used the PUI to evaluate the results. We compared de PUI with the final diagnosis of fever. This diagnosis was done with the available clinical data and the evolution after treatment (antibiotics, steroids or nephrectomy). We considered a positive scan for immunological fever if the PUI was higher than 1.5.

RESULTS

All the controls had a PUI < 1.5 (1.09±0.11). Twenty seven patients with immunological fever had a PUI > 1.5 (1.97±0.80). In 3 patients the fever dissapeared with steroids and in 24 nephrectomy was necessary. Two patients with immunological fever (nephrectomy) were false negative results with a PUI < 1.5 (1.13±0.13). Eleven patients had non immunological fever which dissapeared either with antibiotherapy or spontaneously and they had a PUI < 1.5.

Using as threshold a PUI of 1.5 the sensitivity and specificity of labeled platelets scan to diagnose immunological fever was 93% and 100% whit a positive predictive value of 100% and a negative predictive value of 85%. If we use a PUI of 1.4, the sensitivity increase to 97% and the negative predictive value to 92%.

CONCLUSION

111In-platelets scintigraphy may be a good predictor of immunological activity due to graft rejection in hemodialysis patients with irreversibly non functioning renal graft who present prolonged fever and may allow to take a correct therapeutic option (nephrectomy) whit minimal morbidity and low economical cost.

REFERENCES

1. Setoain J, Lomeña F., Herranz R. et all. Platelets Labeling in Renal Transplantation. Proc. III Wld Congr. Nucl. Med. Biol., pp. 1583- 1585, Pergamon Press, Paris (1982).
2. Thakur M.L., Walsh L., Malech H.L. and Gottschalk A. Indium-111 labeled platelets. Improved method, efficacy and evaluation. *J Nucl Med*, 22:381-385 (1981).
3. Martín Comín J., Lomeña F., Griño J.M. et all. 111In-Oxine-Labeled Platelets in Renal Transplantation. Value in Cyclosporine Therapy. Contr. Nephrol., vol 56, pp. 168-173 . Karger, Basel (1987).
4. Thakur M.L., McKenney S.L. and Park C.H. Simplified and Efficient Labeling of Human Platelets in Plasma Using Indium-111-2-Mercaptopyridine-N-Oxide : Preparation and Evaluation. *J Nucl Med* 26: 510-517,(1985).
5. Piera C., Roca M., Martín Comín J et all. Platelet Labelling with 111-In-Merc. Usefulness in Renal Transplantation. Clinical Application of Radiolabelled Platelets. Kessler C. et all Ed., Kluwer Academic Publishers, Dordrecht (1990), pp. 278-292.
6. Leithner C., Sinzinger H., Schwarz M. and Ulrich W. Possibilities and pitfalls of indium-111 platelet scintigraphy in the monitoring of renal transplant recipients. *The British Journal of Radiology*, 58: 1057-1063, (1985).
7. Leithner C., Schwarz M., Sinzinger H. and Ulrich W. Limited value of 111-Indium platelet scintigraphy in renal transplant pacient receiving cyclosporine. *Clinical Nephrology*, vol 25, N° 3, 141-148, (1986).
8. von Willebrand E., Zola H. and Häyry P. Thrombocyte Aggregates in Renal Allografts. *Transplantation*, 39: 258-262,(1985).
9. Catafau A., Lomeña F., Ricart M.J. et all. Indium-111-labeled platelets in monitoring human pancreatic transplants. *J Nucl Med* 30:1470-1475, (1989).

111In-ANTIMYOSIN ANTIBODIES FOR DETECTION OF HEART TRANSPLANT REJECTION

I. Carrió

Nuclear Medicine Unit
Hospital de Sant Pau
Autonomous University of Barcelona
Barcelona, Spain

HEART TRANSPLANTATION

Detection and treatment for rejection after transplantation are based on the identification of myocyte damage upon endomyocardial biopsies sequentially performed after surgery. The invasive nature of the procedure and the cost of its repeated application in an increasingly larger heart transplant population have lead to the search for alternative methods of detecting early myocardial damage due to rejection. Noninvasive detection of myocardial damage is possible with Indium-111 monoclonal antimyosin antibodies. Binding of these antibodies to myosin takes place only when sarcolemmal disruption occurs and the cell is irreversibly damaged[1]. Detection of rejection-induced myocardial damage in humans was first reported by Frist et al.[2]. In a subsequent report, we described a semiquantitative method of assessing the degree of antimyosin uptake[3] and its usefulness in recognizing variations of such uptake using repeat injections after transplantation[4].

From February 1987 through April 1991, 247 monoclonal antimyosin studies were performed in our institution in 52 patients who were orthotopic allograft recipients. Endomyocardial biopsies were made to coincide with antimyosin studies; from one to 10 biopsy and antimyosin studies (mean, 4.7 ± 2.1) were performed 1-71 months after transplantation. In 33 of these patients, repeat studies were prospectively performed at 1, 2, 3, 6, and 12 months after the surgery and yearly thereafter. Cyclosporine and steroids were administered. Antithymocytic globulin was given for 10 days after transplantation. Diagnosis of acute rejection was made by interpretation of endomyocardial biopsies taken with a Cordis bioptome according to Billingham's criteria: "normal" biopsy, "mild rejection" when cell infiltration without myocyte damage is identified, and "moderate" or "severe rejection" when different degrees of myocyte damage are detected. Treatment for acute rejection was considered only when moderate or severe rejection was detected at biposy.

Radiolabeled Blood Elements, Edited by J. Martin-Comin
Plenum Press, New York, 1994

Antimyosin Studies

0.5 mg of R11-D10-Fab-DTPA (Centocor Europe, Leiden, the Netherlands) labeled with 2 mCi of 111In was administered by slow intravenous injection. Planar scans were obtained 24 and 48 hrs later using a medium energy collimator with a 20% window centered on both peaks of 111In at a preset time of 10 min. Scans were stored in 128x128 frames. The presence of antimyosin uptake in the heart was assessed using a four-step score: 0, no uptake; 1, mild or faint uptake; 2, clear but moderate uptake; and 3, intense myocardial uptake. A quantitative method was then applied. This consisted of drawing a region of interest on the heart and regions on the lungs on the anterior view of the thorax. A heart to lung ratio was obtained dividing average counts per pixel in the heart by average counts per pixel in the lungs. A cutoff point of > 1.55 (normal value 1.43 ± 0.06 + 2 standard deviations) was used to define abnormal studies.

RESULTS

Of the 247 studies, 149 coincided with absent rejection at biopsy, 38 with mild rejection, and 60 with moderate or severe rejection. Heart to lung ratios were were 1.68 ± 0.27, 1.79 ± 0.22, and 1.91 ± 0.32, respectively ($p < 0.0001$).

Sixty biopsies showing cellular damage coexisted with abnormal antimyosin studies in 57 (95%). It is significant than in the biopsy groups with absent or mild rejection a high prevalence of positive antimyosin scans was observed: 62% and 84% respectively. Taking endomyocardial biopsy as a gold standard, sensitivity, specificity and accuracy of antimyosin in the diagnosis of rejection were 95%, 33% and 31%, respectively. When antimyosin studies were taken as the gold standard, the calculated values for biopsy results were 31%, 95% and 95% respectively.

Two hundred thirty-eight of the 247 antimyosin studies coexisted without rejection-related complications; on 9 occasions such complications were detected, with mean heart to lung ratios in the two groups of 1.74 ± 0.3 and 2.1 ± 0.16 respectively ($p < 0.0001$). In none of 193 studies with a heart to lung ratio of less than 2.00 was a complication detected at the time of antimyosin imaging, whereas in 9 of 45 studies with heart to lung ratios of 2.00 or greater, these complications occurred ($p < 0.0001$).

Patterns of Antimyosin Uptake Early After Transplantation: Of 33 patients prospectively followed, a progressive reduction of antimyosin uptake with decrease of the ratio at the third month in relation to that detected at the first ("decreasing" pattern) was associated with an uneventful outcome in 21 of 23 (two died of unrelated cause). In an additional 10 patients, such 3-month reduction of uptake after transplantation did not occur; at 3 months, the heart to lung ratio was equal or higher than that obtained at the first month ("persistent" pattern). In this group 7 patients presented severe rejection related complications (4 deaths from rejection and 3 vascular rejections). Differences between these two patterns in relation to development of complications were significant ($p < 0.001$). Biopsy information from these two groups was non significantly different (percentages of biopsies showing myocyte damage were 37% and 43% respectively).

Long Term Course of Antimyosin Uptake: The 247 antimyosin studies were analyzed according to the time interval at which they were performed after surgery. Studies performed at 1-3, 4-11, 12-23 and more than 24 months showed a prevalence of abnormal antimyosin studies of 95%, 77%, 65% and 46% respectively ($p < 0.0001$). Mean heart to lung ratios were 1.93 ± 0.30, 1.73 ± 0.23, 1.65 ± 0.22 and 1.58 ± 0.20 respectively ($p < 0.001$). Patients with normal antimyosin studies at one year after transplantation seldom presented with subsequent episodes of rejection (1 episode in 9 patients subsequently followed), whereas patients who still had positive antimyosin scans one year after transplantation presented a higher probability of subsequent rejection episodes (17 episodes in 12 patients subsequently followed).

DISCUSSION

The discrepancy between the positivity of antimyosin studies in the absence of myocyte damage at endomyocardial biopsy has been described both in cardiac rejection after heart transplantation and in other types of diffuse myocardial damage[3-6]. Our results indicate that the sampling error is the likely cause of these discrepancies. When individual curves of antimyosin uptake are compared with biopsy results, discrepancies appear to be due to sampling error; this corroborates the lesser sensitivity of endomyocardial biopsy compared with antimyosin studies in the detection of rejection-induced myocardial damage[6].

Antimyosin studies provide information regarding rejection-induced cell damage. Evolution of antimyosin uptake obtained by sequential studies indicates that in most patients a steady state of rejection activity occrs that usually decreases with time. This occurs phenomenon of gradual unresponsiveness to the graft has been referred to as "tolerance". Some patients however, do not appear to attain complete tolerance to the graft. Our results show that the presence of positive antimyosin uptake one year after transplantation correlated with subsequent appearance of biopsy proven rejection during follow-up[7, 8]. In addition, increasing intensities of uptake correlate with a greater probability of detecting biopsy-proven rejection[6,9]. Intense antimyosin uptake, with a heart to lung ratio of 2.00 or greater, can be associated with complications resulting from rejection (death, coronary obstruction), whereas inferior ratios ensure against the occurrence of such complications. In addition, the early 3-month pattern of antimyosin uptake (decreasing or persistent) appears to be of useful prognostic significance. Those patients in whom antimyosin decreased during the first 3 months had an uneventful clinical course, whereas two thirds of those with a persistent pattern showed such complications. This prognostic information is not reflected in the biopsies, as the percentage of patients showing rejection during the first 3 months were similar in the decreasing and persistent groups. A persistent 3-month pattern of antimyosin uptake signals the possibility of rejection-related complications, whereas decreasing uptake pattern ensures against such complications. In the former situation, a closer biopsy surveillance and prompt treatment for rejection based on biopsy results would be required.

After the first year of transplantation, the role of antimyosin studies is to identify patients with normal studies and withdraw them from the biopsy program; biopsy surveillance is required in the remaining patients until normalcy of antimyosin is eventually achieved.

REFERENCES

1. Khaw BA, Scott J, Fallon JT et al. Myocardial injury: Quantitation by cell sorting initiated with antimyosin fluorescent spheres. *Science*; 217: 1050-1053 (1982).
2. Frist W, Yasuda T, Segall G et al. Noninvasive detection of human cardiac transplant rejection with 111In antimyosin (Fab) imaging. *Circulation*; 76: V81-V85 (1987).
3. Carrió I, Bernà Ll, Ballester M, et al. Indium-111 antimyosin scintigraphy to assess myocardial damage in patients with suspected myocarditis and cardiac rejection. *J Nucl Med*; 29: 1893-1900 (1988).
4. Ballester M, Carrió I, Abadal L, et al. Patterns of evolution of myocyte damage after human heart transplantation detected by Indium-111 monoclonal antimyosin. *Am J Cardiol*; 62: 623-627 (1988).

5. Obrador D, Ballester M, Carrió I, et al. High prevalence of myocardial monoclonal antimyosin antibody uptake in patients with chronic idiopathic dilated cardiomyopathy. *J Am Coll Cardiol*; 13: 1289-1293 (1989).

6. Ballester M, Obrador D, Carrió I et al. Early postoperative reduction of monoclonal antimyosin antibody uptake is associated with absent rejection-related complications after heart transplantation. *Circulation*; 85: 61-68 (1992).

7. Carrió I, Berná L, Estorch M et al. Risk stratification of heart transplant patients during long term follow-up by means of indium-111-antimyosin scintigraphy. *J Nucl Med*;5: 782-783 (1990).

8. Ballester M, Obrador D, Carrió I et al. Indium-111-monoclonal antimyosin antibody studies after the first year of heart transplantation. Identification of risk groups and clinical implications. *Circulation*; 82: 2100-2108 (1990).

9. I.Carrió, L.Berná, M.Estorch et al. Risk of rejection related complications after heart transplantation assessed by antimyosin antibody studies. *J Nucl Med*;5: 1019 (1991).

DOSE-DEPENDENT INHIBITION OF ACUTE ARTERIAL THROMBOSIS BY MONOCLONAL ANTIBODY (16N7C2) IN A BABOON MODEL

P.N. Badenhorst, H.F. Kotzé, S. Lamprecht, M. Meiring, V. van Wyk and H. Deckmyn[1]

Department of Haematology
University of the Orange Free State, Bloemfontein, South Africa
[1]Center for Thrombosis and Vascular Research
University of Leuven, Belgium

INTRODUCTION

The pivotal role that blood platelets play in haemostasis and thrombosis caused a keen interest in the development of specific inhibitors of platelet function. The platelet glycoprotein (GP)IIb/IIIa receptor complex for fibrinogen is a particularly attractive target for therapeutic intervention, since it is the exclusive mediator of platelet aggregation. There are about 50,000 GPIIb/IIIa receptors on the surface of normal platelets. When they are reduced to about 10,000 there is a marked decrease in platelet aggregation, a mildly prolonged bleeding time and abolition of in vivo thrombus formation[1]. 16N7C2, a murine monoclonal antibody against human platelets, was developed at the Center for Thrombosis and Vascular Research at the University of Leuven. Preliminary studies showed that it blocks the GPIIb/IIIa receptors of human and baboon platelets, but that it has no effect on cat, dog, pig, rabbit, rat, hamster, mouse and guinea-pig platelets. We therefore decided to evaluate the in vivo potential of this monoclonal antibody in baboons.

METHODS

Thrombosis Model

We measured 111In-platelet deposition onto vascular grafts in a model of acute arterial thrombosis in baboons as previously described[2]. A piece of Dacron vascular graft material (0.5 cm^2) was inserted as an extension segment in a permanent femoral arterio-venous shunt in a baboon and platelet accumulation dynamically imaged with a scintillation camera.

Experimental Protocol

On the first day of the experiment the baboon's platelet were labelled with 111In-tropolone and reinjected as described[3]. The thrombogenic device was inserted and platelet deposition imaged for two hours. The thrombogenic device was then removed and blood-flow re-established. On the second day the monoclonal antibody was injected, the thrombogenic device inserted 15 minutes later and imaged for two hours after which it was removed and blood-flow re-established. The latter procedure was repeated for the next two days.

A dose of 0.3 mg/Kg of antibody was administered to seven baboons and a dose of 0.1 mg/Kg to six baboons.

Quantification of GP IIb/IIIa Receptor Occupation

The number of receptors occupied by the monoclonal antibody was estimated as described[4]. Platelet-rich plasma was incubated with a near saturating dose of 125I-16N7C2 and the number of radiolabelled molecules bound per platelet determined. The number of receptors occupied by the monoclonal antibody was estimated by subtracting the number of molecules of 125I-16N7C2 bound to the platelets after 16N7C2 infusion from that obtained before 16N7C2 infusion.

Other Tests

The following routine coagulation tests were performed: repeated platelet counts; a template bleeding time; platelet aggregation studies with ADP and collagen; a prothrombin time and an activated partial thromboplastin time.

RESULTS

Platelet Deposition on the Thrombogenic Surface

A bolus injection of 0.3 mg/Kg of 16N7C2 virtually abolished platelet deposition on the thrombogenic surface on the first day. Platelet deposition was still inhibited by $\pm$ 79 % after 24 hours and $\pm$ 65 % after 48 hours (Fig. 1a). Injection of 0.1 mg/Kg of the antibody inhibited platelet deposition by $\pm$42 % on the day of injection and by $\pm$ 28 % after 24 hours (Fig. 1b).

Receptor Occupation

Injection of 0.3 mg/Kg of 16N7C2 blocked $\pm$ 64 % of the GPIIb/IIIa receptors 10 minutes after injection (Fig. 2). Receptor occupation then decreased in a linear fashion over the next few days. With the 0.1 mg/Kg dosage, $\pm$ 42 % of the receptors were blocked after 10 minutes, 28 % after 24 hours and 10 % after 48 hours.

Platelet Aggregation

16N7C2 also affected the platelet aggregation response to ADP and collagen. Injection of 0.3 mg/Kg totally inhibited platelet aggregation induced by ADP. Thereafter there was a steady increase in aggregation that returned to normal by the third day. Collagen induced aggregation was markdly decreased but not totally abolished on the first day. Otherwise the pattern was similar to that found with the

344

ADP induced aggregation. The injection of 0.1 mg/Kg of the monoclonal antibody only marginally inhibited platelet aggregation (Fig. 3b)

Coagulation Tests

The bleeding time was only prolonged (20 minutes) on the first day after injection of 0.3 mg/Kg 16N7C2, but returned to normal levels (5 min) by the second day.

The platelet count did not drop following the injection of 16N7C2, nor did it have any effect on the routine coagulation tests.

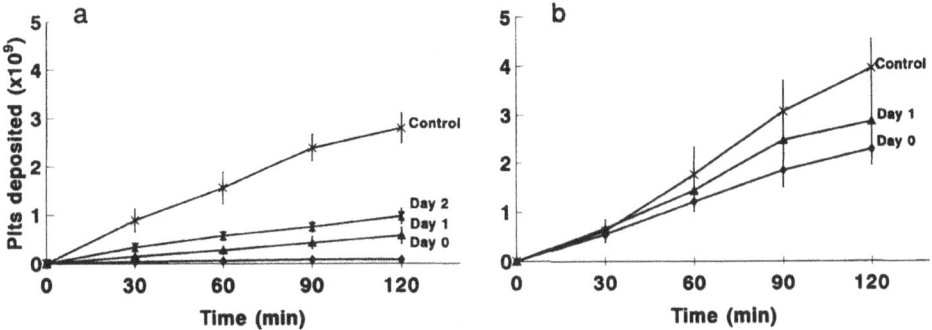

Figure 1. The effects of a bolus injection of 0.3 mg/Kg and 0.1 mg/Kg of 16N7C2 on platelet deposition on a thrombogenic surface are illustrated. The top curve in each graph shows platelet deposition over a 2 hour period before each treatment. A dosage of 0.3 mg of antibody abolished platelet deposition on the first day. Platelet deposition was still inhibited by 79 % after 24 hours and 65 % after 48 hours (a). A dosage of 0.1 mg/Kg resulted in a 42 % reduction in platelet deposition on the first day and 28 % after 24 hours (b).

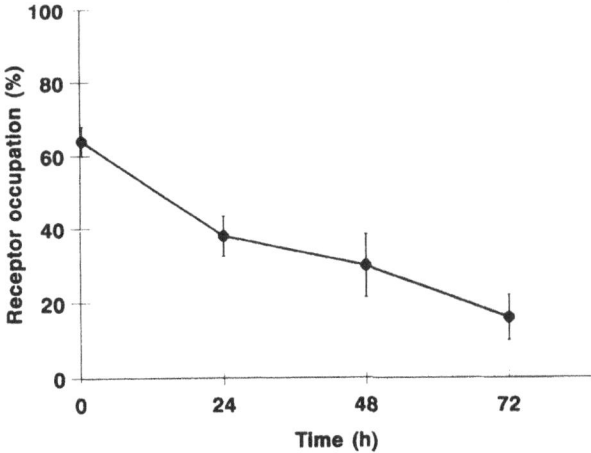

Figure 2. Receptor occupation was measured 10 min after injection of 0.3 mg/Kg of 16N7C2 and then daily for 3 days. Initially 64 % of receptors were blocked. It then decreased in a linear fashion over the next few days.

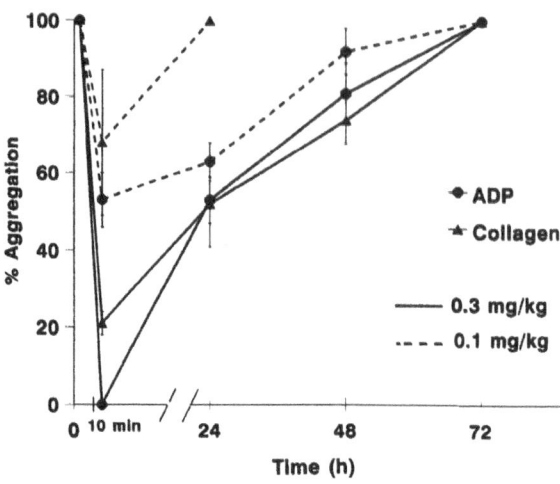

Figure 3. The platelet aggregation responses to 10 μM ADP and 0.05 g/l collagen are shown for both the 0.3 mg/Kg and 0.1 mg/Kg dosages of 16N7C2. The higher dose inhibited platelet aggregation dramatically on the first day. Thereafter there was a steady return to normal by day 2. The effect of 0.1 mg/Kg of the monoclonal antibody was less pronounced but followed a similar pattern.

DISCUSSION

Glycoprotein IIb/IIIa is a two-chain, calcium dependent platelet surface molecule. Its IIb subunit contains the fibrinogen gamma-chain binding region and the amino globular head of the IIIa subunit contains the RGD-binding region. Sequence analysis of the monoclonal antibody 16N7C2, revealed an RGD-sequence in the hypervariable region of the heavy chain that is probably responsible for antibody binding.

The aim was to reduce the number of functional GPIIb/IIIa receptors to a level that would allow an adequate antithrombotic effect without the danger of a bleeding tendency. We calculated that this could be achieved by a dose of 0.3 mg/Kg of the monoclonal antibody to occupy approximately 70 % of the IIb/IIIa receptors. The measured receptor occupancy after injection of 0.3 mg/Kg of 16N7C2 was 64 %, but it was sufficient to abolish platelet deposition on the thrombogenic surface. This dosage of 16N7C2 produced a long term antithrombotic effect with about 65 % of platelet inhibition after 48 hours (Fig 1a). Receptor occupancy decreased in a linear fashion over days and corresponded with the platelet survival of 5 days in the baboon. This could indicate that the increase in unblocked receptors is caused by an influx of new platelets from the bone marrow

No adverse effects were encountered: The platelet count did not fall, blood coagulation was not effected, and the bleeding time was only moderately prolonged on the first day.

Although these experiments with 16N7C2 are promising, at least two factors regarding the use of monoclonal antibodies to GPIIb/IIIa as antithrombotic agents have to be considered. First, there is the question of immunogenicity. We are dealing with a mouse antibody that has the potential to elicit an immune response in man. Although only two out of 16 patients showed an immune response in the Phase 1 study with the 7E3 monoclonal antibody[5], repeat therapy remains a problem. Attempts are being made to modify monoclonal antibodies in such a way that they lose their immunogenicity. Secondly, it must be remembered that GPIIb/IIIa belongs to the super-family of integrin receptors. There is a high homology between the different integrins and one can anticipate some cross-reactivity to develop which could either have a beneficial or harmful effect. This is certainly an aspect that has to be investigated.

These experiments confirmed the usefulness of 111In-labelled platelets and the baboon model to evaluate antithrombotic agents in vivo. They also showed that 16N7C2 is an effective antithrombotic agent with a long term effect in this model of arterial thrombosis. 16N7C2 seems to block the IIb/IIIa receptors permanently because the increase of unblocked receptors over time corresponded with the influx of new platelets into the circulation. Although monoclonal antibodies to GPIIb/IIIa are excellent research tools, much more development is needed before they can be successfully introduced as antithrombotic agents in clinical medicine.

REFERENCES

1. Coller BS, Scudder LE, Beer J, Gold HK, Folts JD, Cavagnaro J, Jordan R, Wagner C, Iuliucci J, Knight D, Ghrayeb J, Smith C, Weisman HF and Berger H. Monoclonal antibodies to platelet glycoprotein IIb/IIIa as antithrombotic agents. *Annals New York Academy of Sciences* 614: 192-213 (1991).
2. Hanson SR, Kotzé HF, Savage B and Harker LA. Platelet interactions with Dacron vascular grafts. A model of acute thrombosis in baboons. *Arteriosclerosis* 5: 595-603 (1985).
3. Kotzé HF, Lötter MG, Badenhorst PN, Heyns A du P. Kinetics of In-111-platelets in the baboon: 1. Isolation and labelling of a viable and representative platelet population. *Thrombosis and Haemostasis* 53: 404-407 (1985).
4. Coller BS and Scudder LE. Inhibition of dog platelet function by in vivo infusion of F(ab)2 fragments of a monoclonal antibody. *Blood* 66: 1456-1459 (1985).
5. Gold HK, Gimple LW, Yasuda T, Leinbach RC, Werner W, Jordan R, Berger H, Collen D and Coller B. Pharmacodynamic study of F(ab')2 fragments of murine monoclonal antibody 7E3 directed against human platelet glycoprotein IIb/IIIa in patients with unstable angina pectoris. *Journal of Clinical Investigation* 86: 651-659 (1990).

HIV-RELATED THROMBOCYTOPENIA: FOUR DIFFERENT CLINICAL SUBSETS

G. Landonio[1], A. Nosari[1], F. Spinelli[2] and R. Vigorelli[2]

[1]Department of Haematology
[2]Department Nuclear of Medicine
Ospedale Niguarda Cà Granda
Milano

INTRODUCTION

The pathogenesis of HIV-related Thrombocytopenias (HIV-rel TP) is still controversial. Many factors have been considered: immunological destruction[1,2,3,4,5,6], retroviral infection of megakaryocytes[7,8,9,10] and altered reticulo-endothelial function [11,12,13]. They perhaps act sinergically in many patients or, conversely, each of them could play a role in different forms of HIV-rel TP. In fact the term "HIV-related Thrombocytopenia" should include more than one kind of TP: in order to confirm this opinion, we reviewed retrospectively 52 cases of HIV-rel TP, evaluating bone marrow morphology, platelet kinetic studies, antiplatelets antibodies and the response to therapy.

PATIENTS AND METHODS

We evaluated 52 patients with HIV-rel TP attending Niguarda Cà Granda Hospital, Milan, in the period Jan 1987-Jan 1992.

They were intravenous drug users, 41 males and 11 females, aging from 21 to 43 yrs (mean 26). They were classified at enrolment in CDC (Center for Disease Control) groups II-9-, III -38-, IVC2 -5-. The mean number of CD4+ lymphocytes was 348+106 while the mean number of CD8+ lymphocytes was 786+152; no patient had detectable serum p-24 antigenemia at enrolment. The platelets count was in the range of 7-83 x 10/l (mean 29). The patients were divided in two groups according to severity of TP: 28 had less than 30 x 10/l and 24 had more than 30 x 10/l.

Bone marrow specimens were examined in all patients at enrolment, evaluating megakaryocytes number and morphology, and other cell lines.

Antiplatelet antibodies were examined in 28 of 52 patients by immunofluorescence test (direct and indirect method on paraformaldeyde-tested -PFA- platelets using fluorescein-conjugates F(ab) anti-human IgG -Dakopatt, Copenhagen, Denmark-)[14,15]. Immunecomplexes were determined only in a few cases (7/52).

Radiolabeled Blood Elements, Edited by J. Martin-Comin
Plenum Press, New York, 1994

Platelet kinetic studies were performed in all patients, using autologous platelets; the lifespan of 111 In-Oxine labelled platelets was studied according to the method of Thakur[16], partially modified. Platelet survival was calculated (normal mean values were 7.20 + 0.80 days): "recovery" (percentage of infused cells circulating at the third hour) was considered as an index of "pooling" (normal mean values: 58.2 + 6.8%). Platelet turnover was calculated according to Harker[17], using the formula: platelet count / platelet survival (days) x 90% / recovery % (normal mean values: 46.4 + 11.2 x 10 platelets per litre per day). External counting was performed simultaneously on spleen, liver and precordium areas at 15 min, 1 h, 3 h and daily thereafter. The following parameters were determined: splenic destruction index (SDI: spleen activity at t x precordium activity at 15 min. / spleen activity at 15 min. x precordium activity at t) and hepatic destruction index (HDI: liver activity at t x precordium activity at 15 min. / liver activity at 15 min. x precordium activity at t); in the normal subjects the ratios are about one.

Patients with moderate TP were followed up without treatment; patients with severe TP were treated in different ways: steroids (1 mg/Kg/day x 4 weeks) and/or High Dose Immunoglobulins (HDIg: 400 mg/Kg/day x 5-7 days) if haemorragic (splenectomy was performed in refractory cases); zidovudine (500-1000 mg/day) if not haemorragic.

The responses were evaluated as complete (CR: platelets > 100x10/l), partial (PR: >50<100x10/l) or failure (F: <50x10/l).

RESULTS

Table 1 shows the results of platelet kinetic studies: they were subdivided in patients with severe and moderate TP. A more significant reduction of platelet survival was observed in patients with "severe" TP; on the contrary the reduction of recovery and platelet turnover was more relevant in patients with "moderate" TP.

Table 1. Kinetic studies with autologous 111In-Oxine labelled platelets.

	"severe" TP ($<30x10^9/$ l)	"moderate" TP ($>30<100x10^9/l$)	"normal" values
Survival (days)	3.1 ± 1.2	4.5 ± 1.4	7.2 ± 0.8
Recovery (%)	32.4 ± 12.1	26.8 ± 11.1	58.2 ± 6.8
SDI (*)	1.5 ± 0.4	1.3 ± 0.3	about one
HDI (**)	1.2 ± 0.2	1.4 ± 0.3	about one
Platelet turnover ($x10^9/$ l / day)	28.3 ± 11.7	22.1 ± 8.9	46.4 ± 11.2

(*)   Splenic Destruction Index
(**) Hepatic Destruction Index

Table 2 cross-references platelet survival (<3 days, 3-6 days, >3 days) with megakaryocytes number and antiplatelet antibodies, in the two groups of patients: a decrease of megakaryocytes number was present in 4/52 patients only; antiplatelets antibodies were not related to severity of TP as direct test (positive in 82% of patients) and as indirect test (positive in 25%).

Table 3 shows the different clinical subsets of TP in the two groups of patients, classified as "acute ITP like" (megakaryocytes normal or increased, platelet survival less than 3 days with normal or reduced recovery), "chronic ITP like" (megakaryocytes

Table 2. Megakaryocytes and anti-platelets antibodies cross-referencewith platelet survival.

	survival (days)	n. cases	megakaryocytes decreased	antiplatelets direct test	antibodies indirect test
"severe" TP	< 3	9	0/9	6/6	2/6
	> 3 < 6	13	1/13	5/6	2/6
	> 6	6	0/6	2/4	1/4
"moderate" TP	< 3	0	--	--	--
	> 3 < 6	10	1/10	4/5	1/5
	> 6	14	2/14	6/7	1/7
Tot		52	4/52 (8%)	23/28 (82%)	7/28 (25%)

normal or increased, platelet survival more than 3 but less than 6 days with normal or reduced recovery), "pooling TP" (megakaryocytes normal, platelet survival more than 6 days with significantly reduced recovery); "hypoplastic TP" (megakaryocytes reduced, independently of platelet survival).

The patients with moderate TP were followed up for a mean time of 27 months. In this group of patients no haemorragic complication was recorded, also in absence of specific therapy.

Table 3. Clinical subsets of HIV-related Thrombocytopenias

	"severe" TP	"moderate" TP	Tot
"acute" ITP-like	9/28 (32%)	0/24 (-)	9/52 (17%)
"chronic" ITP-like	12/28 (43%)	9/24 (38%)	21/52 (40%)
"pooling" TP	6/28 (21%)	12/24 (50%)	18/52 (35%)
"hypoplastic" TP	1/28 (4%)	3/24 (12%)	4/52 (8%)

Table 4 cross-references the reponses to different treatments with the clinical subsets of TP in the patients with severe TP: 3/17 (18%) only responded to steroids and/or HDIg; 10 underwent splenectomy due to persistent haemorragic (7 of them responded); 16 patients, without relevant bleeding, were treated with zidovudine (9/16 - 56% - responded).

Table 4. Response to therapy in "severe" HIV-rel TP

	Steroids and/or HDIg		Splenectomy		Zidovudine	
	n.	CR+PR	n.	CR+PR	n.	CR+PR
"acute" ITP-like	9/9	2/9	5/9	4/5	2/9	1/2
"chronic" ITP-like	7/12	1/7	5/12	3/5	7/12	5/7
"pooling" TP	--	--	--	--	6/6	3/6
"hypoplastic" TP	1/1	0/1	--	--	1/1	0/1
Tot		3/17 (18%)		7/10 (70%)		9/16 (56%)

DISCUSSION

The pathogenesis of HIV rel TP is still controversial, and many factors have been evaluated: 1) immunological destruction of the platelets, 2) retroviral infection of megakaryocytes, 3) alterated reticulo-endothelial function, with "pooling" of the platelets.

1) The immunological mechanism was examined first: high levels of platelets-bound antibodies have been described; nevertheless the mechanism involved is not well known: non specific deposition of complement and immunecomplexes[1,5]; autoantibodies directed agaisnt a specific platelet membrane protein[18,19]; and/or antibodies wich cross-react with viral and platelet antigen[4]; recently the co-existence of immunecomplexes and specific antibodies was also reported[20].

In our study the evaluation of antiplatelet antibodies was not performed in all patients; nevertheless in 28 patients the results were aspecific and neither related to the severity of the TP nor to platelet survival.

2) A direct or indirect effect of HIV infection on megakaryocytes has been postulated by some Authors: evidence of this hypothesis includes suppressed platelet production demonstrated with platelet kinetic studies[7]; improvement of platelet production after zidovudine[21]; and the recent demonstration of HIV infection of megakaryocytes[8,9,10]. We also observed a reduced platelet turnover in most patients: this result was more significant in patients with moderate rather than severe TP. Nevertheless this effect could be explained by a diffuse sequestration of platelets, according to Heyns[22], and not by bone marrow suppression.

3) An alterate reticulo-endothelial function has been postulated by some Authors as another mechanism, due to an increased sequestration, without destruction, of Ig-coated platelets[12,13].

The "pooling" of platelets could be the result of this alterated mechanism. Our results support this idea: 35% of all patients shows a normal platelet survival and other 40% only a slight decrease, with a significant reduction of recovery, as observed in splenic and/or hepatic sequestration. These patients did not show relevant haemorrages during the follow-up.

CONCLUSIONS

The term HIV-related Thrombocytopenia includes more than one form of TP. "Acute ITP-like" TP, "chronic ITP-like" TP, "hypoplastic" TP and "pooling" TP have to be evaluated differently for pathogenesis, clinical manifestations and treatment.

REFERENCES

1. Morris L, Distenfeld A, Amorosi A, et al. Autoimmune thrombocytopenic purpura in homosexual men. *Ann. Intern. Med.*; 96:714-7 (1982).
2. Walsh CM, Nardi MA, Karpatkin S. On the mechanism of thrombocytopenic purpura in sexualy active homosexual men. *N Engl. J. Med.*; 311:635-9 (1984).
3. Savona S, Nardi MA, Lennette ET, et al. Thrombocytopenic purpura in narcotic addicts. *Ann. Intern. Med.*; 102:734-41 (1985).
4. Stricker RB, Abrams DI, Corash L, et al. Target platelet antigen in homosexual men with immune thrombocytopenia. *N. Engl. J. Med.*; 313:1375-80 (1985).
5. Karpatkin S. Immunologic thrombocytopenic purpura in HIV-seropositive homosexual, narcotic addicts ans hemophiliacs. *Sem Hematol*; 25:219-29 (1988).
6. Klaassen RJL, van der Lelie J, Vlekke ABJ, et al. The serology and immunochemistry of HIV-induced platelet-bound immunoglobulin. *Blut*, 59:75-81 (1989).
7. Ballem PJ, Belzberg A, Devine D, et al. Pathophysiology of thrombocytopenia associated with HIV infection in homosexual men. A preliminary report. *Blut*; 59:111-4 (1989).
8. Zucker-Franklin D, Cao YZ, Koury YH. Megakaryocytes of HIV-seropositive individuals express viral RNA (Abstr). V Int. Conf. on AIDS, Montreal; 554 (1989).
9. Raharinivo B, Monté D, Auriault C, et al. Productive HIV-1 infection of the CD4-negative megakaryocytic cell line Dami (Abstr.). VII Int. Conf. on AIDS, Florence; WB 81 (1991).
10. Louache F, Bettaieb A, Henri A, et al. Infection of megakaryocytes by HIV in seropositive patients with ITP. *Blood*; 78:1697-705 (1991).
11. Hymes BK, Greene BJ, Karpatkin, S. The effect of AZT on HIV-related TP. *N. Engl. J. Med.*; 318:516-7 (1988).
12. Ratner L. HIV-associated Autoimmune Thrombocytopenic Purpura: a review. *The Am. J. Med.*; 86:194-8 (1989).
13. Oksenhendler E, Bierling O, Ferchal F, et al. Zidovudine for Thrombocytopenic Purpura related to HIV infection. *Ann. Intern. Med.*; 110:365-8 (1989).
14. van den Borne AEGKr, Helmerhorst FM, Leeuwen EF, et al. Autoimmune Thrombocytopenia: detection of platelet antibodies with the suspension immunofluorescence test. *Br. J. Haematol*; 45:319-27 (1980).
15. van den Borne AEGKr, Verheugt FWA, Dosterhof F, et al. A simple imnunofluorescence test for detection of platelet antibodies. *Br. J. Haematol*; 39:195-207 (1978).
16. Thakur MI, Welch MJ, Joint JH, et al. 111 In labelled platelets: studies on preparation end evaluation of in vitro and vivo functions. *Thromb Res*; 9:354-7 (1976).
17. Harker L. Thrombokinetics in ITP. *Br. J. Haematol*; 19:95-104 (1970).
18. Lelie J, Lange JMAm Vos JJE, et al. Autoimmunity agaisnt blood cells in HIV infection. *Br. J. Haematol*; 67:109-14 (1987).
19. Bettaieb A, Oksenhendler E, Fromont P, et al. Immunochemical analysis of platelet antibodies in HIV-related Thrombocytopenic Purpura: a study of 68 patients. *Br. J. Haematol*; 73:241-7 (1989).
20. Borzini P, Milella AM, Marconi MG. Evidence for the co-existence of immunocomplexes and platelet specific antibodies in HIV infection-related thrombocytopenia in narcotic drug addicts. Experimental results and immunopathogenetic discussion. *Haematologica*; 77:130-6 (1992).
21. Ballem P, Belzberg A, Chambers H, et al. Evidence of a compensated thrombolytic state enhanced by AZT (Abstr.). V Int. Conf. on AIDS, Montreal; 332 (1989).
22. Heyns A, Badenhorst O, Lotter M, et al. Platelet turnover and kinetics in ITP. *Blood*; 67:86-92 (1986).

68Ga MPO PLATELETS IN HUMAN PET THROMBUS IMAGING[a]

D.A. Goodwin[1], E.V. Lang[2], J.E. Atwood[3], R.L. Dalman[4],
C.McK. Ransone[1], C.I. Diamanti[1] and M. McTigue[1]

[1]Departments of Nuclear Medicine
[2]Vascular and Interventional Radiology
[3]Cardiology
[4]Vascular Surgery
 Veterans Administration Medical Center, Palo Alto California
 Stanford University School of Medicine, Stanford California

INTRODUCTION

The excellent immediate results of various interventional techniques for recanalization of peripheral and coronary arterial lesions has highlighted the persistant problem of restenosis, occurring in as many as 30% of patients in 1 year and 66% in 2 years[1]. Platelet deposition and its sequellae are among the most important possible causes of restenosis, and intensive research on the prevention of restenosis has involved many new anti-platelet drugs[2]. A method of measuring platelet deposition *in vivo* would better define the effectiveness of the various anti-platelet protocols, help select patients and permit monitoring of anti-platelet drug activity[3].

In atherosclerosis, a platelet imaging technique might also provide an early diagnostic method that would prompt the initiation of anti-platelet therapy in time to the prevent the occurrence of occlusive vascular events that have a high morbidity and mortality. For example, carotid and coronary artery thrombosis are often diagnosed late in the course of the disease, after serious or fatal complications have occurred[4]. The discovery of effective new specific anti-platelet agents such as GPIIbIIIa (platelet fibrinogen receptor) fibrinogen binding inhibitors (RGD based antagonists)[5], makes early specific diagnosis important. Early detection of the onset of platelet deposition and its location *in vivo* will be valuable for indicating and monitoring these new drugs.

---

[a]Preliminary oral presentation of this work was at the 39th annual meeting of The Society of Nuclear Medicine, Los Angeles, California, June 9 -12, 1992.

While 111In platelets have failed to become widely applied in the clinic, 68Ga labeled platelets offer some potential advantages. The 500 mCi dose limitation due to the 2.8 day half life of 111In and the resulting high radiation dose to the spleen, restricts the counts available for imaging. The ability to use 2-6 mCi of 68Ga and the high sensitivity of the PET scanner will provide more counts and better statistics in the 68Ga image. However it remains to be shown that the high background due to the long 10 day platelet life span in the blood, which necessitates 24 hour images for optimum sensitivity with 111In platelets, can be overcome in the early 1-4 hr images by the higher sensitivity and resolution of 68Ga PET. Of course with 68Ga labeled platelets the PET images must be made in the first 4 hrs after injection due to the 68 minute $T1/2_p$ of 68Ga.

Two encouraging reports, one in rabbits[6] and one in dogs[7], have been published that showed uptake of 68Ga labeled platelets in de-endothelialized arteries *in vivo* by PET. The PET images were made 30 to 60 minutes after injection with 1 to 7 mCi 68Ga labeled platelets. These reports of successful 68Ga thrombus imaging in rabbits and dogs suggest the method might be effectively extended to humans. A Medline search failed to reveal any reports of PET imaging with 68Ga platelets in human to date.

Since our early clinical efforts in 68Ga PET imaging in 1970[8], using the original Anger positron camera, there has been a revolution in PET instrument design. The Siemens/CTI 933/04/20 whole body PET we used has $\approx$ 6 mm in plane resolution, an 8 cm axial field of view and exceptionally high sensitivity and count rate capability[b]. As a result PET is on the threshold of becoming a routine clinical tool, capable of providing quantitative functional information not obtainable from any other source. The 68Ge /68Ga generator[c] is a very cheap source of PET radiopharmaceuticals and a promising alternative to the cyclotron for clinical applications. Among the many potential 68Ga labeled PET agents, 68Ga labeled platelets offers a radiopharmaceutical analog of the well studied 111In oxine platelets, but producing much higher resolution tomographic images having many more counts and improved statistics.

MATERIALS AND METHODS

Synthesis of 68Ga oxine and 68Ga mercaptopyridine-N-oxide (MPO): 68Ga MPO synthesis followed the method of Thakur et al[9] and Yano et al[6]. Four ml ($\sim$20 mCi) of metal-free 68Ga in 1.0N HCl was eluted from a 25 mCi 68Ge /68Ga generator through a Bio-Rex Ag1X8 anion exchange membrane syringe filter (to remove tin) and collected in a metal-free polypropylene conical tube. Using a Rotovap[d] system, the liquid was sucked into a pear shaped acid-washed glass flask and dried in an 80°C water bath under 50 millitor vacuum for approximately 5 minutes. The flask was cooled in a stream of cold water and 300 ml of 0.01N HCl was added while continuing to rotate for 1 minute. The flask was removed from the Rotovap and the 68GaCl$_3$ in 300 ml 0.01N HCl was carefully pipetted from the drying flask into a metal-free polypropylene, conical shaped tube. Following addition of 300 ml of 0.5M sodium acetate buffer (pH 6.0) and vortexing, 300 ml of previously prepared MPO solution (1 mg/ml Na salt[e] in

---

[b]Siemens Gammasonics, Inc., 810 Innovation drive Knoxville, TN 37932.

[c]Dupont Radiopharmaceuticals, 331 Treble Cove Rd., N Billerica, MA 08162

[d]Buchi Ltd. CH 9230 Flawil Switzerland.

[e]Sigma Chemical Co. P.O. Box 14508 St. Louis MO 63178

356

deionized water) was added to the 68Ga acetate and mixed well. The pH was then adjusted to 6.7 to 7.0 with metal-free NaOH. The 68Ga MPO was then added dropwise to the previously prepared platelets.

For determining the labeling yield, 1 ml of chloroform was added to the tube containing a sample of 68Ga MPO and vortexed. The bottom chloroform layer containing the 68Ga MPO complex was removed and assayed in an ion chamber. The mean labeling yield = 95 %.

68Ga oxine was synthesized according to the method of Yano et al[6]. Labeling yields were determined by chromatography on an ITLC plate developed in 95 % chloroform / 5% methanol v/v. In this system free 68Ga stays at the origin and 68Ga oxine runs to the front. Mean labeling yield = 95% was obtained with 100 mg oxine.

Platelet separation and labeling procedure: Platelet preparation was done with a modification of the method we described previously[10]. Two 50 ml syringes, each containing 7.5 ml of NIH ACD[f] solution was used to obtain 85 ml venous blood through a #19 gauge needle after discarding the first 3 ml. In patients that could not tolerate removal of 85 ml blood, the procedure was cut in half ($\approx$ 45 ml). The blood was transfered to 2, 50ml conical polypropylene centrifuge tubes and centrifuged at 220 xG (1100 rpm: Beckman model TJ-6)[g] for 20-25 minutes. Platelet rich plasma (PRP) was carefully pipetted into 2, 50 ml conical polypropylene centrifuge tubes and spun at 1000 xG (2200 rpm) for 15 minutes to obtain a platelet pellet. Platelet poor plasma (PPP) was pipetted off the pellet and saved for later use. The platelets were resuspended in 10 ml of 0.9% saline to dilute out the remaining plasma, gently mixed and repelleted at 1000 x G (2200 rpm) for 10 minutes. The supernatant was removed and the washed platelets resuspended in 1.0ml of 0.9% saline for labeling. The previously prepared 68Ga MPO (or oxine) complex was added to the platelets, gently mixed and incubated at room temperature for 15 minutes. Ten ml of PPP was then added to the platelet - 68Ga MPO incubation mixture to remove any unbound 68Ga, the tube centrifuged at 1000 xG (2200 rpm) for 10 minutes and the washed labeled platelets resuspended in 3 ml PPP for injection. The activity of the supernatent PPP and the platelets was recorded and the labeling yield calculated. With simultaneous 68Ga MPO and platelet preparation (requiring 2 technicians) the 68Ga labeled platelets were ready for injection approximately 1 1/2 hrs after elution of the generator. One operator would require approximately 2 hrs.

Pet imaging of patients: Since the optimum imaging time has not yet been determined, PET scans were begun either immediately after injection or at various times between injection and up to 4 hrs following injection. An average of 2 $\pm$ 0.9 mCi 68Ga labeled platelets was used per patient and 3 patients were studied twice. An early (0-1 hr) and late (2-4 hr) heparinized blood sample was obtained and % activity in the platelets, and recovery were calculated as described previously[10]. The maximum dose per patient, based on dosimetry calculated from 111In human platelet distribution studies[11], was 6 mCi. Images made with 1 to 4 bed positions giving an 8 to 32 cm field of view, depending on the area necessary to cover the region of interest, took from 30 min to 2 hrs. Seven planes were obtained per bed position each usually containing ~1 million coincident events. Transmission images were not obtained. Anticoagulants were not discontinued. Angiography was obtained on all patients.

---

[f]Squibb Diagnostics New Brunswick NJ 08903

[g]Beckman Instruments Inc. Fullerton CA 92634

RESULTS

With the Du Pont generators we are obtaining approximately 68-70 % of the available 68Ga activity which is eluted in the middle 4 , 1 ml fractions of 1 N HCl . With the Rotovap system we routinely evaporated about 1 ml generator eluate per minute for an overall evaporation time of ~5 min. For the last 3 years we have measured the Ge-68 breakthrough, elution efficiency and elution profile of 7 Ga-68 generators. We have found significant Ge-68 breakthrough in only one of them. This occurred slowly with plenty of warning over 2-3 months. Breakthrough is now measured at least 48 hrs after elution on all elutions by simply re-counting a sample after Ga-68 decay to equilibrium with Ge-68. Thus with routine monitoring, 6 of the 7 generators have proven exceptionally safe with little danger of inadvertent administration of large amounts of Ge-68.

The 68Ga MPO platelet labeling and *in vivo* kinetic data are shown in Table 1. Since 68Ga oxine did not label platelets efficiently (10-15%) it was not used for patients[6]. 68Ga MPO labeled platelets more efficiently (36 ± 12%) so it was used in these studies. The 68Ga MPO platelet labeling yield was somewhat lower than we have reported for 111In oxine labeling of platelets (64 + 13% in saline and 34 + 15% in plasma)[10], but stability and platelet viability was equally good. The early recovery (% injected dose circulating in blood) = 31 ± 21% and late (2-4 hrs) recovery = 39 ± 20% indicated good viability and showed the 68Ga MPO platelets were able to circulate with no drop for at least the first 4 hrs. The circulating activity remained mostly in the platelets (64% early, 76% late) indicating stable attachment to platelets for the first 4 hours. Our previous observations with 111In oxine labeled platelets showed good correlation of recovery measured in the first 4 hrs with a normal life span. Damaged platelets dissappeared very rapidly in the first 15 minutes.

The patient studies showed high circulating blood background with the spleen having the highest concentration and the liver concentration about equal to blood. Bone marrow was not evident on any of the images. The 68Ga MPO PET scans resembled the distribution seen in normal 111In oxine platelet images made at early times[12].

There were 2 technically inadequate PET imaging studies. In one patient high lung uptake and low blood pool activity was noted, thought to be due to clumping of damaged platelets during labeling. This patient was included in the kinetic analysis however. In the renal artery stent patient only 370 mCi 68Ga platelets were available which was enough for kinetic measurements, but not for adequate images.

None of the 3 left ventricular clots thought to be present by ultrasound from 1 to 3 months prior to study were visualized. Two patients having carotid endarterectomies; 1 done 1 week prior and one done 24 hrs prior to platelet imaging were both negative. The coronary angioplasty and inguinal angioplasty done 1 day previous to imaging were negative. Thus of the 8 "false negative" images, 2 were technically inadequate, and 4 could be classed as "old clots". No explanation was evident for the remaining 2 negatives other than high blood background.

A 75 yr old male patient who underwent a cranial surgical proceedure 24 hrs earlier, complained of shortness of breath and pleuritic pain and had a positive V/Q mismatch involving a large area in the upper right lung and 2 smaller areas in the left base. The pulmonary angiogram done immediately after the lung scan revealed a large clot in the superior branch of the right main pulmonary artery. A 68Ga platelet PET scan done the following day (mid-thoracic cut) showed the embolus in the same location as the angiogram. Since the patient had an inferior vena cava umbrella also placed the previous day a PET image was made over the lower abdomen. Uptake of 68Ga platelets was seen in the region of the umbrella. A repeat 68Ga platelet scan was done 11 days later which showed disappearance of the activity in the right pulmonary artery.

Table I. Platelet kinetic data on 10 patients: means ± standard deviation. R R Art Stent = Right renal artery stent. AP L P Tib A = Angioplasty of right posterior tibial artery. A P Ing A = Angioplasty of inguinal artery. EA Car = Endarterectomy carotid artery. AP Cor = Angioplasty of coronary artery. LV Clot = Left ventricular clot. PE RPA = Pulmonary embolus in right pulmonary artery.
Reproduced by permission of Nuclear Medicine Communications (14).

Ga-68 PLATELET PATIENT DATA

Patient	Diagnosis	PET Scan	Labeling Yield	Injected (mCi)	15 min-1 hr % Activity in Platelets/mL W.B. (1)	15 min-1 hr Recovery (3)	2-4 hr % Activity in Platelets/mL W.B. (1)	2-4 hr Recovery (2)
E.D.	R R Art Stent	-	14 %	0.37	67 %		64 %	43 %
G.F.	AP L P Tib A	+	43 %	2.27		33 %	75 %	34 %
D.L.	AP Ing A	-	19 %	0.92	12 %	3 %	77 %	25 %
J.H.	EA Car	-	32 %	1.87	72 %	13 %	94 %	20 %
F.R.	AP Cor	-	42 %	2.28	85 %	22 %		
F.F.	LV Clot	-	44 %	3.41	89 %	54 %	89 %	22 %
F.F.	LV Clot	-	47 %	3.63	73 %	36 %		
E.Z.	EA Car	-	31 %	2.26	75 %	37 %		
E.Z.	EA Car	-	28 %	1.84	47 %	29 %	84 %	41 %
H.K.	AP Cor	-	37 %	2.88	59 %	10 %	55 %	32 %
W.M.	PE RPA	-	39 %	0.42	52 %	85 %		
W.M.	PE RPA	+	60 %	1.76	59 %	23 %	52 %	85 %
J.G.	AP Cor	-	35 %	2.03			71 %	27 %
MEAN ± STD DEV:			36 ± 12 %	2.0±0.9 %	64 ± 20 %	31 ± 21 %	76 ± 14 %	39 ± 20 %

A 70 yr old male patient with intermittent claudication in the left calf caused by an atherosclerotic stenosis in the posterior tibial artery underwent percutaneous angioplasty (Figure 1). 68Ga platelets were injected just prior to the proceedure and PET imaging done 4 hrs later. The patient was positioned with the help of skin landmarks made during angioplasty. The angiogram shows the stenotic lesion (Figure 1-Left), the balloon in place (Figure 1-Middle), and the widely patent artery following dilatation (Figure 1-Right). Figure 2 shows coronal cuts through both legs at this level in the PET image. Intense uptake of platelets is seen at the site of the baloon angioplasty in comparison to normal blood background seen in vessels in the left leg and other vessels in the same leg.

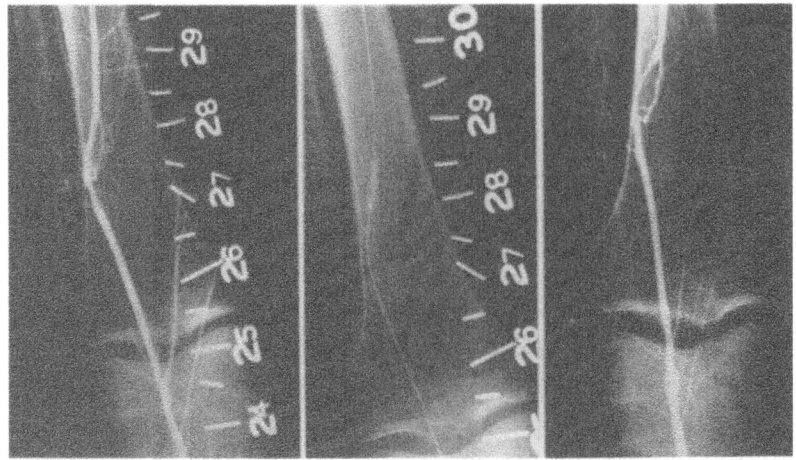

Figure 1. Angiogram of posterior tibial artery. Left: pre-angioplasty showing stenotic lesion, Middle: balloon in place, Right: post-angioplasty showing dilated artery with good flow through the previous stenotic area.

Reproduced by permission of Nuclear Medicine Communications (14).

DISCUSSION

The goal of this investigation was to see if the successful animal studies with 68Ga platelets could be extended to PET imaging in patients. The recent rapid proliferation of interventional procedures coupled with the introduction of new potent specific drugs has made the need for a clinical thrombus imaging agent more urgent.

In-111 platelet scanning has had variable clinical success. In deep pelvic vein thrombosis[10], and intra-cardiac thrombosis[13] it can provide information not available from any other test. However the need to wait 24 hrs for a result and the low count rate preventing good SPECT images, are limitations preventing its widespread use.

In one patient inadequate images were obtained due to low activity and one due to lung uptake of presumably damaged platelets. Of the 6 false negative studies we feel high blood background is the most likely reason for missing platelet deposition.

These preliminary studies show that it is feasable to image platelet deposition within the first 4 hrs after injection. The 68Ga MPO labeled platelets functioned normally as evidenced by the good recovery values and their ability to aggregate on lesions *in vivo*. The images had high enough resolution to sharply define arteries 2-4 mm in diameter. For future improvements, a method with lower background in the first 4 hrs would improve the sensitivity. The quality of the images we obtained with 68Ga platelet PET warrents further research for improved 68Ga platelet radiopharmaceuticals with lower background.

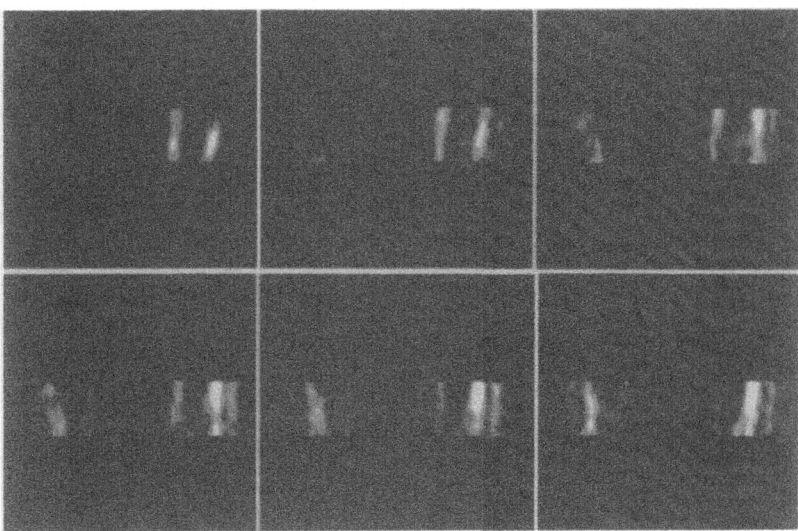

Figure 2. 68Ga platelet PET coronal cuts through both legs at the level of the recently dilated stenotic lesion. Intense uptake of the 68Ga platelets is seen in the dilated segment of the left posterior tibial artery in comparison to the lower normal blood background in the other arteries.

Reproduced by permission of Nuclear Medicine Communications (14).

ACKNOWLEDGMENTS

These studies were supported in part by a merit review grant from the Veterans Administration and PHS grants NIH RO1 CA 28343 and NIH RO1 CA 48282. The authors thank Dr George M. Segall for helpful discussions and Kevin Thomas, VAPA PET Center Technical Director for performing the PET scans and Beth Vertin for excellet technical assistance.

REFERENCES

1. McBride W, Lange Ra, Hillis LD: Restenosis after sucessful coronary angioplasty. *N Engl J Med*; 318: 1734-1737 (1988).
2. Cheesebro JH, Lam JYT, Badimon L, Fuster V: Restenosis after arterial angioplasty: A hemorrheologic response to injury. *An J Cardiol*: 60: 10b-16b (1987).
3. Kaplan AV, Leung L-K, Leung W-H, Grant GW, McDougall IR, Fischell TA: Roles of thrombin and

platelet membrane glycoprotein IIb/IIIa in platelet-subendothelial deposition after angioplasty in an es vivo whole artery model. *Circulation*; 84: 1279-1288 (1991).

4. Rubinstein E: Chap XVIII: Thromboembolism. Scientific American Medicine 1989.

5. Phillips DR, Charo IF, Parise LV, Fitzgerald LA: The platelet membrane glycoprotein IIb-IIIa complex. *Blood*; 4: 831-843.

6. Yano Y, Budinger TF, Ebbe SN et al: Gallium-68 lipophilic complexes for labeling platelets. *J Nuc Med*: 26: 1429-1437 (1985).

7. Welch MJ, Thakur ML, Coleman RE et al: Gallium-68 labeled red cells and platelets: new agents for positron tomography. *J Nucl Med*; 18: 558-562 (1977).

8. Colombetti LG, Goodwin DA, and Togami E: Ga-68-labeled macroaggregates for lung studies. *J Nuc Med*; 11: 704-707 (1970).

9. Thakur ML, McKenney SL and Park CH: Simplified and efficient labeling of human platelets in plasma using indium-111 2 metcaptopyridine-N-oxide: preparation and evaluation. *J Nucl Med*; 26: 510-517 (1985).

10. Goodwin DA, Bushberg JT, Doherty PW et al: Indium-111-labeled autologous platelets for location of vascular thrombi in humans. *J Nuc Med*; 19: 626-634, (1978).

11. Goodwin DA, Finston R and Smith S: The distribution and dosimetry of In-111 labeled leukocytes and platelets in humans. In: Schlafke-Stelson AT & Watson EE, eds. *Proceedings of the third international radiopharmaceutical dosimetry symposium.* Oak Ridge Assoc. Universities, Oak Ridge, Tennessee, 1980; FDA 81-8166, 88-101.

12. Goodwin DA and Lantieri RA: Clinical evaluation of Indium-111 platelet scanning in 60 patients. In: Thakur ML and Gottschalk A, eds. *In-111 labeled neutrophils, platelets and lymphocytes.* Trivirum Pub Co New York NY; 1980: Chap 17 167-170.

13. Ezekowitz MD, Burow RD, Heath PW et al: The diagnostic accuracy of Indium-111 platelet scintigraphy for identifying left ventricular thrombi. *Am J Cardiol* 51: 1712.

14. Goodwin DA, Lang EV, Atwood JE, Dalman RL, Ransone CMc, CI Diamanti, McTigue M. Viability and biodistribution of Ga-68-MPO-labeled human platelets. *Nuc Med Communications: Accepted July, 1993.*

INDEX

The manufacturer's authorised representative in the EU is Springer
Nature Customer Service Centre GmbH, Europaplatz 3, 69115 Heidelberg,
Germany. If you have any concerns regarding our products, please
contact ProductSafety@springernature.com

Printed and bound by CPI Group (UK) Ltd, Croydon, CR0 4YY
23/04/2026
02095623-0010